Pharmaceutics: Development and Applications

Pharmaceutics: Development and Applications

Edited by Mary Durrant

hayle
medical

New York

Hayle Medical,
750 Third Avenue, 9ᵗʰ Floor,
New York, NY 10017, USA

Visit us on the World Wide Web at:
www.haylemedical.com

ISBN: 978-1-63241-474-8

Cataloging-in-Publication Data

Pharmaceutics : development and applications / edited by Mary Durrant.
    p. cm.
Includes bibliographical references and index.
ISBN 978-1-63241-474-8
1. Drugs. 2. Pharmacy. 3. Pharmaceutical technology.
4. Pharmaceutical chemistry. I. Durrant, Mary.
RS92 .P43 2018
615.1--dc23

Table of Contents

Permissions

List of Contributors

Index

Preface

This book aims to highlight the current researches and provides a platform to further the scope of innovations in this area. This book is a product of the combined efforts of many researchers and scientists, after going through thorough studies and analysis from different parts of the world. The objective of this book is to provide the readers with the latest information of the field.

Pharmaceutics refers to the study of old drugs and new chemical entities (NCE) that can be used in treating patients effectively. In other words, it is known as the study of dosage. It includes the practice of formulating drugs into dosage form. Some of the concepts included in this field are pharmaceutical manufacturing, physical pharmacy, pharmaceutical formulation, etc. This book provides comprehensive insights into the field of pharmaceutics. It discusses in detail about the various inventions and revelations of this ever-evolving field. The diverse topics covered in the book address the varied branches that fall under this category. Students, researchers, experts and all associated with pharmaceutics will benefit alike from the text.

I would like to express my sincere thanks to the authors for their dedicated efforts in the completion of this book. I acknowledge the efforts of the publisher for providing constant support. Lastly, I would like to thank my family for their support in all academic endeavors.

Editor

The Genus *Luehea* (Malvaceae-Tiliaceae): Review about Chemical and Pharmacological Aspects

João Tavares Calixto-Júnior,[1] Selene Maia de Morais,[2] Aracélio Viana Colares,[3] and Henrique Douglas Melo Coutinho[4]

[1]*Juazeiro do Norte College (FJN), Juazeiro do Norte, CE, Brazil*
[2]*Biotechnology Postgraduation Programme (RENORBIO), Laboratory of Natural Products, State University of Ceará, Itaperi Campus, Fortaleza, CE, Brazil*
[3]*UNILEAO University Center, Juazeiro do Norte, CE, Brazil*
[4]*Department of Biological Chemistry, Regional University of Cariri, Crato, CE, Brazil*

Correspondence should be addressed to Henrique Douglas Melo Coutinho; hdmcoutinho@gmail.com

Academic Editor: Strahil Berkov

Popularly known as "açoita-cavalo" (whips-horse), *Luehea* species (Malvaceae-Tilioideae) are native to America and are used in folk medicine as anti-inflammatory, antidiarrheal, antiseptic, expectorant, and depurative and against skin infections. Although there are studies showing the chemical constituents of some species, the active substances have not been properly identified. A systematic study was carried out through a computer search of data on CAPES journals, SciELO, ISI Bireme, PubMed, ScienceDirect, ScienceDomain Medline, and Google Scholar from published articles using key words: *Luehea*, açoita-cavalo, and Malvaceae. *Luehea divaricata* was the species with the highest number of studies observed. Triterpenes (9), flavonoids (6), and steroids (4), including saponins, organic acids (4), and one lignan, are the main types of secondary metabolites registered and the most cited flavonoids were rutin and quercetin and among triterpenes there was maslinic acid, which might be associated with the popular indication of its anti-inflammatory action. The vitexin, a C-glycosylated flavone, isolated from three different species, is cited as a possible taxonomic marker of the genus. Studies confirm in part the medicinal uses of plants named as "açoita-cavalo" species. Some pharmacological activities, not assigned to the species of the genus *Luehea* by populations, were observed in laboratory experiments.

1. Introduction

Malvaceae is a family consisting of herbs, subshrubs, shrubs, lianas, and small and large trees, with about 250 genera and 4,200 species, of which, in Brazil, about 80 genera and 400 species are found [1]. According to the List of Species of Flora of Brazil, 69 genera and 754 species are indicated, with 30 genera distributed in 393 taxa of the subfamily Malvoideae [2, 3].

Luehea genus, which belongs to Malvaceae family, is essentially neotropical, existing in southern Mexico, including the West Indies to Uruguay and Argentina. Currently there are about 25 species and 3 varieties, of which 12 species and one variety exist in Brazil, with its highest concentration in the southeast and midwest regions [4]. The genus

Luehea is present in Brazilian Cerrado and thirteen species are registered in Brazilian herbariums: *Luehea altheaeflora* Spruce ex Benth., *Luehea fiebrigii* Burret, *Luehea candicans* Mart., *Luehea candida* (Moc. & Sessé ex DC.) Mart., *Luehea crispa* Krapov., *Luehea cymulosa* Spruce ex Benth., *Luehea divaricata* Martius et Zuccarini, *Luehea grandiflora* Mart. & Zucc., *Luehea paniculata* Mart. & Zucc., *Luehea ochrophylla* Mart., *Luehea rosea* Ducke and *Luehea speciosa* Willd., and *L. conwentzii* K. Schum.

The lectotype of *L. conwentzii* was selected and a new synonym was proposed—*L. eichler* Schum [5]. To Rizzini and Mors [6], the various species are very similar to each other, getting the same common names (horse-whips) and having identical uses.

Among the species of this genus, the most cited are *L. grandiflora* and *L. divaricate*, popularly known as "açoita-cavalo" (whips-horse) [7]. The closest species of *L. divaricata* is *L. paniculata*, which is a tree a little lower, existing in Bolivia, Paraguay, Peru, and several states of Brazil [8]. The herbarium specimens of *L. grandiflora* showed close similarities to those of *L. speciosa* because they are both very polymorphic. However, *L. speciosa* staminodia are profoundly fimbriated, while those of *L. grandiflora* are slightly fimbriated in the apex. So *L. grandiflora* was considered a synonym of *L. speciosa* but was later rehabilitated [9].

A *Luehea* herbal product, composed of dried leaves, is used against dysentery, leucorrhoea, rheumatism, gonorrhea, and tumors; infusion of the flowers is used against bronchitis and the root is depurative [10]. Aerial parts of *L. divaricata* are used popularly for skin wounds and for intimate hygiene [11]. Backes and Irgang [12] reported the use of the bark of this plant as antirheumatic, antidiarrheal, antiseptic, expectorant, and cleanser.

The current state of knowledge of the chemistry and pharmacology of genus *Luehea* indicates its potential for developing anti-inflammatory drugs and antibiotics; however, few studies with species of this genus were reported.

Due to the importance of the genus *Luehea*, as a source of new medicinal agents, a review is worthwhile. The data may support future multidisciplinary studies involving phytochemical studies of the genus species to perform a critical analysis of their use by populations with a view to the preservation of plant species in their respective biomes and promoting rational use of "açoita-cavalo" as a therapeutic resource. A systematic study was carried out through a computer search of data on CAPES journals, SciELO, ISI Bireme, PubMed, ScienceDirect, ScienceDomain Medline, and Google Scholar from published articles using key words: *Luehea*, açoita-cavalo, and Malvaceae. Data was also obtained from theses, proceedings, and book of abstracts and reviews indexed in the databases, used for this work, as well as abstracts and full papers published in scientific events. Dissertations and doctoral theses of Brazilian and international students with relevant data were also examined. Data presented include scientific name and activities of the plants.

2. Development

2.1. Chemical Aspects

2.1.1. Luehea divaricata. Little information is known about the chemical constituents present in the genus *Luehea* [8]. The phytochemical analysis of the leaves of this species showed mainly the presence of flavonoids, saponins, and catechin tannins (condensed tannins) [13]. To a lesser extent, the authors cited the presence of alkaloids, fixed oils, anthocyanins, carotenoids, and polysaccharides. The species presents tannins, essential oil, resin, and mucilage [14].

Portal et al. [15], conducting a phytochemical screening on the extract of *L. divaricata* collected in Belém, Pará State, Northern Brazil, noted the presence in the leaves of reducing sugars, proteins, amino acids, tannins, catechins, flavonoids, carotenoids, steroids, triterpenoids, and saponins. Several

authors performed a phytochemical screening with ethanol extracts of leaf and stem and also observed the presence of flavonoids, tannins, saponins, and triterpenes/steroids [16–18] and Bertucci et al. [19] screening native species of the Uruguay River observed in the hydroalcoholic extract of leaves of *L. divaricata* the presence of these same constituents.

Lopes [18], through phytochemical study of *L. divaricata* collected in Southern Brazil, identified from the alcoholic extract of leaves, tannins, saponins, and flavonoids and isolated by two-dimensional thin-layer chromatography the flavonoids quercetin (**1**), rutin (**2**), and vitexin (**3**) (Figure 1).

Vargas et al. [20] also point out the presence of tannins, flavonoids, and saponins in leaves and bark of *L. divaricata* and also the presence of quercetin (**1**) and kaempferol (**4**) in the extracts. However, Maraschin-Silva and Aqüila [21], investigating the allelopathic potential of this species, only infer about the presence of tannins and saponins in aqueous leaf extract.

Arantes [17] analyzed the ethanol extract of leaves collected in Southern Brazil by HPLC and reported the presence of the flavonoids quercetin (**1**), rutin (**2**), and kaempferol (**4**) and aromatic acids gallic acid (**5**), chlorogenic acid (**6**), and caffeic acid (**7**) (Figure 1).

Tanaka et al. [22] isolated from the methanol extract of leaves of *L. divaricata*, collected in Maringá, Paraná State, Southern Brazil, a new triterpene (basic skeleton of ursene): 3β-p-hydroxybenzoyloxytormentic acid [3β-(p-hydroxybenzoyloxy)-2α-hydroxyurs-12-en-28-oic acid] (**8**), a mixture of tormentic acid ester glucoside (**9**), tormentic acid (**10**), and the maslinic acid (olean-12-ene-2α,3β-diol) (**11**) (basic skeleton of oleanane) (Figure 1).

Tanaka et al. [10], in continuation of previous work, isolated from stem bark and leaves, besides the mentioned triterpenes, the steroid glucopyranosylsitosterol (**12**), (−)-epicatechin (**13**), a flavonoid which belongs to a class of flavan-3-ol, and vitexin (**3**), as already indicated in the same species isolated in previous work [18] (Figure 1).

The presence of flavonoids such as vitexin (**3**) [23, 24] and triterpenes as maslinic acid (**11**) [25, 26] may be associated with the popular indication of its anti-inflammatory action [27].

Besides polyphenols (flavonoids, catechins, anthocyanins, and tannins) the phytochemical screening of the hydroalcoholic extract of bark of *L. divaricata* collected in Leme, São Paulo State, Southeastern Brazil, identified the presence of saponins, triterpenes, steroids, and anthracenes [28]. Walker et al. [29], in histochemical and morphoanatomical study of leaves of *L. divaricata* Mart., reported about the presence of mucilage and calcium oxalate in the form of a prism and drusen in idioblasts.

Luehea ochrophylla. Two papers that focus on the phytochemical analysis of this species are listed in this review. The phytochemical study of skins of *L. ochrophylla* collected in Grão Mogol, Minas Gerais State, Southeastern Brazil, resulted in the isolation of hydrocarbons, aliphatic esters of steroid β-sitosterol (**14**), and pentacyclic triterpenes friedelin (**15**) and β-friedelinol (**16**) [30] (Figure 2).

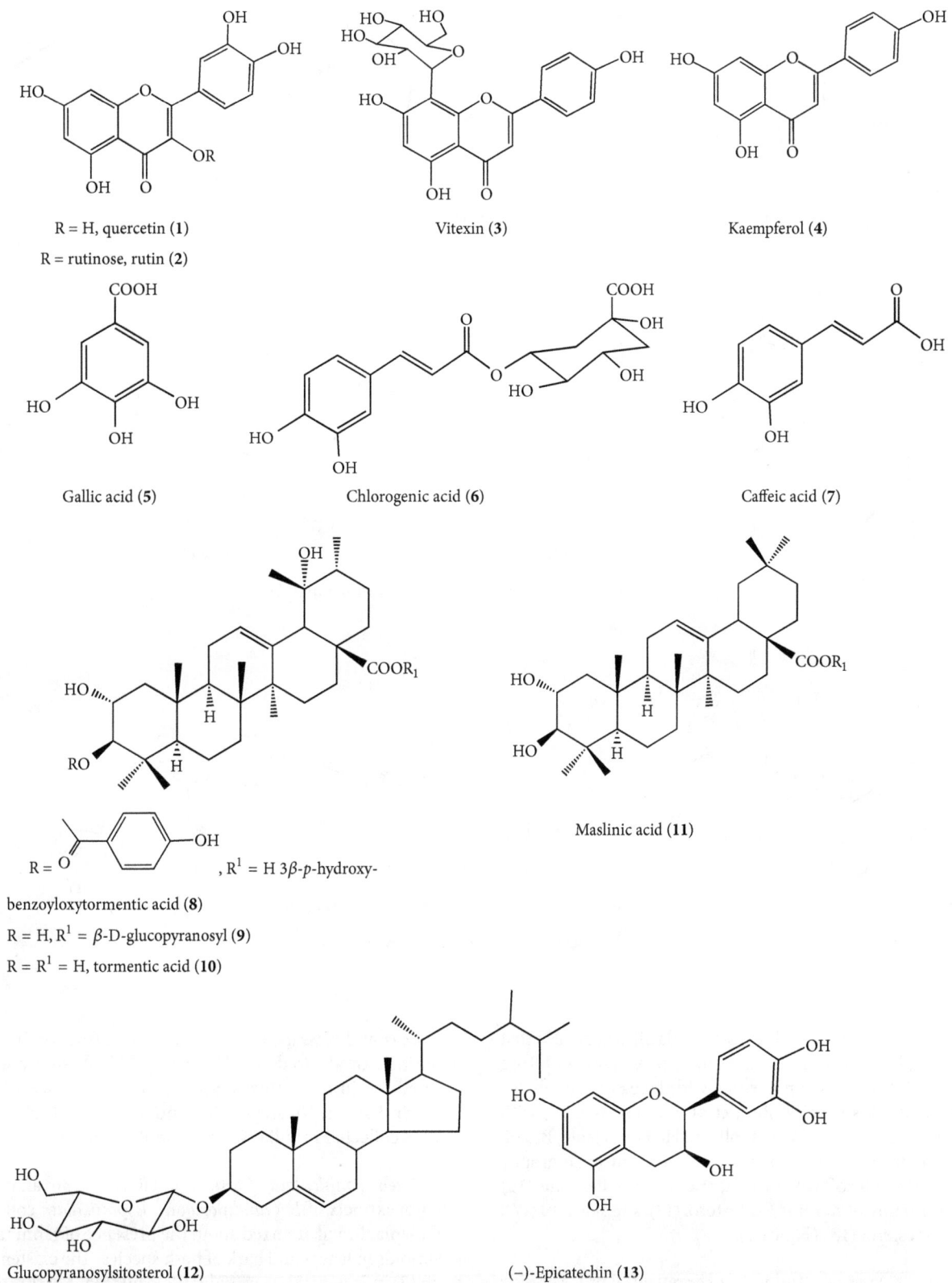

R = H, quercetin (**1**)

R = rutinose, rutin (**2**)

Vitexin (**3**)

Kaempferol (**4**)

Gallic acid (**5**)

Chlorogenic acid (**6**)

Caffeic acid (**7**)

Maslinic acid (**11**)

R = , R^1 = H 3β-p-hydroxy-

benzoyloxytormentic acid (**8**)

R = H, R^1 = β-D-glucopyranosyl (**9**)

R = R^1 = H, tormentic acid (**10**)

Glucopyranosylsitosterol (**12**)

(−)-Epicatechin (**13**)

FIGURE 1: Phytocompounds isolated from *Luehea divaricata*.

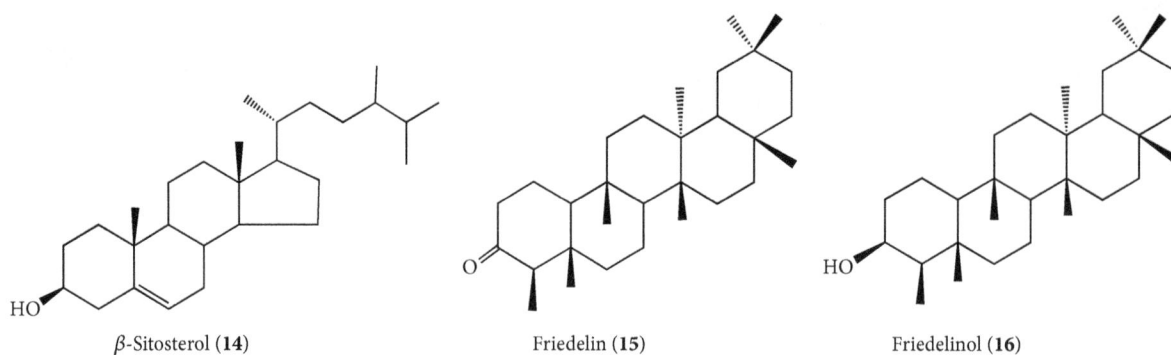

FIGURE 2: Phytocompounds isolated from *Luehea ochrophylla*.

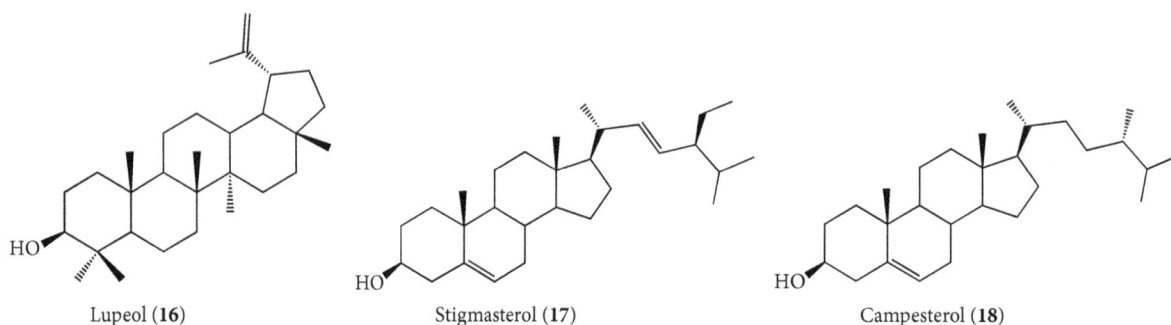

FIGURE 3: Phytocompounds isolated from *Luehea grandiflora*.

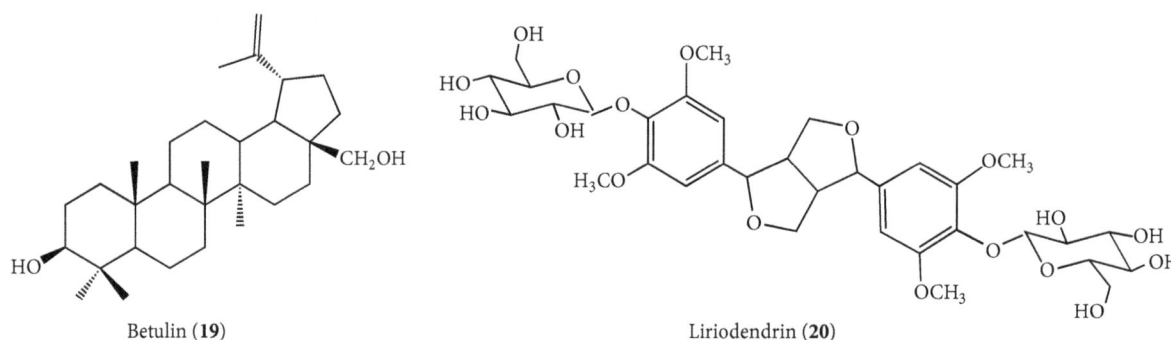

FIGURE 4: Phytocompounds isolated from *Luehea candida*.

2.1.2. Luehea grandiflora. The works of da Silva et al. [30] that indicate polyphenols in the cortex of *L. grandiflora* and Rosa et al. [31, 32] were the only works with focus on the phytochemistry of this species. Rosa et al. [31, 32] working with crude ethanol extract of leaves collected in Goiás State, Brazil, observed, from fractionation by column chromatography isolation, in chloroform fraction, the lupeol triterpene (**16**) and the mixture of steroids β-sitosterol (**14**), stigmasterol (**17**), and campesterol (**18**) (Figure 3).

2.1.3. Luehea candida. The anticancer potential of *L. candida* extracts was evaluated against many cell lines and lupeol (**16**), betulin (**19**), (−)-epicatechin (**13**), vitexin (**3**), and a lignan liriodendrin (**20**) were isolated from the active fractions [8] (Figure 4).

Saénz and Nassar [33] established the presence, in small quantities, of alkaloids in this species. Alkaloids were also pointed out in qualitative studies on *Luehea seemannii* collected in Eastern Nicaragua [34] and leaves and bark in this species collected in Villa Neily, Costa Rica [35, 36].

2.1.4. Luehea paniculata. Barbosa and Reed [35, 36] analyzing ethanol extracts of *L. grandiflora* and *L. paniculata* collected in Goiania, Brazil, inferred about the presence of tannins and flavonoids in leaves and bark of both species. The existence of rutin (**2**) in *L. paniculata* was identified by means of thin-layer chromatography.

Calixto Júnior et al. [37] observed by HPLC-DAD fingerprinting in *L. paniculata* ethanolic extracts (leaves and sapwood) the presence of the gallic acid (**5**), chlorogenic acid

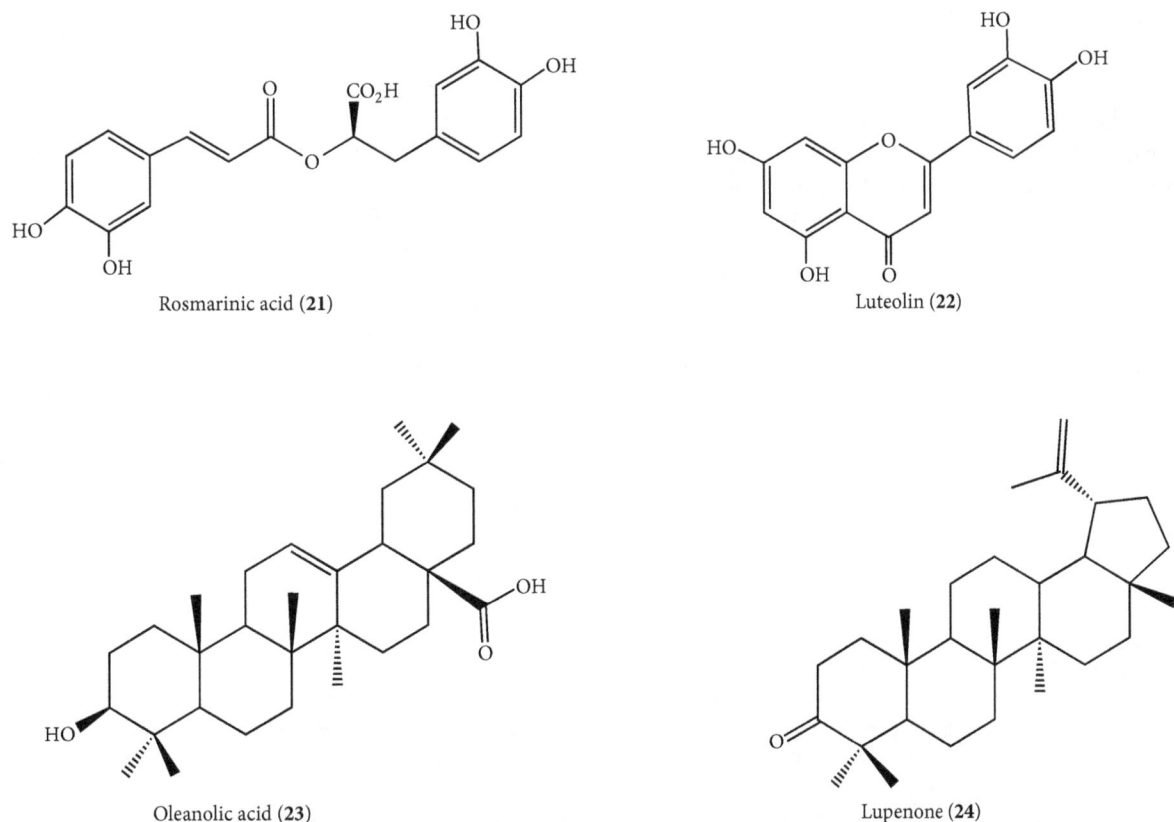

FIGURE 5: Phytocompounds isolated from *Luehea paniculata*.

(6), and rosmarinic acid (21) and flavonoids rutin (2), vitexin (3), and luteolin (22) (Figure 5).

Alves et al. [38] reported the isolation of triterpenes maslinic acid (11) from the chloroform fraction and oleanolic acid (23) and lupenone (24) from the ethyl acetate fraction, as well as evaluating the antiproliferative activity of the crude extract fractions of ethyl acetate and hydromethanol obtained from the leaves of *L. paniculata* collected in the Cerrado, Central Brazil (Figure 5).

2.1.5. Luehea candicans. Silva [39], in a study that involved extraction, isolation, and identification of the chemical constituents of the branches and leaves of *L. candicans* in the Puerto Rico region, Paraná State, Southern Brazil, got the isolation, the crude methanol extract of the stems of two triterpenes belonging to the class of lupins, the lup-20(29)-en-3β-ol (lupeol) (16) and the betulin—3β,28-diidroxilup-20(29)-ene (19). The works of Silva [39] and Da Silva et al. [8] were the only ones found on chemical research in this species.

The presence of vitexin in the leaves of *L. candicans*, *L. divaricata*, and *L. paniculata* species can suggest the hypothesis that this flavone may be a possible taxonomic marker of the genus *Luehea*.

2.2. Ethnopharmacological and Pharmacological Aspects. The popular knowledge about the medicinal uses of horsewhips is reported by several authors [40]; however, there are few studies available on the pharmacological potential

of the species [12]. The highest number of citations on ethnopharmacological information is assigned to the species *L. divaricata*; however, some other species appear in other surveys. *Luehea seemannii* is popularly used against bites and stings (snake, scorpion, and insects) and also as an astringent in Eastern Nicaragua [34].

In a survey conducted about ethnopharmacology of medicinal plants of the Pantanal (Mato Grosso State, Brazil), *L. divaricata* is among the species with the highest relative importance value (1.50) between values ranging from 0.17 to 1.87, among the 261 species mentioned in the work [27]. The authors report citations, by respondents, about the use of *L. divaricata* in the treatment of lung and upper respiratory disease. However, they stress that no scientific evidence exist on the activity of the species in the regulation of cough, while its antibiotic properties also vary. Bessa et al. [41] reported a quote from "açoita-cavalo" as being of use to the treatment of ulcer in rural community of Green Vale Settlement, Tocantins State, Central Brazil.

Several other reports of uses of this species were found: treatment of rheumatism; arthritis; dysentery; internal cleaning of wounds and ulcers; depurative; sore throat; painkiller for toothache; astringent; evils of the bladder; sleep balance; melena (intestinal colic followed by diarrhea with painful bowel movements and presence of blood in the stool); leucorrhea; gonorrhea; bleeding; cough; laryngitis; bronchitis; deworming; gastritis; poor digestion; diarrhea; and cancer and tumors [9, 42–44].

Degen et al. [45] reported medicinal plants traded by their common names and cited "Francisco Álvarez" as *L. divaricata* being employed against diabetes in Argentina and in Paraguay, where the same common name matches *the Banara arguta* Brig. (Flacourtiaceae). The term "Francisco Álvarez" as reference to "açoita-cavalos" in Paraguay is also cited by Carvalho [46], which emphasizes the use of other common names abroad: azota caballo and árbol de San Francisco, Argentina; Francisco Álvarez, Uruguay; and ka'a oveti, Paraguay. In various regions of Brazil the author highlights açoita: açoita-cavalo-do-miúdo, açoita-cavalo-branco, ivantingui, and vatinga in the São Paulo State; açoita-cavalo in Paraná State; in the states of Rio de Janeiro and São Paulo, biatingui, erviteira-do-campo, estibeiro, and estriveira; in Bahia State and São Paulo State, guaxima-do-campo, ibatingui, and ivatingui; in Minas Gerais State, ivitinga; in Bahia State, ivitingui, luitingui, mutamba, and pau-de-canga; in Santa Catarina State, salta-cavalo; in Paraná State and São Paulo State, soita and soita-cavalo; and, in Paraná State, ubatinga.

In folk medicine the "açoita-cavalo" is used in cases of dysentery, bleeding, arthritis, leucorrhoea, rheumatism, and tumors [41]. In ethnodirected work at Quilombo Sangrador, Maranhão State, Northeastern Brazil, the "açoita-cavalo" was one of the species with more valuable importance, with indications for the treatment of diseases of the genitourinary system [47]. Basualdo and Soria [48] included *L. divaricata* Mart. in the list of medicinal plants of Paraguay used in fighting respiratory infections.

The leaves of *Luehea* are marketed as herbal against leucorrhoea, rheumatism, gonorrhea, and tumors; infusion of the flowers is used against bronchitis and the root is depurative [10]. Rai [11] reports that the aerial parts of "açoita-cavalo" (*L. divaricata* Martius et Zuccarini) are used in traditional medicines for skin wounds, grain cleaning, and vaginal washings. Maffei [49] in work on medicinal plants of Uruguay and Chiriani [50] in study about phytotherapy in Argentina inform that the barks are used as antipyretic and antianemic agents, in addition to antidiarrheal, astringent, and antitumor. Quotes on the leaves as herbal against rheumatism, dysentery, gonorrhea, soothing, and antispasmodic are observed in several works [10, 49, 51–53]. The root is pointed out as anti-inflammatory and cleansing by Alice et al. [54], and the flowers are cited, along with bark and leaves, with diuretic, antiarthritic, antileucorrhoea, and wound healing of the skin and vaginal washings [22, 40, 49, 55, 56]. The bath of the stem bark was quoted in ethnobotanical survey in the Upper Rio Grande, Minas Gerais State, Southeastern Brazil, [57] as being of use for dysentery, as antirheumatic and antihemorrhagic agent.

According to Alice et al. [58], the bark of the *L. divaricata* is also used to combat the fever and is also suitable for gastrointestinal and liver disorders. The leaves are used as anti-inflammatory and employed in disorders of the respiratory tract and bronchitis. In popular phytotherapy the cortex of stems of *L. divaricata* is used in decoctions and infusions by tonic and antidiarrheal characteristics [59]. The resin of the fruit is applied as antiodontalgic; 1% flowers infusion is used as sedative and the infusion of the leaves as anti-inflammatory [60, 61].

2.3. Microbiological Activities. Five studies have reported effects against microorganisms in this species. The antifungal activity of *L. divaricata* was evaluated by Zacchino et al. [62]. As a result, the authors pointed out the moderate action of dichloromethane extract in inhibiting the growth of hyphae of some species of dermatophytes; however, this inhibitory effect is not observed for other fungal species [10, 40]. However, the extract of *L. divaricata* showed strong inhibition of the growth of *Staphylococcus aureus*, *Staphylococcus epidermidis*, *Klebsiella pneumonia*, and *Escherichia coli* in one study [40] but showed only moderate inhibition in another study and another collection site [10].

Montovani et al. [63] also investigated antimicrobial action in extract of *L. divaricata*. Collected in São Pedro do Iguaçu, Paraná State, Southern Brazil, the authors obtained extracts of leaves from three solvents (hexane, ethyl acetate, and ethanol) and diagnosed positive effects in inhibiting *S. aureus*, *Bacillus cereus*, *E. coli*, and *Salmonella typhi*. However, for the fungus *Aspergillus niger*, they obtained negative result; Coelho De Souza et al. [64], as a result of ethnopharmacological study, evaluated the antimicrobial potential of some plants in common use in the Rio Grande do Sul State (Southern Brazil) using the agar diffusion method; the authors found that the methanol extract of *L. divaricata* showed activity against the *Micrococcus luteus* bacteria. The extract showed no activity against other bacteria such as *S. aureus*, *S. epidermidis*, and *E. coli*, even against yeast *Candida albicans*.

Marques et al. [65] reported the biological activities study of *L. paniculata* of the Brazilian Cerrado, which showed inhibitory effect of ethanol extract of *L. paniculata* leaves on *S. aureus* bacteria.

Calixto Júnior et al. [37] pointed out as irrelevant the activity of *L. paniculata* leaf ethanolic extract (LEELP) tested against six strains of *Candida* (MIC $\geq$ 1024). This work is the first recorded piece of research on the potentialization of Fluconazole using extracts of *L. paniculata* against three strains of *Candida*, in particular, *C. tropicalis* and *C. albicans*, and there was, therefore, a synergism when the extracts were combined with Fluconazole.

2.4. Anti-Inflammation and Toxicity. Lopes [18] investigated the anti-inflammatory action of *L. divaricata*. From an experiment using the aqueous extract obtained from the dried leaves of the plant, the authors used the test of rat paw edema induced by carrageenan. The extract was administered intraperitoneally at doses of 100 and 150 mg/kg and orally, using a stomach tube at a dose of 300 mg/kg. According to the authors, the dose of 150 mg/kg administered intraperitoneally obtained the peak reduction of the edema. Siqueira [28] claims to have the hydroalcoholic extract of *L. divaricata* that reduced the rate of ulcerative lesions produced by indomethacin and ethanol. The author indicates that the mechanism of action antiulcerogenic is partly related to the activity of sulfhydryl radicals and by the precipitation of proteins produced by the presence of polyphenols present in the plant.

Bianchi [66] conducted studies of acute and subacute toxicity with extracts of this species. In both tests Swiss mice, males, were used. The alcoholic extract administered intraperitoneally at doses of 250 mg/kg and 500 mg/kg triggered diarrhea and bristling fur, within 72 hours, that were observed in the acute toxicity test. 50% of deaths of the animals were seen using a dose of 500 mg/kg for 48 hours. In the subacute toxicity test, the authors administered a dose of 25 mg/kg of aqueous and alcoholic extract by means intraperitoneally, once a week for 8 days. The aqueous extract triggered the death of an animal after the 8th dose, unlike the alcoholic extract that at this dose did not cause any deaths [67]. Vargas et al. [20] showed genotoxic (mutagenic) activity in aqueous leaf extract of *L. divaricata* in the Ames test (*Salmonella*/microsome) with microsomal activation. This fact can be explained by the presence of tannins and flavones in the leaves of the species that present patterns of hydroxylation, which could possibly cause damage to the DNA structure [54].

The phytotoxic activity of *L. divaricata* was shown clearly by Souza et al. [68]. The authors point out the test with aqueous extract of leaves collected in Pelotas, Southern Brazil, which showed an inhibitory effect on the germination of *Lactuca sativa*. Nevertheless, *L. divaricata* extracts demonstrate *in vivo* lack of toxicity or mutagenicity [69, 70].

2.5. Antioxidant Potential. Good antioxidant activity and analgesic properties in leaves of *L. divaricata* were pointed out by Müller [40]. By DPPH method, the author observed the crude extract and ethyl acetate and butanol fractions with similar antioxidant with the quercetin. Arantes [17] showed antioxidant activity at low concentrations of ethanol extract of the leaves of this species, observed by reducing basal levels of lipid peroxidation by the extract and its protective effect against lipid peroxidation and decreased cell viability induced by nitroprusside sodium in rat brain *in vitro*.

Antioxidant effect of the ethanol extract of *Luehea paniculata* roots was evaluated by the method of scavenging free radical DPPH [37]. This extract demonstrated an antioxidant potential almost similar to the value associated with the flavonoid quercetin (EC_{50} = 0.85 and 0.01 mg/mL, resp.). Calixto Júnior et al. [37] showed good results in antioxidant test of leaf extract and bark with IC_{50} values: 0.32 and 0.24 mg/mL, respectively.

2.6. Antiproliferative Activity. Alves et al. [38] analyzed the antiproliferative activity of the crude extract and ethyl acetate and hydromethanol fractions of *L. paniculata* leaves. The evaluation was performed at concentrations from 0.25 to 250 mg/mL against three human tumor cell lines, breast (MCF-7), lung (NCI-H460), and glioma (U251), by the colorimetric method with sulforhodamine B. The results showed moderate antiproliferative potential for those fractions.

The crude methanolic extracts of the branches and leaves of *Luehea candicans* were evaluated using the following cancer cell lines: MCF-7 (breast), NCI-ADR (breast expressing the multidrug resistance phenotype), NCI-460 (lung), UACC-62 (melanoma), 786-0 (kidney), OVCAR (ovarian), PCO-3 (prostate), HT-29 (colon), and K-562 (leukaemia). The crude methanolic extracts from the branches (B) and leaves (L) were able to inhibit the growth of the K-562 and 786-0 cell lines in a dose-dependent manner, with GI_{50} values

of 8.1 and 5.4 µg/mL, respectively. The hexane (L1), chloroform (L2), and methanol (L4) fractions derived from extract L showed a high selectivity and pronounced cytostatic activity against 786-0 (GI_{50} ~40 µg/mL). A significant amount of lupeol was isolated from fraction L2. The chloroform (B2) and methanol (B3) fractions derived from extract (B) exhibited less selectivity, showing the highest cytostatic activity against K-562, NCI-ADR, OVCAR, MCF-7, and NCI-460 cells, with GI_{50} values between 27 and 40 µg/mL [8].

Silva [39] studied *L. candicans* in the region of Puerto Rico, Paraná State, Southern Brazil, and assessed, by biological tests, the antibacterial, antifungal, and antiproliferative crude extracts, fractions, and isolated compounds. None of the extracts, however, showed significant antibacterial activity; however, the crude extract of the leaves showed antifungal activity against *Candida krusei* strain with a fungicide at a concentration of 125 mg/mL (CMF) and fungistatic concentration of 62.5 mg/mL (CIM). The crude extract of *L. candicans* still showed antiproliferative activity with cytostatic effect of 85% (25 µg/mL) and cytocidal effect by 25%, the highest concentration used for cell kidney cancer. The hexane, CHCl_3, and MeOH fractions demonstrated a cytostatic effect of 100% against kidney cancer cells. The crude extract of the stems showed cytostatic and antiproliferative activity with little selectivity among the studied strains (25% cell death at the highest concentration) effects, since the crude extract of *L. candicans* and hexane, CHCl_3 and MeOH fractions were selective for cells of kidney cancer exhibiting antiproliferative activity with cytostatic effect (growth inhibition) by 85% at a concentration of 25 mg/mL for the crude extract and 100% (250 µg/mL) for fractions. The antifungal activity of triterpenes, steroids, and flavonoids isolated was also tested, but without any substances presenting activity.

3. Conclusion

Studies confirm in part the medicinal uses of plants named as "açoita-cavalo" species. Some pharmacological activities not assigned to the species of the genus *Luehea* by populations were observed in laboratory experiments.

28 papers focusing on phytochemical studies with species of the genus were observed. The most studied in this regard are *L. divaricata*, *L. paniculata*, and *L. candicans*. The chemical composition of the leaf and stem is similar in different species, leading to the assertion that similar actions relate to common components in different representatives of the genus. Several secondary metabolites were found as triterpenes, steroids, flavonoids, lignans, organic acids, and flavone vitexin.

The vitexin, a C-glycosylated flavone, isolated from three different species of *Luehea* is cited as a possible marker of taxonomic genus and to prove this hypothesis further chemical research studies are required to find it in other species. The flavone vitexin and triterpene maslinic acid may be associated with anti-inflammatory action, which is considered the main popular indication for the genus.

Disclosure

All research is done by the authors.

Competing Interests

The authors declare that they have no competing interests.

Acknowledgments

The authors are grateful to the governmental agencies CNPq and CAPES for the financial support.

References

[1] V. C. Souza and H. Lorenzi, *Botânica Sistemática: Guia Ilustrado para Identificação das Famílias de Angiospermas da Flora Brasileira*, Plantarum, Nova Odessa, Brazil, 2005.

[2] M. G. Bovini, "Malvaceae na reserva rio das pedras, mangaratiba, Rio de Janeiro, Brasil," *Rodriguesia*, vol. 61, pp. 289–301, 2010.

[3] M. G. Bovini, G. Esteves, and M. C. Duarte, "Malvaceae," in *Lista de Espécies da Flora do Brasil*, JBRJ, Rio de Janeiro, Brazil, 2013.

[4] M. C. D. S. Cunha, "Revisão das espécies de gênero *Luehea* Willd. (Tiliaceae) ocorrentes no Estado do Rio de Janeiro," *Sellowia*, vol. 37, pp. 5–41, 1985.

[5] M. C. D. S. Cunha, "Contribution to the study of the genus *Luehea* in Brazil a new synonym for *Luehea conwentzii*," *Bradea*, vol. 1, pp. 232–233, 1982.

[6] C. T. Rizzini and W. B. Mors, *Botânica Econômica Brasileira*, USP, São Paulo, Brazil, 1976.

[7] M. P. Pio Corrêa, *Dicionário das Plantas Úteis do Brasil e das Exóticas Cultivadas*, Ministério da Agricultura, Brasília, Brazil, 1984.

[8] D. A. Da Silva, V. G. Alves, D. M. M. Franco et al., "Antiproliferative activity of *Luehea candicans* Mart. et Zucc. (Tiliaceae)," *Natural Product Research*, vol. 26, no. 4, pp. 364–369, 2012.

[9] M. Brandão, "Plantas medicamentosas do cerrado mineiro," *Informe Agropecuário*, vol. 15, pp. 15–21, 1991.

[10] J. C. A. Tanaka, C. C. da Silva, B. P. Dias Filho, C. V. Nakamura, J. E. de Carvalho, and M. A. Foglio, "Chemical constituents of *Luehea divaricata* Mart. (Tiliaceae)," *Química Nova*, vol. 28, no. 5, pp. 834–837, 2005.

[11] M. K. Rai, *Plant-Derived Antimycotics*, Haworth Press, London, UK, 2003.

[12] P. Backes and B. Irgang, *Árvores do Sul: Guia de Identificação e Interesse Ecológico*, Instituto Souza Cruz, Porto Alegre, Brazil, 2002.

[13] R. C. Bortoluzzi, C. I. B. Walker, and M. P. Manfron, "Análise química qualitativa e morfo-histológica de Luehea divaricata Mart," in *XVIII Simpósio de Plantas Medicinais do Brasil*, Manaus, Brazil, 2002.

[14] H. Lorenzi, *Árvores Brasileiras: Manual de Identificação e Cultivo de Plantas Arbóreas Nativas do Brasil*, Plantarum, Nova Odessa, Brazil, 1988.

[15] R. K. V. P. Portal, A. O. Lameira, and F. N. S. Ribeiro, "Fenologia e Screening fitoquímico do Açoita-cavalo," in *Manaus, 17° Seminário de Iniciação Científica e 1° Seminário de Pós-Graduação da Embrapa Amazônia Oriental*, 2013.

[16] C. B. Alice, G. A. A. B. Silva, N. C. S. Siqueira, and L. A. Mentz, "Levantamento fitoquímico de alguns vegetais utilizados na medicina popular do Rio Grande do Sul (Parte I)," *Cadernos de Farmácia*, vol. 1, no. 2, pp. 83–94, 1985.

[17] L. P. Arantes, *Atividade antioxidante in vitro do extrato etanólico das folhas de Luehea divaricata Mart [M.S. thesis]*, UFSM, Santa Maria, Brazil, 2012.

[18] E. Lopes, *Avaliação das Atividades Biológicas de Luehea divaricata*, Semana Acadêmica de Estudos Farmacêuticos. Faculdade de Farmácia, São Paulo, Brazil, 1990.

[19] A. Bertucci, F. Haretche, C. Olivaro, and A. Vázquez, "Prospección química del bosque de galería del río Uruguay," *Revista Brasileira de Farmacognosia*, vol. 18, no. 1, pp. 21–25, 2008.

[20] V. M. Vargas, R. R. Guidobono, and J. A. Henriques, "Genotoxicity of plant extracts," *Memórias do Instituto Oswaldo Cruz*, vol. 86, pp. 67–70, 1991.

[21] F. Maraschin-Silva and M. E. A. Aqüila, "Contribuição ao estudo do potencial alelopático de espécies nativas," *Revista Árvore*, vol. 30, no. 4, pp. 547–555, 2006.

[22] J. C. A. Tanaka, G. J. Vidotti, and C. C. Da Silva, "A new tormentic acid derivative from *Luehea divaricata* Mart. (Tiliaceae)," *Journal of the Brazilian Chemical Society*, vol. 14, no. 3, pp. 475–478, 2003.

[23] H. J. Choi, J. S. Eun, and B. G. Kim, "Vitexin, an HIF-1α has anti-metastatic potential in PC12 cells," *Molecular Cell Biology*, vol. 22, pp. 291–299, 2006.

[24] J. H. Kim, B. C. Lee, J. H. Kim et al., "The isolation and antioxidative effects of vitexin from *Acer palmatum*," *Archives of Pharmacal Research*, vol. 28, no. 2, pp. 195–202, 2005.

[25] Y. W. Hsum, W. T. Yew, P. L. V. Hong et al., "Cancer chemopreventive activity of maslinic acid: suppression of COX-2 expression and inhibition of NF-KB and AP-1 activation in raji cells," *Planta Medica*, vol. 77, no. 2, pp. 152–157, 2011.

[26] C. Li, Z. Yang, C. Zhai et al., "Maslinic acid potentiates the antitumor activity of tumor necrosis factor α by inhibiting NF-κB signaling pathway," *Molecular Cancer*, vol. 9, article 73, 2010.

[27] I. G. C. Bieski, F. R. Santos, R. M. de Oliveira et al., "Ethnopharmacology of medicinal plants of the pantanal region (Mato Grosso, Brazil)," *Evidence-Based Complementary and Alternative Medicine*, vol. 2012, Article ID 272749, 36 pages, 2012.

[28] M. G. Siqueira, *Atividade antiulcerogênica do extrato bruto hidroalcoólico da Luehea divaricata Martus et Zuccarini [M.S. thesis]*, Campinas, UNICAMP, 2006.

[29] C. I. B. Walker, G. D. Zanetti, and C. S. Ceron, "Morfoanatomia e Histoquimica das folhas de *Luehea divaricata* Mart," *Latin American Journal of Pharmacy*, vol. 27, pp. 203–210, 2008.

[30] D. A. da Silva, V. G. Alves, D. M. M. Franco et al., "Antiproliferative activity of *Luehea candicans* Mart. et Zucc. (Tiliaceae)," *Natural Product Research*, vol. 26, no. 4, pp. 364–369, 2012.

[31] R. Hegnauer, *Chemotaxonomie der Pflanzen. Band 6*, Birk Häuser, Zürich, Switzerland, 1973.

[32] E. A. Rosa, C. C. Silva, and C. M. A. Oliveira, "Estudo fitoquímico preliminar da espécie vegetal Luehea grandiflora (Tiliaceae)," I Jornada Paranaense dos Grupos PET, UNICENTRO, 2006.

[33] J. A. Saénz and M. C. Nassar, "Phytochemical screening of Costa Rica plants: alkaloid analysis III," *Revista de Biologia Tropical*, vol. 15, pp. 195–202, 1968.

[34] F. G. Coe, D. M. Parikh, and C. A. Johnson, "Alkaloid presence and brine shrimp (Artemia salina) bioassay of medicinal species of eastern Nicaragua," *Pharmaceutical Biology*, vol. 48, no. 4, pp. 439–445, 2010.

[35] D. F. S. Barbosa and E. Reed, "Caracterização química das drogas obtidas a partir das folhas do açoita-cavalo," 57a Reunião Anual da SBPC, 2005.

[36] J. A. Sáenz and M. Nassar, "Phytochemical screening of Costa Rican plants: alkaloid analysis. IV," *Revista de Biologia Tropical*, vol. 18, no. 1, pp. 129–138, 1970.

[37] J. T. Calixto Júnior, S. M. Morais, C. G. Martins et al., "Phytochemical analysis and modulation of antibiotic activity by *Luehea paniculata* Mart. & Zucc. (Malvaceae) in multiresistant clinical isolates of *Candida* spp.," *BioMed Research International*, vol. 2015, Article ID 807670, 10 pages, 2015.

[38] V. G. Alves, F. Vandresen, and E. A. Rosa, *Triterpenos e Atividade Antiproliferativa de Luehea paniculata (Tiliaceae)*, I Simpósio Iberoamericano de Investigação em Câncer, 2013.

[39] D. A. Silva, *Estudo Químico e Avaliacão de Atividade Antifúngica e Antiproliferativa da Espécie Luehea candicans MART et ZUCC, (Tiliaceae) [M.S. thesis]*, UEM, Maringá, Brazil, 2004.

[40] J. B. Müller, *Avaliação das atividades antimicrobiana, antioxidante e antinociceptiva das folhas da Luehea divaricata Martius [M.S. thesis]*, UFSM, Santa Maria, Brazil, 2006.

[41] N. Bessa, J. Borges, F. Beserra et al., "Prospecção fitoquímica preliminar de plantas nativas do cerrado de uso popular medicinal pela comunidade rural do assentamento vale verde—Tocantins," *Revista Brasileira de Plantas Medicinais*, vol. 15, no. 4, pp. 692–707, 2013.

[42] R. A. Longhi, "Lista das árvores: árvores e arvoretas do sul," L&PM, 1995.

[43] M. R. Ritter, G. R. Sobierajski, E. P. Schenkel, and L. A. Mentz, "Plantas usadas como medicinais no município de Ipê, RS, Brasil," *Revista Brasileira de Farmacognosia*, vol. 12, no. 2, pp. 51–62, 2002.

[44] P. E. R. Carvalho, *Espécies Arbóreas Brasileiras*, Embrapa Florestas, 2006.

[45] R. Degen, N. Soria, and M. Ortiz, "Problemática de nombres comunes de plantas medicinales comercializadas en Paraguay," *Dominguezia*, vol. 21, pp. 11–16, 2005.

[46] J. E. Carvalho, "Atividade antiulcerogênica e anticâncer de produtos naturais e de síntese," *Multiciência*, vol. 7, pp. 1–18, 2006.

[47] R. Monteles and B. U. C. Pinheiro, "Plantas medicinais em um quilombo maranhense: uma perspectiva etnobotânica," *Revista de Biologia e Ciências da Terra*, vol. 7, pp. 17–37, 2007.

[48] I. Basualdo and N. Soria, "Farmacopea Herbolaria Paraguaya: especies de la medicina Folklrica utilizada para combatir enfermedades del aparato respiratorio," *Rojasiana*, vol. 32, pp. 197–238, 1996.

[49] B. R. A. Maffei, *Plantas Medicinales*, Nuestra Tierra, Montevideo, Uruguay, 1969.

[50] C. H. B. Chiriani, *La Vuelta a los Vegetales—Tratado Moderno de Fitoterapia*, Hachette, 1982.

[51] F. W. Freire, "Plantas medicinais brasileiras," *Boletin Agricola*, vol. 34, pp. 252–494, 1933.

[52] M. González, A. Lombardo, and A. J. Vallarino, "Plantas de la medicina vulgar del Uruguay," *Cérrito*, 1937.

[53] M. Toursarkissian, *Plantas Medicinales de la Argentina*, Hemisferio Sur, 1980.

[54] C. B. Alice, V. M. F. Vargas, G. A. A. B. Silva et al., "Screening of plants used in south Brazilian folk medicine," *Journal of Ethnopharmacology*, vol. 35, no. 2, pp. 165–171, 1991.

[55] Y. Roig and J. T. Mesa, *Plantas Medicinales Aromáticas o Venenosas de Cuba*, Cultural, 1945.

[56] R. Reitz, "Plantas medicinais de Santa Catarina," *Anais Botanicos do Herbário Barbosa Rodrigues*, vol. 2, pp. 71–116, 1950.

[57] R. L. da Rosa, G. M. Nardi, A. G. F. Januário et al., "Anti-inflammatory, analgesic, and immunostimulatory effects of *Luehea divaricata* Mart. & Zucc. (Malvaceae) bark," *Brazilian Journal of Pharmaceutical Sciences*, vol. 50, no. 3, pp. 599–610, 2014.

[58] C. B. Alice, N. C. S. Siqueira, and L. A. Mentz, *Plantas Medicinais de Uso Popular: Atlas Farmacognóstico*, Ulbra, 1995.

[59] D. Saggesi, *Yerbas Medicinales Argentinas*, Rosario, 1959.

[60] H. B. Lahitte, M. J. B. Hurrell, L. Jankowski et al., *Plantas Medicinales Rioplatenses*, Ed. LOLA, 1998.

[61] J. Alonso and C. Desmarchelier, *Plantas Autóctonas Medicinales de la Argentina*, Buenos Aires, Argentina, LOLA, 2005.

[62] S. Zacchino, C. Santecchia, S. López et al., "*In vitro* antifungal evaluation and studies on mode of action of eight selected species from the Argentine flora," *Phytomedicine*, vol. 5, no. 5, pp. 389–395, 1998.

[63] P. A. B. Montovani, A. C. Gonçalves Jr., and A. Moraes, "Atividade antimicrobiana do extrato de Açoita-cavalo (*Luehea sp.*)," *Revista Brasileira de Agroecologia*, vol. 4, pp. 3731–3735, 2009.

[64] G. Coelho De Souza, A. P. S. Haas, G. L. Von Poser, E. E. S. Schapoval, and E. Elisabetsky, "Ethnopharmacological studies of antimicrobial remedies in the south of Brazil," *Journal of Ethnopharmacology*, vol. 90, no. 1, pp. 135–143, 2004.

[65] M. C. S. Marques, L. Hamerski, and F. R. Garcez, "*In vitro* biological screening and evaluation of free radical scavenging activities of medicinal plants from the Brazilian Cerrado," *Journal of Medicinal Plant Research*, vol. 15, pp. 957–962, 2013.

[66] N. R. Bianchi, "Estudo da toxicidade de *Luehea divaricata*," *Revista Brasileira de Farmácia*, vol. 77, pp. 49–50, 1996.

[67] C. Rauber, F. B. Mello, and J. R. B. Mello, "Avaliação toxicológica pré-clínica do fitoterápico contendo *Aristolochia cymbifera*, *Plantago major*, *Luehea grandiflora*, *Myrocarpus frondosus*, *Piptadenia colubrina* (Cassaú Composto) em ratos Wistar," *Acta Scientiarum Veterinária*, vol. 34, pp. 15–21, 2006.

[68] S. A. M. Souza, L. V. Cattelaia, and D. P. Vargas, "Efeitos de extratos aquosos de plantas medicinais nativas do Rio Grande do Sul sobre a germinação de sementes de alface," *Biologia & Saúde*, vol. 11, pp. 29–38, 2005.

[69] A. E. Bighetti, M. A. Ant, A. Possent, and M. A. Antônio, "Efeitos da administração aguda e subcrônica da *Luehea divaricata* Martus et Zuccarini," *Lecta*, vol. 22, no. 1-2, pp. 53–58, 2004.

[70] L. P. Felício, E. M. Silva, V. Ribeiro et al., "Mutagenic potential and modulatory effects of the medicinal plant *Luehea divaricata* (Malvaceae) in somatic cells of Drosophila melanogaster: SMART/wing," *Genetics & Molecular Research*, vol. 10, no. 1, pp. 16–24, 2011.

High-Throughput Screening of Potential Skin Penetration-Enhancers Using Stratum Corneum Lipid Liposomes: Preliminary Evaluation for Different Concentrations of Ethanol

Pajaree Sakdiset,[1,2] Yuki Kitao,[1] Hiroaki Todo,[1] and Kenji Sugibayashi[1]

[1]*Faculty of Pharmaceutical Sciences, Josai University, 1-1 Keyakidai, Sakado, Saitama 350-0295, Japan*
[2]*School of Pharmacy, Walailak University, 222 Thai Buri, Tha Sala, Nakhon Si Thammarat 80160, Thailand*

Correspondence should be addressed to Kenji Sugibayashi; sugib@josai.ac.jp

Academic Editor: Srinivas Mutalik

In this study, we developed a technique for high-throughput screening (HTS) of skin penetration-enhancers using stratum corneum lipid liposomes (SCLLs). A fluorescent marker, sodium fluorescein (FL), entrapped in SCLLs was prepared to provide a preliminary evaluation of the effect of different concentrations of ethanol on the disruption effect of SCLLs, which is an alternative for skin penetration-enhancing effects. In addition, SCLLs containing a fluorescent probe (DPH, TMA-DPH, or ANS) were also prepared and utilized to investigate SCLL fluidity. The results using SCLL-based techniques were compared with conventional skin permeation and skin impedance test using hairless rat skin. The obtained correlations were validated between FL leakage, SCLL fluidity with various probes, or skin impedance and increases in the skin permeation enhancement ratio (ER) of caffeine as a model penetrant. As a result, FL leakage and SCLL fluidity using ANS were considered to be good indices for the skin penetration-enhancing effect, suggesting that the action of ethanol on the SC lipid and penetration-enhancing is mainly on the polar head group of intercellular lipids. In addition, this screening method using SCLL could be utilized as an alternative HTS technique for conventional animal tests. Simultaneously, the method was found to be time-saving and sensitive compared with a direct assay using human and animal skins.

1. Introduction

Skin is of considerable interest as an administration route for drugs with both local and systemic effects. However, the main obstacle for drugs to pass through the skin and exert their pharmacological activities is the intrinsic barrier function of the stratum corneum (SC). The SC is the uppermost layer of the skin which consists of keratin-filled corneocytes and intercellular lipids [1, 2]. Generally, drugs in vehicles applied topically onto the skin firstly distribute into the SC and then diffuse mainly through the intercellular lipid domain [3]. Because the intercellular lipids organize into multilamellar complexes filling the intercellular spaces to provide a strong barrier against the entry of the exogenous drugs [4], approaches to overcome the skin barrier function have been investigated extensively to improve the skin permeability of drugs.

Use of chemical penetration enhancers (CPEs) is a conventional and effective approach to overcome the high barrier function of the SC. They promote the skin permeation of drugs by reducing skin barrier resistance [5]. CPEs may disrupt intercellular lipids or interact with intracellular proteins or with both regions in the SC [6]. Conventional CPEs have been screened using skin permeation experiments to determine the cumulative amount of skin permeation, flux, and permeability coefficient of drugs in the presence and absence of CPEs [7]. However, these conventional approaches are time-consuming, complicated, and resource-expensive. These methods are not practical for high-throughput screening (HTS) with various types and concentrations of CPEs as part of their discovery and development. In addition, increasing awareness of animal welfare issues nowadays has brought about a reduction in animal-based experiments, especially in the cosmetics industry. This situation gives rise to a need to develop an effective replacement approach that can provide HTS for effective CPEs and avoid the use of experimental animals.

SC lipid liposomes (SCLLs) consist of a lipid mixture similar to multilamellar lipid bilayers that are composed of ceramides, cholesterol, cholesterol esters, and fatty acids [4, 8]. SCLLs have been used as an SC intercellular lipid mimicking model to investigate the effect of agents on the skin permeability and the mechanism of enhanced skin delivery [9, 10]. One of the determination procedures is based on the change in transition temperature of SCLLs due to the chemicals determined by DSC [9]. However, this technique is also time-consuming and cannot simultaneously determine various samples, and it is difficult to obtain quantitative data. SCLLs containing entrapped marker(s) (e.g., glucose, mannitol, and calcein) have been applied to determine the release rate of the markers [9, 11–13]. In addition, labeled fluorescent probes are also used to measure the fluidizing effect of CPEs on SCLLs [14]. However, these methods are still not appropriate for HTS of CPEs because of the complicated analytical methods and rather long experimental time.

Thus, the aim of the present study was to establish a simple, quantitative, fast, and practical approach for HTS of potential CPEs. Ethanol was used as a model CPE to firstly investigate the potential of SCLLs based on the HTS methodology, because it is well known and is already in use to increase the skin penetration of various drugs such as hydrocortisone, 5-fluorouracil, and estradiol [15–17]. SCLLs entrapping a hydrophilic fluorescent probe, sodium fluorescein (FL), and incubating with three fluorescent probes with different lipophilicities were used to observe SCLL leakage and fluidity, respectively, and compared with conventional *in vitro* skin permeation tests as well as skin impedance test to determine the effectiveness of this HTS technology.

2. Materials and Methods

2.1. Materials. FL, lignoceric acid, palmitic acid, boric acid, potassium chloride, sodium hydroxide, chloroform, methanol, and ethanol were purchased from Wako Pure Chemicals Industries, Ltd. (Osaka, Japan). Cholesterol, cholesteryl sulfate, octacosanoic acid, 1,6-diphenyl-1,3,5-hexatriene (DPH), N,N, N-trimethyl-4-(6-phenyl-1,3,5-hexatrien-1-yl)phenyl-ammonium *p*-toluenesulfonate (TMA-DPH), and 8-anilino-1-naphthalenesulfonic acid ammonium salt (ANS) were from Sigma-Aldrich (St. Louis, MO, USA). Ceramide type III and ceramide type VI were from Evonik Industries AG (Essen, Germany). These reagents were used without further purification.

2.2. Experimental Animals. Male WBN/ILA-Ht hairless rats, weighing between 200 and 260 g, were obtained from the Life Science Research Center, Josai University (Saitama, Japan), and Ishikawa Experimental Animal Laboratories (Saitama, Japan). Rats were bred in a room maintained at $25 \pm 2°C$, in

which the on and off times for the lighting were 07:00 and 19:00, respectively. Animals had free access to water and food (MF, Oriental Yeast Co., Ltd., Tokyo, Japan).

All breeding procedures and experiments on the animals were performed in accordance with the guidelines of the Animal Experiment Committee of Josai University.

2.3. Methods

2.3.1. Preparation of Stratum Corneum Lipid Liposomes. SCLLs were prepared by a thin film hydration method reported by Hatfield and Fung [18] with a slight modification. The SCLLs had 5.5 mg/mL of total lipids including 33% ceramide type III, 22% ceramide type VI, 25% cholesterol, 5% cholesteryl sulfate, 7.5% lignoceric acid, 3.75% palmitic acid, and 3.75% octacosanoic acid. FL was used as an entrapped agent, and 0.1 M borate buffer (pH 9.0) was used as a dispersing medium. First, all lipid components were dissolved in the mixture of chloroform : methanol (2 : 1) in a round-bottomed flask. The solvent was then evaporated at 60°C under reduced pressure using a rotary evaporator until the thin film was obtained on the flask wall. The flask was then purged with N_2 gas and allowed to stand overnight. Next, the flask was placed in a water bath at 90°C for 30 min for annealing of the thin lipid film. Then, 2.5 mg/mL FL in 0.1 M borate buffer was added to the flask and vortexed until the thin lipid film was completely dissolved. An ultrasonic probe (VCX-750, Sonics & Materials Inc., Newtown, CT, USA) was then immersed in the liposome suspension at an amplitude of 20% for 30 s. A freeze-thaw process was then performed by immersing the flask in liquid N_2 followed by a 90°C water bath, each for 3 min for 4 cycles. The obtained liposomes were further extruded with a Lipex™ Extruder (Northern Lipids Inc., Burnaby, BC, Canada) using a membrane filter with pore sizes of 400, 200, and 100 nm (Nuclepore® track-etched membranes, GE Healthcare, Tokyo, Japan) (twice for each size of membrane filter). After preparation of the liposomes, they were centrifuged in an ultracentrifuge (Hitachi CS100GXL, Hitachi Koki Co., Ltd., Tokyo, Japan) at 289,000 ×g, 4°C twice for 15 min, twice for 10 min, and 5 times for 5 min. At each centrifugation process, the supernatant was removed and the same volume of 0.1 M borate buffer was added and mixed to prepare test liposome suspensions with removed free FL. The blank SCLLs were also prepared by previously explained process, without adding FL.

2.3.2. Determination of Sodium Fluorescein Leakage from Stratum Corneum Lipid Liposomes. SCLLs containing FL (FL-SCLLs) and different concentrations of ethanol (0–100% ethanol in 0.1 M borate buffer) were placed at a ratio of 1 : 9 v/v in an ultracentrifuge tube and mixed 5 times by pipetting. The samples were allowed to stand for 30 min and immediately ultracentrifuged at 289,000 ×g, 4°C for 5 min. The supernatant was collected to determine the FL content using a microplate reader (SpectraMax® M2^e, Molecular Devices, LLC., Sunnyvale, CA, USA) at excitation and emission wavelengths of 485 and 535 nm, respectively. This study was also performed using 75% ethanol and 0.1 M borate buffer to represent the total and background FL leakage, respectively.

The FL leakage from SCLLs was then calculated using the following equation:

$$\text{FL leakage (\%)} = \left(\frac{\text{FL}_{\text{sample}} - \text{FL}_{\text{background}}}{\text{FL}_{\text{total}} - \text{FL}_{\text{background}}} \right) \times 100. \quad (1)$$

2.3.3. Measurement of Stratum Corneum Lipid Liposome Membrane Fluidity.

The fluorescent probes DPH, TMA-DPH, and ANS were solubilized in phosphate-buffered saline (PBS) at concentrations of 2×10^{-5}, 1×10^{-5}, and 6×10^{-3} M, respectively. The fluidity of SCLL membranes was determined by incubating blank SCLLs and each fluorescent solution ($25:75\ \mu$L) in a 96-well plate and then shaking using an orbital shaker (IKA® MS 1 Minishaker, Sigma-Aldrich, Wilmington, NC, USA) at 500 rpm for 30 min in the absence of light. Next, different concentrations of ethanol in 0.1 M borate buffer ($100\ \mu$L) were added and shaken in the same conditions. The fluorescence polarization (P_f) was measured at 25°C using a microplate reader (SpectraMax M5^{e}, Molecular Devices, LLC., Sunnyvale, CA, USA). The respective excitation and emission wavelengths were 358 nm and 425 nm for DPH, 365 nm and 430 nm for TMA-DPH, and 337 nm and 480 nm for ANS. P_f value was calculated using the following equation:

$$P_f = \left(\frac{I_{0,0} - GI_{0,90}}{I_{0,0} + GI_{0,90}} \right), \quad (2)$$

where G was the grating correction coefficient; $G = I_{90,0}/I_{90,90}$. In addition, the decrease in P_f indicating the degree of membrane fluidity was calculated using the following equation.

$$\text{Decrease in } P_f = \left(\frac{P_{f,\text{control}} - P_{f,\text{sample}}}{P_{f,\text{control}}} \right) \times 100, \quad (3)$$

where $P_{f,\text{control}}$ was obtained from blank SCLLs incubated with fluorescent probe and 0.1 M borate buffer.

2.3.4. Measurement of Skin Impedance Reduction Rate.

The mixture of three types of anesthesia (medetomidine, 0.375 mg/kg; butorphanol, 2.5 mg/kg; and midazolam, 2 mg/kg) was injected intraperitoneally into hairless rats. Hairs were removed from the back under anesthesia. The treated back skin was excised, and subcutaneous fat was removed carefully using scissors. The skin was mounted with the SC side up on a square-type diffusion cell with an effective area of 19.5 cm^2 and a receiver volume of 45 mL. Eight donor cells with an effective diffusion area of 0.795 cm^2 were glued with cyanoacrylate bond (Aron Alpha®, Konishi Co. Ltd., Osaka, Japan) onto the skin. Then, 1.0 and 45 mL of physiological saline were added to the donor and receiver cells, respectively, to hydrate the skin. Skin impedance was then determined using an impedance meter (Asahi Techno Lab., Ltd., Kanagawa, Japan) 1 h after hydration. Thereafter, the physiological saline was removed from the donor cell and 1.0 mL of different concentrations of ethanol was applied for 1 h. At the end of the experiment, the donor solution was removed, the same volume of fresh saline was added, and skin impedance was determined again. The skin impedance reduction (%) was calculated from the following equation.

$$\begin{aligned} &\text{Skin impedance reduction (\%)} \\ &= \left(1 - \frac{\text{Impedance after ethanol pretreatment}}{\text{Impedance after hydration}} \right) \\ &\quad \times 100. \end{aligned} \quad (4)$$

2.3.5. In Vitro Skin Permeation Experiments.

Excised abdominal skin from hairless rat was mounted in a vertical-type Franz diffusion cell (receiver cell volume is 6.0 mL and effective permeation area is 1.77 cm^2) with the SC side facing the donor cells and the dermal side facing the receiver cell. The receiver cell was filled with 6.0 mL PBS (pH 7.4). PBS was also added to the donor cells for 1 h for skin hydration. Then, 0.5 mL of 2 mg/mL caffeine solution in 0, 10, 20, 30, 40, 50, 75, or 100% ethanol in PBS was applied to determine the skin permeation of caffeine at 32°C over 8 h, while the receiver solution was agitated at 500 rpm using a magnetic stirrer. At predetermined times, 0.5 mL aliquots were collected and the same volume of PBS was added to keep the volume constant.

2.3.6. Determination of Caffeine Permeation.

The concentration of caffeine was determined using a high-performance liquid chromatography (HPLC) system (Prominence, Shimadzu Corporation, Kyoto, Japan) equipped with a UV detector (SPD-M20A, Shimadzu Corporation). Briefly, the receiving solutions were mixed with the same volume of methanol. After centrifugation at 21,500 ×g at 4°C for 5 min, the resulting supernatant ($20\ \mu$L) was injected directly into the HPLC system. Chromatographic separation was performed at 40°C using an Inertsil ODS-3, $5\ \mu$m in diameter, 4.6 mm I.D. × 150 mm (GL Sciences Inc., Tokyo, Japan). The mobile phase was 0.1% phosphoric acid : methanol 7 : 3 v/v and the flow rate was 1.0 mL/min. UV absorbance detection was performed at 280 nm.

2.3.7. Calculation of Skin Permeation Parameter.

Skin permeation flux of 5 to 8 h after starting the experiment was calculated by linear regression of the skin permeation profile of caffeine. Skin permeation coefficient was obtained by dividing the skin permeation flux with the initial concentration of the applied caffeine in the donor compartment. The increase in the skin-penetration-enhancement ratio (ER) after an 8 h permeation experiment was calculated with a following equation.

$$\text{Increase in ER} = \left(\frac{Q_{\text{sample}} - Q_{\text{control}}}{Q_{\text{control}}} \right), \quad (5)$$

where Q_{sample} and Q_{control} are the cumulative amounts of caffeine permeated per unit area of skin over 8 h from different concentrations of ethanol and PBS, respectively.

2.3.8. Statistics.

The differences among the obtained data were analyzed using unpaired t-test. The differences were considered significant when $p < 0.05$. Pearson's correlation

TABLE 1: Flux, permeability coefficient, and enhancement ratio of caffeine from different concentrations of ethanol.

Formulation	Flux ($\mu g/cm^2/h$)	Permeability coefficient ($\times 10^{-7}$ cm/s)	Enhancement ratio
0% ethanol	0.81 ± 0.17	1.12 ± 0.24	1.00 ± 0.22
10% ethanol	0.88 ± 0.15	1.22 ± 0.21	1.07 ± 0.19
20% ethanol	1.52 ± 0.29	2.12 ± 0.40	1.60 ± 0.32
30% ethanol	1.95 ± 0.35	2.71 ± 0.49	2.02 ± 0.34
40% ethanol	2.94 ± 0.19	4.08 ± 0.26	2.82 ± 0.15
50% ethanol	3.82 ± 0.40	5.31 ± 0.55	4.33 ± 0.52
75% ethanol	3.67 ± 0.13	5.10 ± 0.19	4.85 ± 0.19
100% ethanol	4.22 ± 0.62	5.86 ± 0.86	4.26 ± 0.47

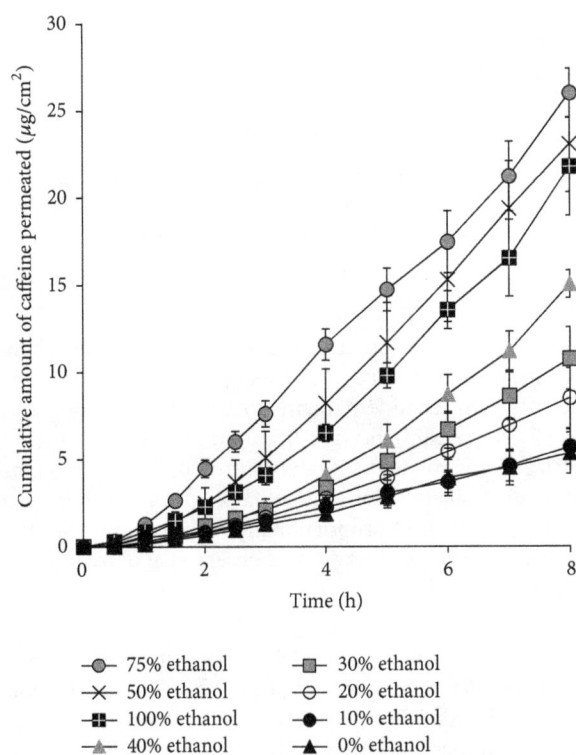

Legend:
- 75% ethanol
- 50% ethanol
- 100% ethanol
- 40% ethanol
- 30% ethanol
- 20% ethanol
- 10% ethanol
- 0% ethanol

FIGURE 1: Time course of cumulative amount of caffeine permeated through full-thickness hairless rat skin after application with different concentrations of ethanol. Each value represents the mean ± SE ($n = 3$–5).

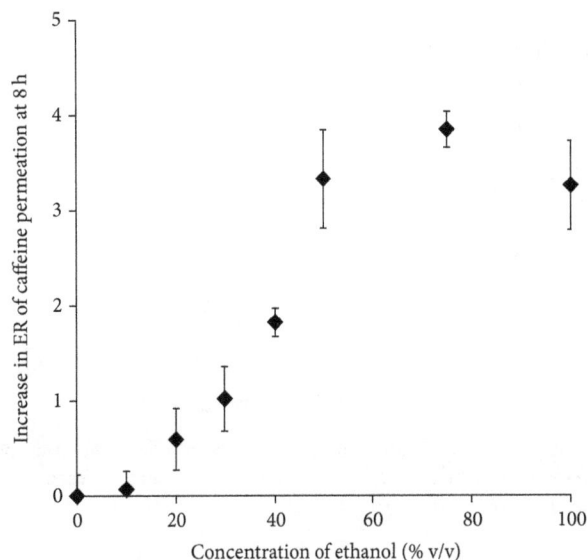

FIGURE 2: Effect of ethanol concentration on the increase in the skin-penetration-enhancement ratio (ER) of caffeine permeated over 8 h. Each value represents the mean ± SE ($n = 3$–5).

coefficient was used to determine the relationship between the results from SCLL test and skin permeation study.

3. Results and Discussion

3.1. Results

3.1.1. Effect of Ethanol on In Vitro Skin Permeation of Caffeine.
In the present study, caffeine was selected as a hydrophilic model drug to evaluate the relationship between its skin permeation rate and the effect of different concentrations of ethanol on SC lipid disruption. Figure 1 shows the cumulative amounts of caffeine permeated through the excised hairless rat skin. Typical *in vitro* skin permeation profiles of caffeine

(lag time and following almost steady-state profiles) were observed in all cases when using 0–100% ethanol as in the donor solution. Figure 2 illustrates the relationship between the increase in ER and the ethanol concentration in the donor solution. Figures 1 and 2 show that the skin permeation of caffeine was strongly dependent on the ethanol concentration in the caffeine solution. When the ethanol concentration increased from 0% to 50%, the skin permeation rate of caffeine also increased. However, at 100% ethanol, caffeine permeation was rather decreased compared with the samples with 50% and 75% ethanol. The maximum skin permeation of caffeine was observed with 75% ethanol in the present study. The skin permeation flux, permeability coefficient, and enhancement ratio of caffeine obtained from different concentrations of ethanol are also summarized in Table 1.

3.1.2. Effect of Ethanol on the Skin Impedance.
Skin impedance has been used as an index of the skin permeation rate of drugs, especially of hydrophilic drugs, because the decrease in skin impedance is related to decreased barrier function of the skin. Therefore, we determined skin impedance after

TABLE 2: Characteristics of blank stratum corneum lipid liposomes (SCLLs) and sodium fluorescein entrapped in SCLLs (FL-SCLLs).

	Blank SCLLs	FL-SCLLs
Size (nm)	221.1 ± 8.6	282.8 ± 3.2
Polydispersity index	0.556 ± 0.017	0.215 ± 0.014
Zeta potential (mV)	-87.0 ± 2.3	-99.6 ± 3.3

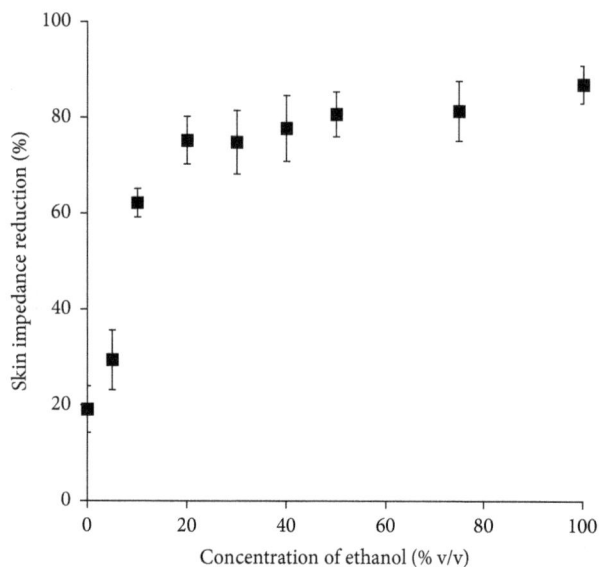

FIGURE 3: Effect of different concentrations of ethanol on the percentage of skin impedance reduction. Each value represents the mean $\pm$ SE ($n = 3$–5).

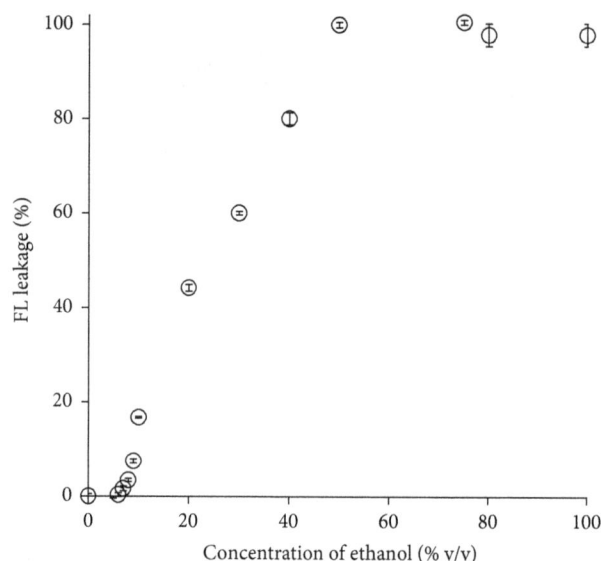

FIGURE 4: Effect of different concentrations of ethanol on the sodium fluorescein (FL) leakage from stratum corneum lipid liposomes (SCLLs). Each value represents the mean $\pm$ SE ($n = 3$).

pretreatment with different concentrations of ethanol. Figure 3 shows the decrease in skin impedance with different concentrations of ethanol on excised back skin of hairless rats. Ethanol treatment changed the skin impedance even at a low concentration. Ethanol solution at a concentration of 5% reduced skin impedance by about 30%, and 20–100% ethanol could reduce skin impedance about 75–80%.

3.1.3. Stratum Corneum Lipid Liposomes Characteristics.
Table 2 summarizes the characteristics of blank SCLLs and FL-SCLLs prepared in the present study. The vesicle size and distribution of FL-SCLLs were a little larger but narrower, respectively, than the blank SCLLs, indicating that the vesicle dispersion was homogeneous. Both the liposome formulations showed highly negative surface charge of -87.0 ± 2.3 and -99.6 ± 3.3 mV, respectively, because of the ionized fraction of fatty acids at pH 9.0. The presence of FL anions inside the SCLLs leads to higher negative surface charge. The zeta potential of both SCLL formulations indicated high electrostatic repulsion among the particles and excellent kinetic stability [19].

3.1.4. Effect of Ethanol on the Sodium Fluorescein Leakage from Stratum Corneum Lipid Liposomes.
Next, the effect of different concentrations of ethanol was tested on the disruption of SCLLs. Figure 4 shows the relation between the

FL leakage (%) and ethanol concentration. As the ethanol concentration increased, FL leakage also increased in a concentration-dependent manner. At low ethanol concentrations (0–5% ethanol), no significant promotion was observed in FL leakage compared with the control (0.1 M borate buffer). At higher concentrations of ethanol, on the other hand, FL leakage increased proportionally with the concentration. However, no more FL leakage was observed at more than 50% ethanol.

3.1.5. Effect of Ethanol on Membrane Fluidity of Stratum Corneum Lipid Liposomes.
Figure 5 shows the membrane fluidity of blank SCLLs incubated with fluorescent probes with different lipophilicities. The decrease in P_f was used as an index of membrane fluidity of SCLLs. The results with DPH and TMA-DPH as fluorescent probes showed relatively low membrane fluidity. The maximum decrease was observed at 100% ethanol, which provided 37.8% and 17.9% decreases in P_f for DPH and TMA-DPH, respectively. High membrane fluidity was observed when using ANS probe at low concentrations of ethanol.

3.1.6. Relationship between Sodium Fluorescein Leakage and Increase in Skin-Penetration-Enhancement Ratio.
SCLLs were used as an SC lipid model to investigate the enhancing effect of ethanol on the skin permeation of caffeine. The correlation was evaluated between the present SCLL-based HTS data and the conventional skin-penetration-enhancing profiles of caffeine. Figure 6(a) shows the relationship between the increase in ER of the cumulative amount of caffeine permeated through skin over 8 h (x-axis) and FL leakage (%) from SCLLs (y-axis). The correlation coefficient of this relationship was 0.888. The obtained profile was concave relative to x-axis, indicating that ethanol more markedly

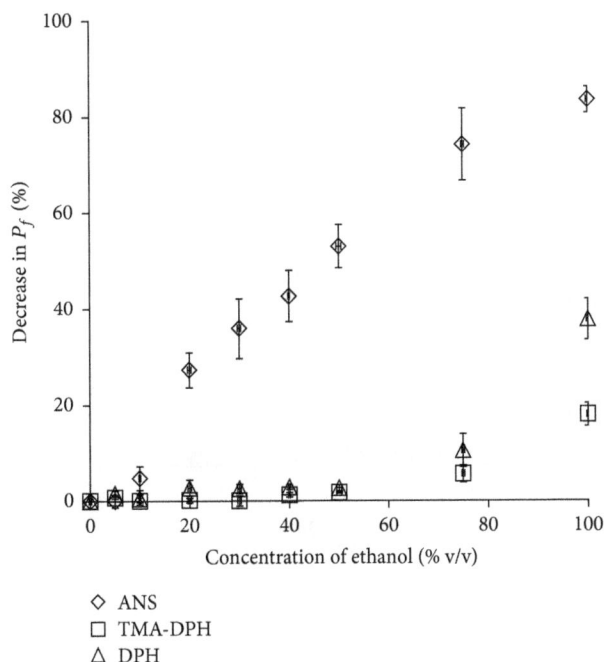

FIGURE 5: Effect of different concentrations of ethanol on the percentage decrease in fluorescence polarization (P_f) using three fluorescent probes: 1,6-diphenyl-1,3,5-hexatriene (DPH), N,N,N-trimethyl-4-(6-phenyl-1,3,5-hexatrien-1-yl)phenyl-ammonium p-toluenesulfonate (TMA-DPH), and 8-anilino-1-naphthalenesulfonic acid ammonium salt (ANS). Each value represents the mean ± SE ($n = 3$).

affected SCLL disruption than the skin permeation of caffeine, especially at low concentrations of ethanol. Almost linear relationship could be observed at higher concentrations of ethanol. The semilog plot, as shown in Figure 6(b), shows a very high correlation coefficient of 0.974.

3.1.7. Relationship between Stratum Corneum Lipid Liposome Membrane Fluidity and Increase in Skin Penetration-Enhancement Ratio. Figure 7(a) shows a relationship between SCLL membrane fluidity and the increase in the ER. The data from 100% ethanol were not included in this correlation, because the reduction in the ER might be an exceptional case, with such a high concentration of ethanol having a reversed effect on the skin permeation of caffeine. The linear relationship could be obtained in SCLL membrane fluidity measured using the ANS probe with a correlation coefficient of 0.899, whereas DPH and TMA-DPH showed poorer correlations (R^2 of DPH and TMA-DPH: 0.638 and 0.748, resp.). In the data using ANS probe, a higher correlation was obtained in the semilog plot as shown in Figure 7(b), similar to Figure 6(b).

3.1.8. Relationship between Skin Impedance Reduction and Increase in Skin Penetration-Enhancement Ratio. Figure 8 shows a relation between skin impedance reduction and increase in ER. No good relationships were observed; the correlation coefficient was 0.456 between the increase in ER at 8 h and impedance reduction, although such skin impedance

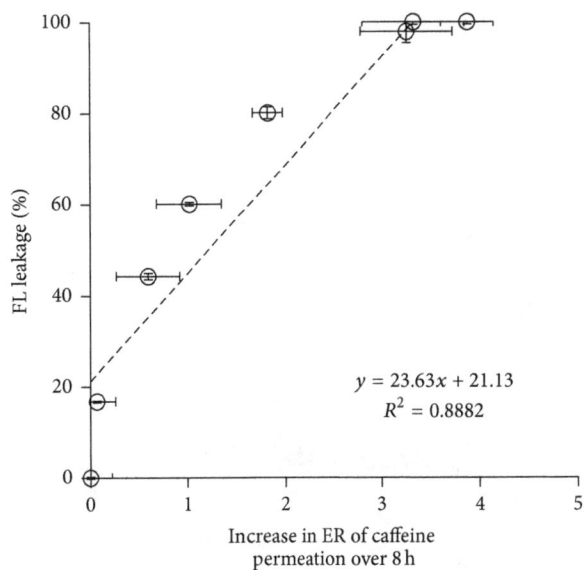

(a)

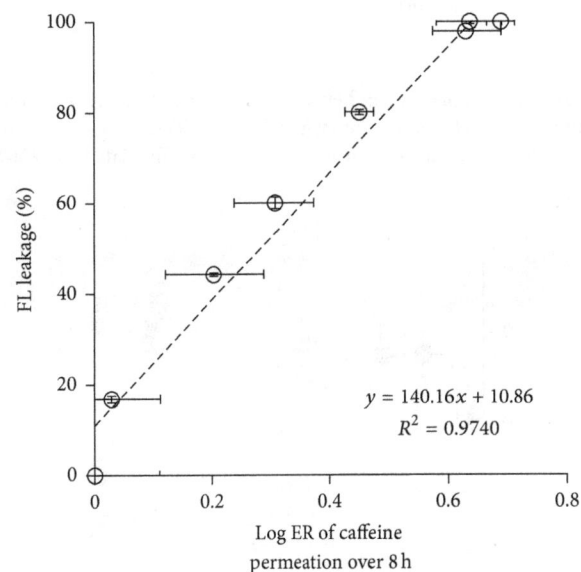

(b)

FIGURE 6: The relationship between sodium fluorescein (FL) leakage and increase in the skin penetration-enhancement ratio (ER) (a); log ER of caffeine permeated over 8 h from each concentration of ethanol solution (b). Each value represents the mean ± SE ($n = 3$–5).

was reported to be correlated with a big amount of skin permeation data of drugs.

3.2. Discussion. In the present study, an HTS approach for searching for effective CPEs was established based on using SCLLs as a model membrane mimicking the primary skin-penetration domain of the SC lipid bilayer. Different concentrations of ethanol were used in the first step, because this is a well-known CPE contained in many topical and transdermal formulations. The composition of lipids used in SCLLs, closely similar to the lipid composition of intercellular

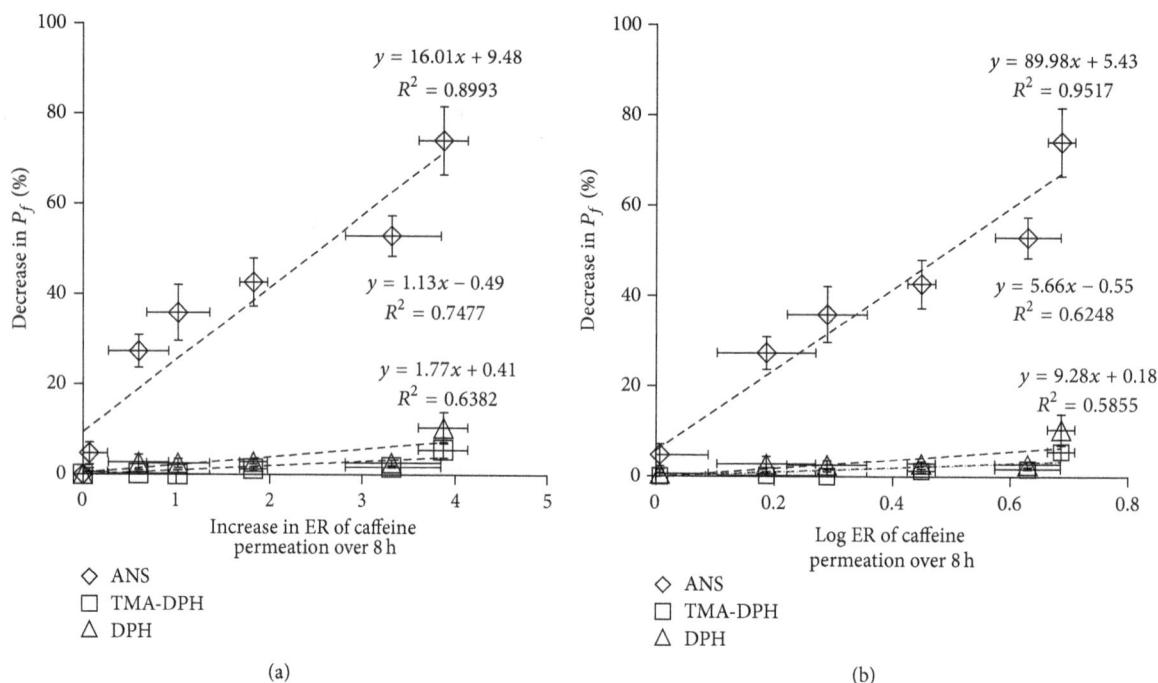

$$y = 16.01x + 9.48$$
$$R^2 = 0.8993$$

$$y = 1.13x - 0.49$$
$$R^2 = 0.7477$$

$$y = 1.77x + 0.41$$
$$R^2 = 0.6382$$

◇ ANS
□ TMA-DPH
△ DPH

(a)

$$y = 89.98x + 5.43$$
$$R^2 = 0.9517$$

$$y = 5.66x - 0.55$$
$$R^2 = 0.6248$$

$$y = 9.28x + 0.18$$
$$R^2 = 0.5855$$

◇ ANS
□ TMA-DPH
△ DPH

(b)

FIGURE 7: The relationship between percentage of decrease in fluorescence polarization (P_f) using various fluorescent probes and increase in the skin penetration-enhancement ratio (ER) (a); log ER of caffeine permeated over 8 h from each concentration of ethanol solution (b). Each value represents the mean ± SE ($n = 3$–5). The data from 100% ethanol was excluded in this figure.

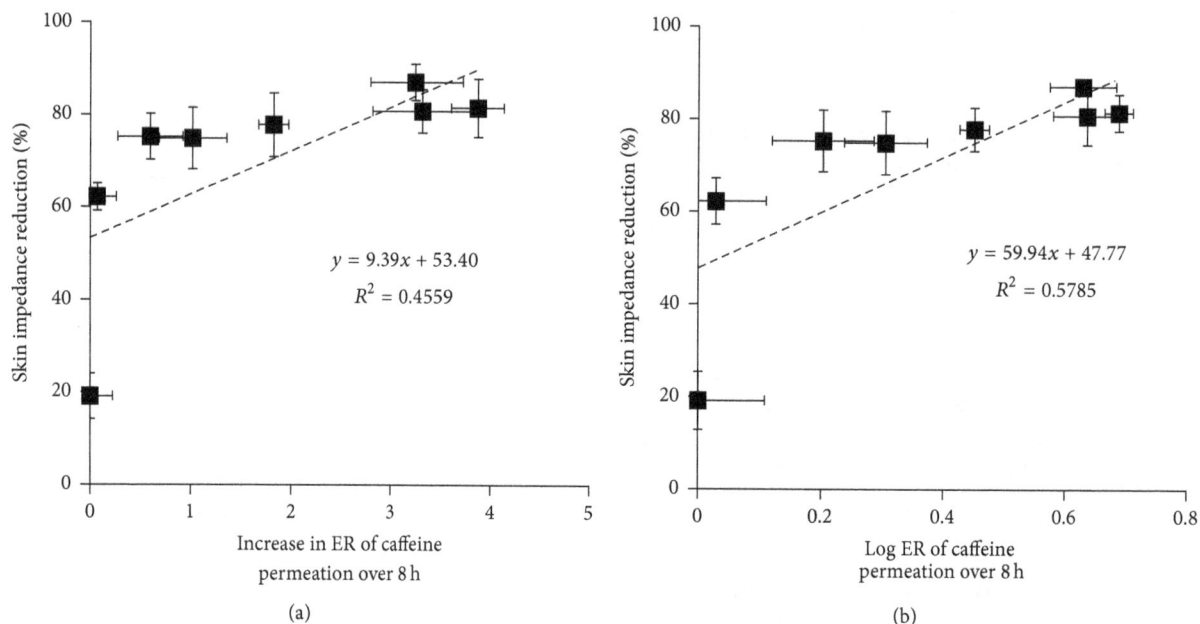

$$y = 9.39x + 53.40$$
$$R^2 = 0.4559$$

(a)

$$y = 59.94x + 47.77$$
$$R^2 = 0.5785$$

(b)

FIGURE 8: The relationship between skin impedance reduction and increase in the skin penetration-enhancement ratio (ER) (a); log ER of caffeine permeated over 8 h from each concentration of ethanol solution (b). Each value represents the mean ± SE ($n = 3$–5).

lipids, was comprised of 33% ceramide type III, 22% ceramide type IV, 15% fatty acids (palmitic : lignoceric : octacosanoic acid: 1 : 2 : 1), 25% cholesterol, and 5% cholesteryl sulfate and buffer (pH, 9.0), which was reported to enhance the stability of SCLL vesicles [18]. A fluorescent hydrophilic marker, FL, was entrapped in SCLLs in order to monitor the degree

of its membrane rupture by ethanol. Furthermore, SCLL membrane fluidity using probe of various lipophilicities was also measured in an HTS manner. These experiments were compared with conventional methods for the determination of skin penetration-enhancing effect of chemicals: *in vitro* permeation and impedance studies using hairless rat skin.

Skin permeation experiments with caffeine were conducted in asymmetric conditions to determine the penetration-enhancing effect of ethanol. The increase in ER by ethanol was concentration-dependent (Figures 1 and 2). A similar ethanol concentration-dependent effect was observed when using indomethacin in our previous study [20]. However, the permeation of caffeine decreased at the highest ethanol concentration, because highly concentrated ethanol dehydrates the skin membrane and reduces the skin permeation of drugs [21]. Our previous study also found that the skin permeability of hydrophilic drugs was increased but inversely decreased by low and high concentration of ethanol, respectively [22]. In addition, X-ray diffraction data confirmed that low concentrations of ethanol disturbed the short lamellar structure of SC lipids, but the high concentration caused an aligned structure [23].

Skin impedance has been reported to correlate with drug permeability through skin [22, 24]. Then, we determined the back skin impedance to increase the sensitivity of ethanol on impedance and to reduce the number of rats sacrificed. Ethanol could reduce the skin impedance and clearly alter the flux of low molecular weight ions through the skin [22]. Nevertheless, the relationship was not linear between the reduction in skin impedance and the increase in ER (Figure 8). This is because low concentrations of ethanol could greatly reduce the skin impedance but higher concentrations remained stable (Figure 3). Therefore, the reduction in skin impedance by ethanol might not be a good indicator for the skin penetration-enhancement effect. This may be because of different thermodynamic activities of caffeine in different concentrations of ethanol when using the same concentration of caffeine in different ethanol concentrations. In other words, the thermodynamic activity of a certain concentration of caffeine is low in high concentrations of ethanol, resulting in lower skin permeation of caffeine from higher concentrations of ethanol solution. Another possibility is that lower skin impedance may be obtained from the same concentration of caffeine at low ethanol concentrations because skin impedance is also dependent on the ethanol concentration in skin. When checking other CPEs rather than solvent types such as ethanol, skin impedance may be dependent on the penetration-enhancing effect, because little contribution is expected by nonsolvent type enhancers on the thermodynamic activity of penetrants.

Using SCLL leakage tests, FL leakage was observed from low (≥5%) to high (~100%) concentrations of ethanol and the degree was ethanol concentration-dependent (Figure 4), suggesting that the disruption effect on the SCLL membrane was closely related to ethanol concentration. Ethanol has been reported as a markedly effective skin penetration-enhancer by various mechanisms because of an increase in drug solubility, improvement in drug partitioning into the SC, modification of thermodynamic activity of drugs, solvent (ethanol) drag effect across the skin, fluidization and extraction of SC lipids, and the structure modification of SC keratin [21, 25]. SCLLs used in the present experiment are a model representing only the SC lipids with lack of cellular proteins such as keratin [6]. Therefore, the present SCLL leakage results might

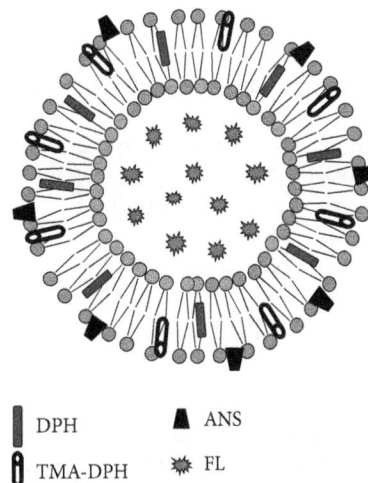

FIGURE 9: Location of fluorescent probes in stratum corneum lipid liposomes (SCLLs).

not be totally predictive for all mechanisms associated with the skin penetration-enhancing effects of ethanol.

SCLLs mimic SC lipids in the intercellular domain where CPEs act. Then, three different fluorescent probes, DPH, TMA-DPH, and ANS, were used to determine the SCLL membrane fluidity in order to better understand the effect of ethanol on lipid packing. High fluidity in the SCLL membrane represents a high degree of lipid molecule disorganization, which provides high permeability of drugs through the bilayer [26]. The ethanol effect on the fluidity of SCLL was determined, especially in the region where each fluorescent probe was contained, as depicted in Figure 9. DPH and TMA-DPH serve as markers for molecular movement in the hydrophobic core and superficial surface of SCLLs [27], respectively. The effect of ethanol on SCLL fluidity using DPH and TMA-DPH showed similar patterns (Figure 5). Although lower ethanol concentrations could not promote SCLL fluidity, the effect was clearly found with more than 50% ethanol. On the other hand, ANS, a marker of molecular movement on the exterior membrane surface [27], changed membrane fluidity even at low ethanol concentrations, and good linearity was observed between SCLL fluidity and ethanol concentration (Figure 5). The results using these three fluorescent probes provided a possible effect of ethanol on SCLL membranes, suggesting that ethanol disrupted mainly the polar head region outside the liposome membrane similar to a previous report [28]. The use of ANS may be the most suitable for evaluating the skin penetration-enhancement effects from ethanol.

Good correlations were obtained especially in the FL leakage test (Figure 6) and SCLL fluidity detected using the ANS probe (Figure 7), indicating that SCLLs could be an optional model to investigate the skin penetration-enhancing effects of CPEs as well as their mode of actions. Furthermore, our approach was able to determine the enhancing effect by ethanol in a very short period. Thus, time-consuming skin permeation experiments, which normally take about 8 h to a few days, could be markedly reduced to only 30–60 min incubation times using SCLLs with probes and CPEs. Various samples could be simply and simultaneously evaluated using a 96-well plate fluorescence spectroscopy microplate reader. In addition, our method could avoid the use of animal membranes in comparison with typical skin permeation approaches. Despite the observation that this method was quite sensitive even at low concentrations of ethanol, which vary from the actual results of skin permeation experiments, this approach could be a practical tool to discover effective CPEs for use in topical and transdermal formulations.

4. Conclusions

The present HTS approach using SCLLs could be a promising model to determine the effect of ethanol on the skin permeability of drugs, because a good correlation was obtained from SCLL-based experiments and a skin permeation study. The ease of handling of the various fluorescent probes could also identify the possible mechanism of action of ethanol for enhancing skin permeation. Although skin impedance tests have been reported to correlate with skin permeability, SCLL results showed better predictability for the skin penetration-enhancement effect by ethanol, for which the primary action is on the disruption of SC intercellular lipids. The present findings could clarify the advantages of SCLLs not only for screening approaches to investigate the potential of CPEs but also for drug delivery systems.

Competing Interests

The authors declare that there is no conflict of interests.

References

[1] A. Naik, Y. N. Kalia, and R. H. Guy, "Transdermal drug delivery: overcoming the skin's barrier function," *Pharmaceutical Science and Technology Today*, vol. 3, no. 9, pp. 318–326, 2000.

[2] J. Van Smeden, M. Janssens, G. S. Gooris, and J. A. Bouwstra, "The important role of stratum corneum lipids for the cutaneous barrier function," *Biochimica et Biophysica Acta—Molecular and Cell Biology of Lipids*, vol. 1841, no. 3, pp. 295–313, 2014.

[3] P. W. Wertz and B. Van Den Bergh, "The physical, chemical and functional properties of lipids in the skin and other biological barriers," *Chemistry and Physics of Lipids*, vol. 91, no. 2, pp. 85–96, 1998.

[4] P. W. Wertz, "Lipids and barrier function of the skin," *Acta Dermato-Venereologica Supplement*, no. 208, pp. 7–11, 2000.

[5] B. W. Barry, "Mode of action of penetration enhancers in human skin," *Journal of Controlled Release*, vol. 6, no. 1, pp. 85–97, 1987.

[6] G. M. El Maghraby, B. W. Barry, and A. C. Williams, "Liposomes and skin: from drug delivery to model membranes," *European Journal of Pharmaceutical Sciences*, vol. 34, no. 4-5, pp. 203–222, 2008.

[7] K. Sugibayashi, K. Hosoya, Y. Morimoto, and W. I. Higuchi, "Effect of the absorption enhancer, Azone, on the transport of 5–fluorouracil across hairless rat skin," *Journal of Pharmacy and Pharmacology*, vol. 37, no. 8, pp. 578–580, 1985.

[8] P. W. Wertz, W. Abraham, L. Landmann, and D. T. Downing, "Preparation of liposomes from stratum corneum lipids," *Journal of Investigative Dermatology*, vol. 87, no. 5, pp. 582–584, 1986.

[9] C.-K. Kim, M.-S. Hong, Y.-B. Kim, and S.-K. Han, "Effect of penetration enhancers (pyrrolidone derivatives) on multilamellar liposomes of stratum corneum lipid: a study by UV spectroscopy and differential scanning calorimetry," *International Journal of Pharmaceutics*, vol. 95, no. 1–3, pp. 43–50, 1993.

[10] G. M. M. E. Maghraby, M. Campbell, and B. C. Finnin, "Mechanisms of action of novel skin penetration enhancers: phospholipid versus skin lipid liposomes," *International Journal of Pharmaceutics*, vol. 305, no. 1-2, pp. 90–104, 2005.

[11] K. Yoneto, S. K. Li, A. Ghanem, W. I. Higuchi, and D. J. A. Crommelin, "A mechanistic study of the effects of the 1–Alkyl–2–pyrrolidones on bilayer permeability of stratum corneum lipid liposomes: a comparison with hairless mouse skin studies," *Journal of Pharmaceutical Sciences*, vol. 84, no. 7, pp. 853–861, 1995.

[12] T. M. Suhonen, L. Pirskanen, M. Räisänen et al., "Transepidermal delivery of β-blocking agents: evaluation of enhancer effects using stratum corneum lipid liposomes," *Journal of Controlled Release*, vol. 43, no. 2-3, pp. 251–259, 1997.

[13] M. Suhonen, S. K. Li, W. I. Higuchi, and J. N. Herron, "A liposome permeability model for stratum corneum lipid bilayers based on commercial lipids," *Journal of Pharmaceutical Sciences*, vol. 97, no. 10, pp. 4278–4293, 2008.

[14] K. Yoneto, S. K. Li, W. I. Higuchi, W. Jiskoot, and J. N. Herron, "Fluorescent probe studies of the interactions of 1-alkyl-2-pyrrolidones with stratum corneum lipid liposomes," *Journal of Pharmaceutical Sciences*, vol. 85, no. 5, pp. 511–517, 1996.

[15] B. Berner, G. C. Mazzenga, J. H. Otte, R. J. Steffens, R. Juang, and C. D. Ebert, "Ethanol: water mutually enhanced transdermal therapeutic system II: skin permeation of ethanol and nitroglycerin," *Journal of Pharmaceutical Sciences*, vol. 78, no. 5, pp. 402–407, 1989.

[16] D. Friend, P. Catz, J. Heller, J. Reid, and R. Baker, "Transdermal delivery of levonorgestrel I. Alkanols as permeation enhancers in vitro," *Journal of Controlled Release*, vol. 7, no. 3, pp. 243–250, 1988.

[17] L. K. Pershing, L. D. Lambert, and K. Knutson, "Mechanism of ethanol-enhanced estradiol permeation across human skin in vivo," *Pharmaceutical Research*, vol. 7, no. 2, pp. 170–175, 1990.

[18] R. M. Hatfield and L. W.-M. Fung, "A new model system for lipid interactions in stratum corneum vesicles: effects of lipid composition, calcium, and pH," *Biochemistry*, vol. 38, no. 2, pp. 784–791, 1999.

[19] C. Freitas and R. H. Müller, "Effect of light and temperature on zeta potential and physical stability in solid lipid nanoparticle (SLN®) dispersions," *International Journal of Pharmaceutics*, vol. 168, no. 2, pp. 221–229, 1998.

[20] K. Sugibayashi, M. Nemoto, and Y. Morimoto, "Effect of several penetration enhancers on the percutaneous absorption of indomethacin in hairless rats," *Chemical and Pharmaceutical Bulletin*, vol. 36, no. 4, pp. 1519–1528, 1988.

[21] A. C. Williams and B. W. Barry, "Penetration enhancers," *Advanced Drug Delivery Reviews*, vol. 64, pp. 128–137, 2012.

[22] D. Horita, H. Todo, and K. Sugibayashi, "Effect of ethanol pretreatment on skin permeation of drugs," *Biological and Pharmaceutical Bulletin*, vol. 35, no. 8, pp. 1343–1348, 2012.

[23] D. Horita, I. Hatta, M. Yoshimoto, Y. Kitao, H. Todo, and K. Sugibayashi, "Molecular mechanisms of action of different

concentrations of ethanol in water on ordered structures of intercellular lipids and soft keratin in the stratum corneum," *Biochimica et Biophysica Acta—Biomembranes*, vol. 1848, no. 5, pp. 1196–1202, 2015.

[24] P. Karande, A. Jain, and S. Mitragotri, "Relationships between skin's electrical impedance and permeability in the presence of chemical enhancers," *Journal of Controlled Release*, vol. 110, no. 2, pp. 307–313, 2006.

[25] M. E. Lane, "Skin penetration enhancers," *International Journal of Pharmaceutics*, vol. 447, no. 1-2, pp. 12–21, 2013.

[26] M. Michelon, R. A. Mantovani, R. Sinigaglia-Coimbra, L. G. de la Torre, and R. L. Cunha, "Structural characterization of β-carotene-incorporated nanovesicles produced with non-purified phospholipids," *Food Research International*, vol. 79, pp. 95–105, 2016.

[27] C. Tan, B. Feng, X. Zhang, W. Xia, and S. Xia, "Biopolymer-coated liposomes by electrostatic adsorption of chitosan (chitosomes) as novel delivery systems for carotenoids," *Food Hydrocolloids*, vol. 52, pp. 774–784, 2016.

[28] N. Dayan and E. Touitou, "Carriers for skin delivery of trihexyphenidyl HCl: ethosomes vs. liposomes," *Biomaterials*, vol. 21, no. 18, pp. 1879–1885, 2000.

3

Application of Cerium (IV) as an Oxidimetric Agent for the Determination of Ethionamide in Pharmaceutical Formulations

Kanakapura Basavaiah,[1] **Nagib A. S. Qarah,**[1] **and Sameer A. M. Abdulrahman**[2]

[1]*Department of Chemistry, University of Mysore, Manasagangotri, Mysore 570 006, India*
[2]*Department of Chemistry, Faculty of Education and Sciences Rada'a, Al-Baydha University, Al Bayda, Yemen*

Correspondence should be addressed to Kanakapura Basavaiah; kanakapurabasavaiah@gmail.com

Academic Editor: Rama Pati Tripathi

Two simple methods are described for the determination of ethionamide (ETM) in bulk drug and tablets using cerium (IV) sulphate as the oxidimetric agent. In both methods, the sample solution is treated with a measured excess of cerium (IV) solution in H_2SO_4 medium, and after a fixed standing time, the residual oxidant is determined either by back titration with standard iron (II) solution to a ferroin end point in titrimetry or by reacting with o-dianisidine followed by measurement of the absorbance of the orange-red coloured product at 470 nm in spectrophotometry. In titrimetry, the reaction proceeded with a stoichiometry of 1 : 2 (ETM : Ce (IV)) and the amount of cerium (IV) consumed by ETM was related to the latter's amount, and the method was applicable over 1.0–8.0 mg of drug. In spectrophotometry, Beer's law was obeyed over the concentration range of 0.5–5.0 μg/mL ETM with a molar absorptivity value of 2.66×10^4 L/(mol·cm). The limits of detection (LOD) and quantification (LOQ) calculated according to ICH guidelines were 0.013 and 0.043 μg/mL, respectively. The proposed titrimetric and spectrophotometric methods were found to yield reliable results when applied to bulk drug and tablets analysis, and hence they can be applied in quality control laboratories.

1. Introduction

Ethionamide (ETM), chemically known as 2-ethylthioisonicotinamide, is a second-line orally administered drug that is used for the treatment of multidrug resistant tuberculosis [1]. The drug has been in use since 1960s, because it is cheap, easily available, relatively nontoxic, and efficacious [2]. ETM is a structural analog of isoniazid [3, 4] and is found to inhibit mycolic acid biosynthesis [5] with good bioavailability [6].

The drug is official in the British Pharmacopoeia [7], which describes a titrimetric assay with acetous perchloric acid in anhydrous acetic acid medium. Other methods based on fluorometric [8] and spectrophotometric [9–19] techniques have been reported for its assay in pharmaceuticals. Other than the official method [7], three more titrimetric methods are found in the literature for the assay of ETM in pharmaceuticals [20–22]. Reddy et al. [20] titrated ETM with N-bromosuccinamide using several anthraquinones as indicators. The drug in 25–500 μmol levels was assayed by Ciesielski et al. [21] by titrating it with iodine in alkaline medium.

Employing AgS-ion-selective electrode as the sensor, Obtemperanskaya et al. [22] have reported a micro method by titration of the drug solution with 0.01 M $AgNO_3$. The titrant used in the previously reported method [20] is unstable and requires daily standardization whereas the method employing membrane electrode [22] is tedious and time-consuming. It is desirable that the methods used in routine analysis should be simple and rapid with minimum experimental operations. Though ETM is prone to oxidation, a stable and strong oxidant such as cerium (IV) did not figure among the several titrimetric or spectrophotometric reagents that have been employed earlier for the assay of ETM. The reported spectrophotometric methods suffer from some disadvantages such as need for longer contact time, pH adjustment, multistep reactions, extraction step, and dependence on critical experimental variables.

In this paper, we describe two simple, rapid, and sensitive methods for the determination of ETM in pharmaceuticals using cerium (IV) as the oxidant. The methods are based on the oxidation of ETM by a measured excess of cerium (IV)

in H_2SO_4 medium followed by the determination of the unreacted oxidant either by titration with iron (II) visually (titrimetry) or by reacting it with ortho-dianisidine and measuring the absorbance of the orange-red coloured product at 470 nm (spectrophotometry). The two methods were found to be fairly accurate and precise in addition to being more sensitive compared to the previously reported methods.

2. Materials and Methods

2.1. Materials. Pharmaceutical grade ethionamide, certified to be 99.84% pure, was received as gift from Panacea Biotic Ltd. and used as received. Three brands of tablets, namely, Ethide (Lupin Ltd., Mumbai, India), Ethiokox (Radicura Private Ltd., New Delhi, India), and Myobid (Panacea Biotic, New Delhi, India) labeled to contain 250 mg of ETM per tablet, were purchased from local commercial sources.

2.2. Apparatus. A Systronics model 166 digital spectrophotometer (Systronics, Ahmedabad, Gujarat, India) with matched 1 cm quartz cells was used for absorbance measurements.

2.3. Chemicals and Reagents. All chemicals used were of analytical reagent grade. Double distilled water was used throughout the investigation.

Cerium (IV) Solution (0.01 M). An approximately 0.01 M cerium (IV) solution was prepared by dissolving the required quantity of cerium (IV) sulphate (Loba Chemie, Mumbai, India) in 0.5 M H_2SO_4 with the aid heat and filtered using glass wool; the solution was standardized [23] with pure ferrous ammonium sulphate (Loba Chemie, Mumbai, India) and used in titrimetry. The stock standard solution was diluted appropriately with 0.5 M H_2SO_4 to get 100 μg/mL cerium (IV) for use in spectrophotometry.

Ferrous Ammonium Sulphate, FAS (0.01 M). It is prepared by dissolving the calculated amount of the chemical in water in the presence of few drops of dilute H_2SO_4 and standardized using pure potassium dichromate [23].

Ortho-Dianisidine, ODS (0.05%). It is prepared by dissolving the calculated amount of the chemical (Loba Chemie, Mumbai, India) in ethanol.

Sulphuric Acid (5 M). Concentrated acid (98%; sp. gr. 1.82, Merck, Mumbai, India) was diluted appropriately with water to get 5 M acid and used in spectrophotometry, and the same solution was diluted to 2 M level for use in titrimetry.

Ferroin Indicator. Prepared by dissolving 0.695 g of $FeSO_4 \cdot 7H_2O$ (Alpha Chemicals, India, assay 99%) and 1.485 g of 1,10-phenanthroline monohydrate (Qualigens Fine Chemicals, Mumbai, India, assay 100%) in water and diluted to volume in a 100 mL calibrated flask.

Standard Drug Solution. A solution of 1 mg/mL ETM was prepared by dissolving 250 mg of pure drug in 0.1 M H_2SO_4 and diluted to volume in a 250 mL calibration flask with the

same solvent and used in titrimetric assay. The stock solution was diluted stepwise with 0.1 M H_2SO_4 to get a working concentration of 20 μg/mL for spectrophotometry.

2.4. General Procedures

2.4.1. Titrimetric Assay. A 10 mL aliquot of the drug solution containing 1.0–8.0 mg of ETM was placed in a 100 mL titration flask and acidified with 5 mL of 2 M H_2SO_4. Ten milliliters of 0.01 M cerium (IV) solution was pipetted into the flask and the contents were mixed well. After a standing time of 5 min, the residual oxidant was titrated with ferrous ammonium sulphate (FAS) solution using a drop of ferroin indicator. A blank titration was performed, and the amount in the aliquot was computed from the amount of cerium (IV) that reacted with ETM.

2.4.2. Spectrophotometric Assay. Different aliquots (0.0, 0.25, 0.5, . . . , 2.5 mL) of 20 μg/mL ETM solution were accurately transferred into a series of 10 mL calibrated flasks. To each flask 3 mL of 5 M H_2SO_4 was added, followed by 1 mL of 100 μg/mL Ce(IV) solution. The contents were mixed well and the flasks were set aside for 10 min. Finally, 1 mL of 0.05% ODS solution was added to each flask, and the volume was brought to the mark with 5 M H_2SO_4. The absorbance of each solution was measured after 5 min at 470 nm against a water blank.

A standard graph was prepared by plotting the difference between blank absorbance and sample absorbance as a function of concentration of the drug, and the concentration of the unknown was computed using the regression equation derived from the absorbance-concentration data.

2.4.3. Procedure for Tablets. Twenty tablets were weighed accurately and ground into a fine powder. A portion of the powder equivalent to 100 mg of ETM was weighed accurately and transferred into a 100 mL calibrated flask, 60 mL of 0.1 M H_2SO_4 was added, and the content was shaken for 20 min; the volume was diluted to the mark with 0.1 M H_2SO_4, mixed well, and filtered using Whatman 42 filter paper. The filtrate (1 mg/mL in ETM) was used in assay by titrimetry, and the same solution was diluted to 20 μg/mL level for assay by spectrophotometry.

2.4.4. Procedures for Method Validation. The assay validation procedures were carried out according to the current ICH guidelines [24], which include linear range, limits of detection (LOD) and quantification (LOQ), precision, accuracy, robustness, ruggedness, and selectivity.

(1) Linear Range, LOD, and LOQ. In titrimetry, the range was determined by titrating different amounts of drug under optimized conditions and the "n" value (number of moles of cerium (IV) reacting with each mole of ETM) was calculated. In spectrophotometry, the linearity was assessed by the calibration graph, which was constructed by plotting the absorbance versus concentration of ETM and the regression equation was calculated. The LOD and LOQ were calculated using the relation ks/b, where $k = 3$ for LOD and 10 for

LOQ, s is the standard deviation of seven blank absorbance readings, and b is the slope of the calibration curve [25].

(2) Accuracy and Precision. The accuracy of the proposed methods was determined on the basis of the difference in mean calculated and amount/concentration taken (% deviation from the actual concentration, DFA); and the precision was determined by calculating the intraday and interday relative standard deviation. These were computed by analyzing standard solution of ETM at three levels seven times on the same day (intraday) and on five consecutive days (interday).

(3) Robustness and Ruggedness. Robustness was evaluated by assaying the standard solutions after slight but deliberate variations in the analytical conditions like contact time and volume of H_2SO_4. Ruggedness, on the other hand, was assessed by a study in which the determination was performed by three analysts and also by a single analyst using three different burettes (titrimetry) and cuvettes (spectrophotometry).

(4) Selectivity. The placebo blank and synthetic mixture were analyzed by the developed methods and the results compared with those obtained on standard drug solution. A placebo blank of the composition: 20 mg talc, 30 mg starch, 20 mg sucrose, 20 mg lactose, 10 mg gelatin, 20 mg sodium alginate, 30 mg magnesium stearate, and 20 mg methyl cellulose was prepared by homogeneous mixing in a mortar. Ten milligrams of placebo was placed in a 50 mL calibration flask and its extract was prepared as described under Section 2.4.3. To 50 mg of the placebo blank prepared above, 100 mg of pure ETM was added and mixed thoroughly and the mixture was

quantitatively transferred into a 100 mL calibrated flask; and then steps described under Section 2.4.3 were followed.

(5) Application to Tablets. Tablet solution prepared as described earlier was subjected to analysis by applying the developed procedures by taking 5 mL aliquot (titrimetry) and 3 mL aliquot (spectrophotometry) in five replicates, and the measured analytical signal was used to calculate the percent of the label claim. For comparison, the tablet extract in glacial acetic acid was titrated potentiometrically with acetous perchloric acid [7].

(6) Recovery Test. Preanalyzed tablet powder was spiked with pure drug at three levels and the total quantity of the drug was calculated, and finally the percent recovery of the pure drug added was calculated.

3. Results and Discussion

Cerium (IV) sulphate is a chemical compound which is frequently used as an oxidizing agent in titrimetric methods. The orange colour of cerium (IV) ion is reduced to the colourless cerium (III) ion.

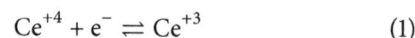

$$Ce^{+4} + e^{-} \rightleftharpoons Ce^{+3} \tag{1}$$

Cerium (IV) is a powerful oxidizing agent which finds immense applications in the analysis of several pharmaceuticals [26–32]. This property of the oxidant was used in the present assay. The drug (ETM) was allowed to react with cerium (IV) in H_2SO_4 medium and gets oxidizing to its sulphoxide.

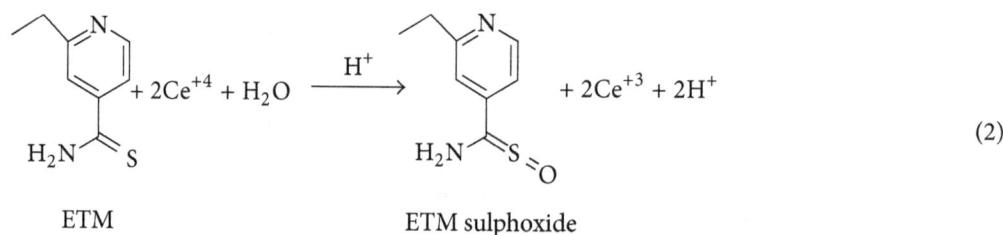

$$\text{(2)}$$

ETM   ETM sulphoxide

After an appropriate reaction time, the residual oxidant was determined by two approaches. In titrimetry, the unreacted oxidant was determined by titration with FAS using ferroin indicator.

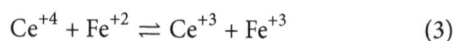

$$Ce^{+4} + Fe^{+2} \rightleftharpoons Ce^{+3} + Fe^{+3} \tag{3}$$

The amount of cerium (IV) reacted was related to the amount of drug, and the drug-oxidant reaction followed a $1:2$ stoichiometry which served as the basis of the calculations. In spectrophotometry, the unconsumed oxidant was determined by reacting with ODS as shown in (4) and measuring the absorbance of the coloured species of the oxidation product of ODS at 470 nm (Figure 1).

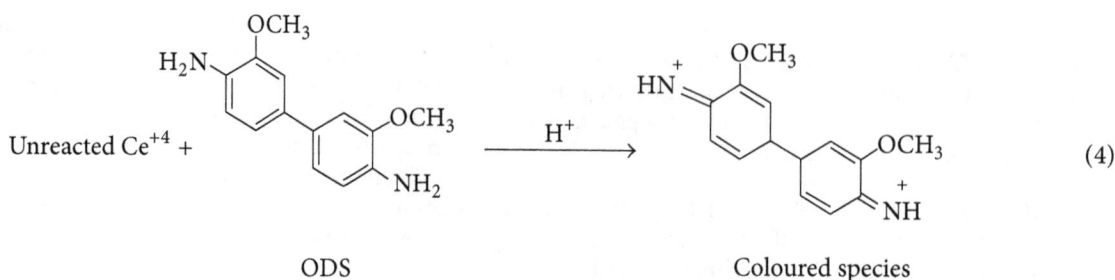

$$\text{(4)}$$

ODS   Coloured species

$$ETM + Ce\ (IV) \xrightarrow{\ H^+\ } Oxidation\ product\ of\ ETM + unreacted\ Ce\ (IV)$$

$$Unreacted\ Ce\ (IV) \longrightarrow Titrated\ with\ standard\ FAS\ using\ ferroin\ indicator\ (titrimetric\ method)$$

$$Unreacted\ Ce\ (IV) + ODS \xrightarrow{\ H^+\ } Oxidatio\ product\ of\ ODS$$
$$Orange\ coloured\ product\ measuered\ at\ 470\ nm$$
$$(Spectrophotometric\ method)$$

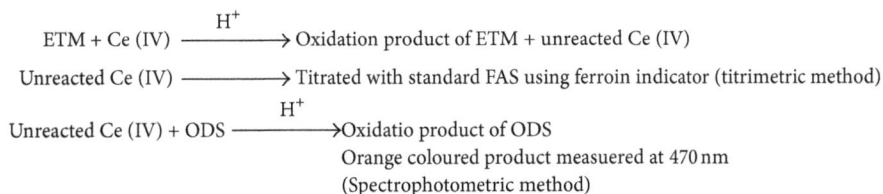

SCHEME 1: The possible reaction pathways and basis of assays.

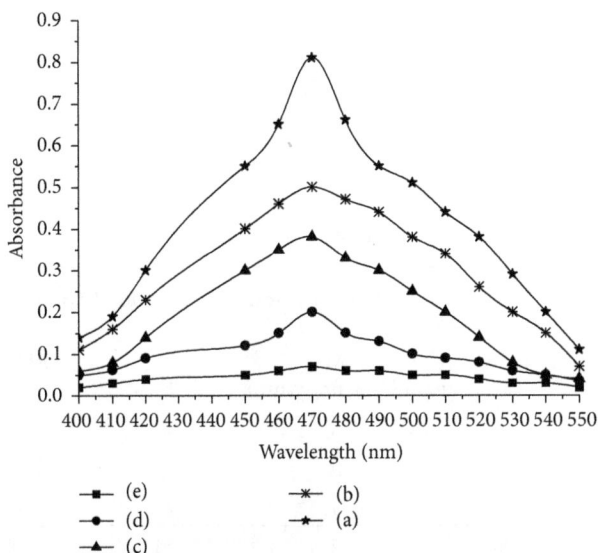

FIGURE 1: Absorption spectra of the reaction product in the presence of (a) 0.0; (b) 2.0; (c) 3.0; (d) 4.0; and (e) 5.0 μg/mL ETM; the amount of other reactants remained constant.

TABLE 1: Sensitivity and regression parameters.

Parameter	Spectrophotometric method
λ_{max}, nm	470
Colour stability	30 min
Linear range, μg/mL	0.5–5.0
Molar absorptivity (ε), L/(mol·cm)	2.66×10^4
Sandell sensitivity*, μg/cm^2	0.0063
Limit of detection (LOD), μg/mL	0.013
Limit of quantification (LOQ), μg/mL	0.043
Regression equation, Y**	
Intercept (a)	0.0038
Slope (b)	0.1591
Standard deviation of a (S_a)	9.89×10^{-2}
Standard deviation of b (S_b)	2.18×10^{-2}
Regression coefficient (r)	0.9989

*Limit of determination as the weight in μg/mL of solution, which corresponds to an absorbance of $A = 0.001$ measured in a cuvette of cross-sectional area 1 cm^2 and $l = 1$ cm. **$Y = a + bX$, where Y is the absorbance, X is the concentration in μg/mL, a is intercept, and b is slope.

The calibration graph is a plot of the difference in absorbance of the reagent blank and sample solution versus the concentration of ETM (Figure 2), and this served as basis for the quantification. The possible reaction pathways and basis of assays are shown in Scheme 1.

In spectrophotometric method, three blanks were prepared. The first blank which contained all reactants except ETM gave maximum absorbance. The second blank contained only Ce (IV) and H_2SO_4. The third blank contained optimum amounts of ODS and acid. Since the last two blanks had negligible absorbance at 470 nm, measurements were made against double distilled water.

3.1. Method Development.
Direct titration of ETM with cerium (IV) in different H_2SO_4 concentrations was not successful. Back titrimetric assay was possible in the presence of 5 mL of 2 M H_2SO_4 in a total volume of 25 mL (net, 0.4 M).

A contact time of 5 min was found optimum for the range (1–8 mg) studied with 0.01 M cerium (IV) solution. A fixed reaction stoichiometry of 1 : 2 (drug : oxidant) was found for the investigated range of ETM. Beyond these limits (<1 and >8 mg), slightly inconsistent reaction ratios were obtained.

The ability of cerium (IV) to oxidize ETM and also ODS to an orange-red coloured product was exploited for the indirect

spectrophotometric assay. A slightly higher concentration of H_2SO_4 was required for the twin oxidation steps involved, and to stabilize the coloured product. The oxidation of drug took somewhat a longer time (10 min) as compared to titrimetry (5 min), and a further 5 min was required to stabilize the oxidation product of ODS, which was stable for the next 30 min thereafter.

3.2. Method Validation

3.2.1. Linearity, LOD, and LOQ of Spectrophotometric Method.
The absorbance-concentration plot was linear with a good correlation coefficient (0.9989) in the 0.5–5.0 μg/mL range. Sensitivity parameters such as molar absorptivity (ε), Sandell's sensitivity, LOD, and LOQ along with the slope and intercept of the regression equation are compiled in Table 1. Low values of LOD and LOQ and high value of (ε) confirm the sensitivity of the method for the determination of ETM in bulk drug as well in drug product.

3.2.2. Accuracy and Precision.
Replicate determination of ETM in pure drug solution at three levels was performed on an intraday and interday basis as a part of the accuracy and precision evaluation of the proposed methods. Relative standard deviation (% RSD), a measure of precision, and

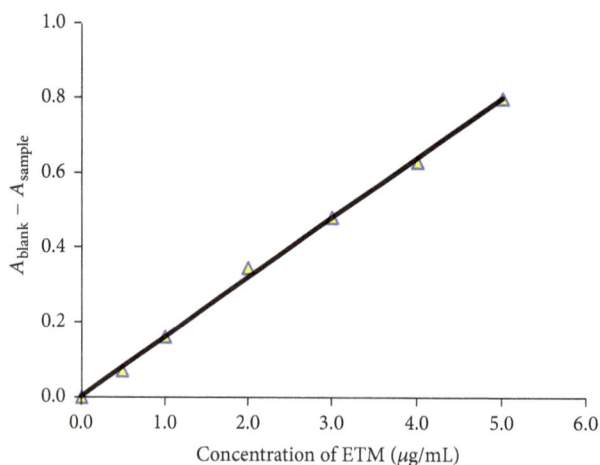

FIGURE 2: Calibration graph.

TABLE 2: Evaluation of intraday and interday accuracy and precision.

Method	ETM taken (mg or μg/mL)	Intraday accuracy and precision ($n = 7$)			Interday accuracy and precision ($n = 5$)		
		ETM found[a] (mg or μg/mL)	RSD[b] %	RE[c] %	ETM found (mg or μg/mL)	RSD[b] %	RE[c] %
Titrimetry	2.0	2.01	1.12	0.50	1.97	1.74	1.50
	4.0	3.94	1.35	1.50	4.03	2.03	0.75
	6.0	6.08	1.55	1.33	6.11	1.69	1.83
Spectrophotometry	1.0	0.98	1.41	2.00	1.02	1.81	2.00
	2.0	1.97	1.38	1.50	2.03	1.57	1.50
	3.0	3.04	1.65	1.33	2.95	1.93	1.67

[a]Mean value of seven determinations; [b]relative standard deviation (%); [c]relative error (%).

relative error (% RE), an indicator of accuracy values, were calculated to be $\leq$2% (intraday) and <2.1% (interday), as shown in Table 2.

3.2.3. Robustness and Ruggedness.
To evaluate the robustness, two experimental variables, namely, contact time and acid concentration, were altered slightly deliberately, and the influence of these changes was studied on the performance of the methods. The performance remained unaffected as shown by small values of % RSD ($\leq$2.31). Determination of drug in solution at three levels was done by using three different burettes in titrimetric method and three cuvettes in spectrophotometric method and also by three persons using the same equipment. The person-to-person and equipment-to-equipment variations did not significantly affect the results as shown in Table 3.

3.2.4. Selectivity.
To determine the selectivity of the described methods, placebo and synthetic mixture analyses were performed. Replicate analyses of placebo blank gave a titer value almost equal to that blank titration in titrimetry and absorbance value very much the same as the reagent blank in spectrophotometry. When the synthetic mixture was subjected to analysis, at three amount/concentration levels

by the proposed methods, the percent recoveries of pure drug ranged from 99.34 $\pm$ 1.12 to 101.7 $\pm$ 2.34 indicating noninterference from the inactive ingredients.

3.2.5. Application to Tablets.
Three brands of tablets of 250 mg strength were analyzed by the proposed methods and the results are presented in Table 4. The same tablets were also analyzed by the reference method [7] for comparison. The results revealed that there is a close agreement between the results obtained by the proposed methods and those of the reference method, besides the label claim. When the results were statistically evaluated by applying Student's t-test for accuracy and variance ratio F-test for precision, the calculated t- and F-values did not exceed the tabulated values at the 95% confidence level and four degrees of freedom, suggesting that the proposed methods and the reference method have similar accuracy and precision.

3.2.6. Accuracy by Recovery Study.
Accuracy of the proposed methods was further confirmed by recovery study following the standard-addition procedure. The percent recovery values of pure drug added shown in Table 5 unambiguously demonstrate that inactive ingredients such as talc, gelatin, starch,

TABLE 3: Method robustness and ruggedness expressed as intermediate precision (% RSD).

| Method | ETM taken (mg or μg/mL) | Robustness (% RSD) Parameters altered | | Ruggedness (% RSD) | |
		Contact time[*]	Volume of H_2SO_4[**]	Inter-analysts ($n = 3$)	Interburettes/cuvettes ($n = 3$)
Titrimetry	2.0	0.88	0.67	1.33	1.91
	4.0	1.05	0.88	1.66	1.83
	6.0	1.24	1.58	1.11	2.11
Spectrophotometry	1.0	1.53	1.85	1.44	1.97
	2.0	2.31	1.17	0.97	1.73
	3.0	2.24	1.74	1.47	1.65

In titrimetry, ETM taken/found is in mg and the same was in μg/mL in spectrophotometry. [*]Contact time used: 4, 5, and 6 min in titrimetric method; 8, 10, and 12 min in spectrophotometric method. [**]Volumes of H_2SO_4 were 4, 5, and 6 mL (2 M) in titrimetric method and 2.5, 3.0, and 3.5 mL (5 M) in spectrophotometric method.

TABLE 4: Results of analysis of tablets by the proposed methods and statistical comparison of the results with the reference method.

| Tablet brand name | Nominal amount | Found[*] (% of nominal amount ± SD) | | |
| | | Reference method | Proposed methods | |
			Titrimetry	Spectrophotometry
Ethide	250	100.2 ± 1.23	99.88 ± 1.02 $t = 0.45$ $F = 1.45$	100.44 ± 1.86 $t = 0.24$ $F = 2.29$
Ethiokox	250	96.22 ± 1.45	98.4 ± 1.71 $t = 2.17$ $F = 1.39$	98.06 ± 2.46 $t = 1.44$ $F = 2.88$
Myobid	250	97.34 ± 1.54	98.96 ± 1.85 $t = 1.51$ $F = 1.44$	95.84 ± 1.78 $t = 1.43$ $F = 1.34$

[*]Mean value of five determinations.
(Tabulated t-value at the 95% confidence level and for four degrees of freedom is 2.78).
(Tabulated F-value at the 95% confidence level and for four degrees of freedom is 6.39).

TABLE 5: Results of recovery experiment through standard-addition method.

Method	Tablet studied	ETM in tablet (mg; μg/mL)	Pure ETM added (mg; μg/mL)	Total found (mg; μg/mL)	Pure ETM recovered (percent ± SD[*])
Titrimetry	Ethide 250	2.99	1.5	4.55	101.43 ± 1.42
		2.99	3.0	5.92	98.97 ± 0.84
		2.99	4.5	7.48	100.11 ± 0.68
Spectrophotometry	Ethide 250	1.51	0.75	2.33	103.22 ± 2.44
		1.51	1.50	3.21	104.82 ± 2.53
		1.51	2.25	3.82	102.14 ± 2.35

[*]Mean value of three determinations.

magnesium stearate, sodium alginate, and methylcellulose do not interfere in the determination of the active ingredient.

4. Conclusions

The oxidation reaction between the ETM and cerium (IV) in acid medium was advantageously exploited for the development of two simple, rapid, cost-effective, and sensitive methods for the determination of ETM in pharmaceuticals. The methods use cheap and easily available chemicals and an inexpensive instrument which can be accessed in any industrial quality control laboratory. The methods employ a stable oxidant unlike the previously reported titrimetric and spectrophotometric methods. Titrimetry is applicable over a micro scale (<10 mg) compared to the reported titrimetric methods including the official method, which would require 300–500 mg per trial. The proposed spectrophotometric method has a molar absorptivity value of 2.66×10^4 L/(mol·cm) with a linear dynamic range of 0.5–5.0 μg/mL and is one of the most sensitive methods ever developed for ETM (Table 6). Hence, the proposed methods can be

TABLE 6: Comparison of the proposed and the existing spectrophotometric and titrimetric methods for the determination of ETM.

(a) Spectrophotometry

SL number	Reagent/s	Methodology	Linear range (μg/mL)	Remark	Ref.
1	DCNQ	Orange coloured product in ethanol measured at 440 nm	—	—	[9]
2	DCNQ	Red coloured product formed in the presence of ammonia in alcoholic medium measured at 540 nm	6–42	20 min contact time	[10]
3	Iron (III)	Purple-violet colour complex in acid medium measured at 510 nm	0–36	Less sensitive and the molar absorptivity is equal to 2.48×10^3 L/(mol·cm)	[11]
4	Iron (III) PPD	Thionine compound measured at 600 nm	—	Multiple step reaction involved	[12]
5	Sodium nitroprusside	Orange coloured product in basic medium measured at 510 nm	—	—	[13]
6	Sodium nitroprusside	Orange-red complex measured at 490 nm	5–32	—	[14]
7	PAR-V^{+5}	Ternary complex (1:1:1) extracted into chloroform and measured at 560 nm	0.2–20	30 min contact time, extraction step is required	[15]
8	Osmic acid	Light yellow coloured product formed at pH4 measured at 375 nm	0.25–40	60 min contact time, pH adjustment is required	[16]
9	NBS-CB	Unbleached dye colour measured in acid medium at 540 nm	0.2–5.0	Critical acid conc.; less stable reagent used	[17]
10	KMnO$_4$	Blue coloured manganate in alkaline medium measured at 610 nm (direct method)	1–10	Critical NaOH conc. Reaction rate precariously dependent on experimental variables	[18]
		Absorbance at a fixed time of 20 min measured (kinetic method)	1–10		
11	Sodium azide-iodine	Decrease in absorbance at the 5th min measured at 348 nm (kinetic method)	10–100	Reaction rate precariously dependent on experimental conditions	[19]
12	*Ce(IV)/ODS*	*Orange-red coloured species measured at 470 nm*	*0.5–5.0*	*Nondrastic experimental conditions, no critical pH adjust, no heating or extraction step. Shorter contact time (15 min), no use of organic solvent*	*Present work*

(b) Titrimetry

SL number	Reagent/s	End point detection	Linear range	Remark	Ref.
1	NBS	Visually	—	Less stable oxidant used	[20]
2	I$_2$-NaOH	Potentiometrically	25–500 μ mol	Critically dependent on alkaline concentration	[21]
3	AgNO$_3$	Potentiometrically	—	Preparation of AgS-sensor is tedious & cumbersome, expensive titrant used	[22]
4	*Ce(IV)/FAS*	*Unreacted Ce^{4+} titrated versus FAS*	*1–8 mg*	*Stable titrant used, facile working conditions employed*	*Present work*

DCNQ: Dichloronaphthoquinone; PAR: 4-(2-pyridylazo) resorcinol; PPD: p-phenylenediamine; NBS: N-bromosuccinimide; CB: Celestine blue; ODS: ortho-dianisidine; FAS: ferrous ammonium sulphate.

conveniently employed in laboratories which can ill-afford costly chromatographic techniques.

Competing Interests

The authors declare that there is no conflict of interests regarding the publication of this paper.

Acknowledgments

The authors are thankful to Panacea Biotec Ltd. for their generous gift sample of ethionamide. Professor Kanakapura Basavaiah wishes to thank the University Grants Commission, New Delhi, India, for the award of BSR faculty fellowship. The author Nagib A. S. Qarah is thankful to the UGC New Delhi, India, for supporting research.

References

[1] J. E. Conte Jr., J. A. Golden, M. Mcquitty, J. Kipps, E. T. Lin, and E. Zurlinden, "Effects of AIDS and gender on steady-state plasma and intrapulmonary ethionamide concentrations," *Antimicrobial Agents and Chemotherapy*, vol. 44, no. 5, pp. 1337–1341, 2000.

[2] V. A. Ongaya, W. A. Githui, H. Meme, C. Kiiyukia, and E. Juma, "High ethionamide resistance in Mycobacterium tuberculosis strains isolated in Kenya," *African Journal of Health Sciences*, vol. 20, no. 1-2, pp. 37–41, 2012.

[3] J. Crofton, P. Chaulet, and D. Maher, *Guidelines for the Management of Multidrug-Resistant Tuberculosis*, World Health Organization, Geneva, Switzerland, 1997.

[4] J. S. Blanchard, "Molecular mechanisms of drug resistance in *Mycobacterium tuberculosis*," *Annual Review of Biochemistry*, vol. 65, pp. 215–239, 1996.

[5] K. Takayama, L. Wang, and H. L. David, "Effect of isoniazid on the in vivo mycolic acid synthesis, cell growth, and viability of *Mycobacterium tuberculosis*," *Antimicrobial Agents and Chemotherapy*, vol. 2, no. 1, pp. 29–35, 1972.

[6] J. N. Delgado and W. A. Remers, *Wilson and Gisvold's Textbook of Organic Medicinal and Pharmaceutical Chemistry*, Lippincott-Raven, New York, NY, USA, 10th edition, 1998.

[7] The British Pharmacopeia, *Volume I & II Monographs: Medicinal and Pharmaceutical Substances, Ethionamide*, The British Pharmacopeia, London, UK, 2009.

[8] M. I. Walash, A. M. El-Brashy, M. E.-S. Metwally, and A. A. Abdelal, "FLuorimetric determination of carbocisteine and ethionamide in drug formulation," *Acta Chimica Slovenica*, vol. 51, no. 2, pp. 283–291, 2004.

[9] M. M. Bedair, "Use of 2,3-dichloro-1,4-naphthoquinone for the spectrophotometric assay of five thio compounds of pharmaceutical importance," *Alexandria Journal of Pharmaceutical Sciences*, vol. 5, pp. 64–67, 1991.

[10] M. B. Devani, C. J. Shishoo, H. J. Mody, and P. K. Raja, "Detection of thioamides: determination of ethionamide with 2,3-dichloro-1,4-naphthoquinone," *Journal of Pharmaceutical Sciences*, vol. 63, no. 9, pp. 1471–1473, 1974.

[11] A. K. Shah, Y. K. Agrawal, and S. K. Banerjee, "Spectrophotometric method for the rapid determination of microgram amounts of ethionamide," *Analytical Letters*, vol. 14, no. 17-18, pp. 1449–1464, 1981.

[12] M. S. El-Din, F. Belal, and S. Hassan, "Spectrophotometric determination of some pharmaceutically important thione-containing compounds," *Zentralblatt für Pharmazie, Pharmakotherapie und Laboratoriumsdiagnostik*, vol. 127, no. 3, pp. 133–135, 1988.

[13] F. A. Ibrahim, "Colorimetric estimation of certain thione-compounds of pharmaceutical importance," *Mansoura Journal of Pharmaceutical Sciences*, vol. 10, pp. 334–344, 1994.

[14] M. B. Devani, C. J. Shishoo, and K. Doshi, "A spectrophotometric determination of ethionamide in tablets," *Indian Journal of Pharmaceutical Sciences*, vol. 43, no. 4, pp. 149–150, 1981.

[15] H. Sikorska-Tomicka, "Spectrophotometric determination of ethionamide and thionicotinamide with 4-(2-pyridylazo) resorcinol and vanadium," *Chemia Analityczna (Warsaw)*, vol. 38, pp. 745–751, 1993.

[16] H. Sikorska-Tomicka, "Spectrophotometric determination of ethionamide and thionicotinamide with osmic acid," *Mikrochimica Acta*, vol. 87, no. 3, pp. 151–157, 1985.

[17] C. S. P. Sastry, K. R. Srinivas, and K. M. M. K. Prasad, "Spectrophotometric determination of drugs in pharmaceutical formulations with N-bromosuccinimide and Celestine blue," *Mikrochimica Acta*, vol. 122, no. 1-2, pp. 77–86, 1996.

[18] M. I. Walash, A. M. El-Brashy, M. S. Metwally, and A. A. Abdelal, "Spectrophotometric and kinetic determination of some sulphur containing drugs in bulk and drug formulations," *Bulletin of the Korean Chemical Society*, vol. 25, no. 4, pp. 517–524, 2004.

[19] M. I. Walash, M. E.-S. Metwally, A. M. El-Brashy, and A. A. Abdelal, "Kinetic spectrophotometric determination of some sulfur containing compounds in pharmaceutical preparations and human serum," *Il Farmaco*, vol. 58, no. 12, pp. 1325–1332, 2003.

[20] B. S. Reddy, R. R. Krishna, and C. S. P. Sastry, "Titrimetric determination of some antitubercular drugs by sodium nitrite and N-bromosuccinimide (NBS) using internal indicators," *Indian Drugs*, vol. 20, pp. 28–29, 1982.

[21] W. Ciesielski, A. Krenc, and U. Złłobińska, "Potentiometric titration of thioamides and mercaptoacids with iodine in alkaline medium," *Chemia Analityczna*, vol. 50, no. 2, pp. 397–405, 2005.

[22] S. I. Obtemperanskaya, M. M. Buzlanova, I. V. Karandi, R. Shakhid, and A. N. Kashin, "Potentiometric determination of some drugs and other physiologically active substances using a silver sulfide ion-selective electrode," *Journal of Analytical Chemistry*, vol. 51, no. 4, pp. 419–423, 1996.

[23] A. I. Vogel, *A Textbook of Quantitative Inorganic Analysis*, The English Language Book Society and Longman, London, UK, 3rd edition, 1961.

[24] ICH, International conference on hormonisation of technical requirement for registration of pharmaceuticals for human use, ICH harmonised tripartite guideline: validation of analytical procedures: text and methodology Q2(R1), Complementary Guideline on Methodology dated 06 November 1996, incorporated in November 2005, London.

[25] J. C. Miller and J. N. Miller, *Statistic for Analytical Chemistry*, Ellis Horwood, New York, NY, USA, 4th edition, 1994.

[26] I. A. Darwish, A. S. Khedr, H. F. Askal, and R. M. Mahmoud, "Simple fluorimetric method for determination of certain antiviral drugs via their oxidation with cerium (IV)," *Il Farmaco*, vol. 60, no. 6-7, pp. 555–562, 2005.

[27] N. Rajendraprasad, K. Basavaiah, and K. B. Vinay, "Volumetric and spectrophotometric determination of oxcarbazepine in tablets," *Acta Chimica Slovenica*, vol. 58, no. 3, pp. 621–628, 2011.

[28] H. D. Revanasiddappa, H. N. Deepakumari, and S. M. Mallegowda, "Development and validation of indirect spectrophotometric methods for lamotrigine in pure and the tablet dosage forms," *Analele Universitatii din Bucuresti-Chimie*, vol. 20, no. 1, pp. 49–55, 2011.

[29] K. Basavaiah, U. Chandrashekar, and H. C. Prameela, "Cerimetric determination of propranolol in bulk drug form and in tablets," *Turkish Journal of Chemistry*, vol. 27, no. 5, pp. 591–599, 2003.

[30] M. S. Raghu, K. Basavaiah, K. N. Prashanth, and K. B. Vinay, "Titrimetric and spectrophotometric methods for the assay of ketotifen using cerium(IV) and two reagents," *International Journal of Analytical Chemistry*, vol. 2013, Article ID 697651, 9 pages, 2013.

[31] H. F. Askal, O. H. Abdelmegeed, S. M. S. Ali, and M. A. El-Hamd, "Spectrophotometric and spectrofluorimetric determination of 1,4-dihydropyridine drugs using potassium permanganate and cerium (IV) ammonium sulphate," *Bulletin of Pharmaceutical Sciences*, vol. 33, no. 2, pp. 201–215, 2010.

[32] K. Basavaiah, O. Z. Devi, K. Tharpa, and K. B. Vinay, "Oxidimetric assay of simvastatin in pharmaceuticals using cerium (IV) and three dyes as reagents," *Proceedings of the Indian National Science Academy*, vol. 74, no. 3, pp. 119–124, 2008.

4

Structural Alteration in Dermal Vessels and Collagen Bundles following Exposure of Skin Wound to Zeolite–Bentonite Compound

Shahram Paydar,[1,2] **Ali Noorafshan,**[3] **Behnam Dalfardi,**[4,5]
Shahram Jahanabadi,[6] **Seyed Mohammad Javad Mortazavi,**[7,8]
Seyedeh-Saeedeh Yahyavi,[3] **and Hadi Khoshmohabat**[9]

[1]*Trauma Research Center, Shahid Rajaee (Emtiaz) Trauma Hospital, Shiraz University of Medical Sciences, Shiraz, Iran*
[2]*Department of General Surgery, School of Medicine, Shiraz University of Medical Sciences, Shiraz, Iran*
[3]*Histomorphometry and Stereology Research Centre, Shiraz University of Medical Sciences, Shiraz, Iran*
[4]*Student Research Committee, Shiraz University of Medical Sciences, Shiraz, Iran*
[5]*Department of Internal Medicine, Shiraz University of Medical Sciences, Shiraz, Iran*
[6]*International Branch, Shiraz University of Medical Sciences, Shiraz, Iran*
[7]*Medical Physics Department, School of Medicine, Shiraz University of Medical Sciences, Shiraz, Iran*
[8]*Ionizing and Non-Ionizing Radiation Protection Research Center (INIRPRC), Shiraz University of Medical Sciences, Shiraz, Iran*
[9]*Trauma Research Center, Baqiyatallah University of Medical Sciences, Tehran, Iran*

Correspondence should be addressed to Behnam Dalfardi; dalfardibeh@gmail.com

Academic Editor: Srinivas Mutalik

Background. This study examines the impact of one-time direct application of haemostatic agent zeolite–bentonite powder to wounded skin on the healing process in rats. *Materials and Methods.* 24 male Sprague-Dawley rats were randomly allocated into two groups ($n = 12$): (1) the rats whose wounds were washed only with sterile normal saline (NS-treated) and (2) those treated with zeolite–bentonite compound (ZEO-treated). The wound was circular, full-thickness, and 2 cm in diameter. At the end of the 12th day, six animals from each group were randomly selected and terminated. The remaining rats were terminated after 21 days. Just after scarification, skin samples were excised and sent for stereological evaluation. *Results.* The results showed a significant difference between the two groups regarding the length density of the blood vessels and diameter of the large and small vessels on the 12th day after the wound was inflicted. Besides, volume density of both the dermis and collagen bundles was reduced by 25% in the ZEO-treated rats in comparison to the NS-treated animals after 21 days. *Conclusions.* One-time topical usage of zeolite–bentonite haemostatic powder on an animal skin wound might negatively affect the healing process through vasoconstriction and inhibition of neoangiogenesis.

1. Introduction

High bleeding still accounts for up to 40% of preventable deaths following traumatic injuries [1]. Haemostatic agents can considerably contribute to stopping such uncontrolled haemorrhage in trauma patients and reduce the possibility of its undesirable consequences [1, 2]. However, in spite of their usefulness in emergency cases, haemostatic materials are not available in all parts of the world. Moreover, an ideal haemostat has not been produced yet. Hence, improvement of the available haemostatic agents and production of new ones have remained in focus [2, 3].

One haemostatic agent that was recently produced in Iran (called CoolClot) is a compound mainly composed of zeolite (one third of the weight) and bentonite (two thirds of the weight) clays, two minerals which are widely available in the country [3, 4]. This recently introduced product was originally made in powder form and has been proven to control life-threatening arterial bleeding. Another advantage of this product is that it does not have the potential burn effects caused by other zeolite-based haemostatic agents [3–5].

The criteria for the idealness of haemostatic agents include the ability to stop haemorrhage from making large arteries or veins actively bleed within two minutes of application; being ready to use with no requirement for on-site preparation; the ability to deliver and act through a pool of blood; being risk-free; causing no further tissue injury; having no negative impact on the wound; having no risk of viral disease transmission; being easy to use for the casualty, medical staff, and nonmedical first responders; being lightweight and durable; having wide temperature storage capabilities (ideally –10 to +55°C); having a minimum of two years shelf-life; and being inexpensive [1–3]. Considering these criteria, it seems reasonable to assess different aspects of any newly introduced haemostatic agent, particularly its impact on wound healing and tissue safety.

According to the aforementioned criteria, an ideal haemostatic material should have no negative impact on the fresh wound (site of topical application) and its healing process [3]. A method that is used in dermatological research, particularly for assessment of wound healing, is stereology. This technique is defined as a set of mathematical and statistical tools that estimate three-dimensional features of objects from their regular two-dimensional sections and provide the examiner with a better understanding of the tissue morphology [6–9].

This study aims to stereologically evaluate the impact of one-time topical application of zeolite–bentonite compound on the skin wound healing process in an animal model and assess its tissue safety.

2. Materials and Methods

2.1. Animals and Wound Creation.

To conduct this research, according to a previously used method [3], 24 healthy adult male Sprague-Dawley rats (mean weight: 230 g) were chosen and randomly divided into two groups ($n = 12$): (1) normal saline-treated group (NS-treated) and (2) zeolite–bentonite compound-treated group (ZEO-treated). The animals were housed in temperature- and humidity-controlled rooms with 12-hour light/dark photoperiods and had free access to similar amounts of standard food (provided from the Centre of Comparative and Experimental Medicine, Shiraz University of Medical Sciences, Fars province, Shiraz, Iran) and water. The rats were adapted to their environment 10 days prior to the start of the study. The research protocol was approved by the Animal Ethics Committee of Shiraz University of Medical Sciences, Shiraz, Iran.

To begin the experiment under general anaesthesia (through the intramuscular injection of ketamine [50 mg per kg; Alfasan International, Woerden, The Netherlands] and xylazine [10 mg per kg; Alfasan International]) in a clean but not sterile condition, a circular full thickness cutaneous wound with 2 cm diameter was generated on the dorsum

of each animal using forceps and scissors. Just after wound creation, a single dose of zeolite–bentonite powder (in dry form; with a mean weight of 8 gr) was applied on the skin wound of the rats in the ZEO-treated group. The powder was spread as uniformly as possible on the wound site using a sterile applicator stick. The cutaneous wounds of the animals in the NS-treated group were only washed with sterile normal saline. From the second day of the research, the skin wounds of both groups of animals were washed daily with normal saline. The wounds were left completely open during the study time span.

At the end of the 12th day, six animals per group were randomly selected and terminated with a high dose of inhaled ether. After 21 days, the remaining animals were also terminated by a similar method. Just after scarification, full thickness skin samples were excised from the site of the wounded skin. The samples were fixed in buffered formaldehyde and sent for further processing.

2.2. Stereological Analysis.

We used stereological analysis to examine tissue samples [10]. The samples were sectioned into $0.5 \times 0.5 \, \text{mm}^2$ and nine to 10 pieces were sampled in a systematic uniform random pattern. Isotropic uniform random sectioning is necessary for the estimation of the vessels' length. Therefore, the samples were embedded in a cylindrical block and sectioned using a microtome after choosing random orientation according to the orientator method. In this way, four-micrometer sections were obtained and stained with Heidenhain's AZAN trichrome stain.

Microscopic analyses of the skin were performed using a video-microscopy system composed of a microscope (Nikon E-200, Tokyo, Japan) linked to a digital camera and a flat monitor. The volume densities (the fraction of the tissue which was occupied by the favoured structure)—of parts including epidermis, dermis, hypodermis, collagen bundles, and vessels—were estimated using the point-counting method. Briefly, a point grid was overlaid on the images of the skin and the density was obtained using the following formula:

$$V_v \,(\text{structure, reference}) = \frac{\Sigma P \,(\text{structure})}{\Sigma P \,(\text{reference})}, \quad (1)$$

where "$\Sigma P(\text{structure})$" and "$\Sigma P(\text{reference})$" were the total points hitting the favoured structure and the whole skin sections, respectively.

The length density (L_v, the length of the vessels in the unit volume of the dermis and hypodermis) and the mean diameter of a vessel were estimated using a counting frame at a final magnification of 1380x and 130x to differentiate the capillaries (up to 10 μm) and larger vessels (more than 10.1 micrometer), respectively.

The following formula was used to estimate the length density:

$$L_v = 2 \times \frac{\Sigma Q}{[(a/f) \times \Sigma P]}, \quad (2)$$

where "ΣQ", "(a/f)", and "ΣP" were the total profiles of the vessels, area per counting frame and the total hitting of central point of the frame with the reference tissue.

TABLE 1: The mean and standard deviation of the animal weight, volume density (mm^3/mm^3, ×100) of the different layers of the skin, collagen bundle, length density (mm/mm^3), and diameter (μm) of the vessels, 12 and 21 days after treating the rats with NS and ZEO. ($n = 6$).

Groups	Volume density				Length density	Diameter	
	Epidermis	Dermis	Hypodermis	Collagen	Vessels	>10 μm	<10 μm
NS-treated (12)	2.6 ± 0.6	17.6 ± 6.4	79.6 ± 6.7	45.1 ± 6.0	6.8 ± 0.9	37.5 ± 10.1	6.1 ± 0.7
ZEO-treated (12)	2.1 ± 0.8	20.0 ± 0.4	77.8 ± 4.5	45.9 ± 9.9	4.7 ± 1.2*	23.3 ± 7.8*	5.0 ± 0.7*
NS-treated (21)	3.6 ± 0.7	49.8 ± 8.9	46.4 ± 9.1	45.6 ± 9.3	5.0 ± 2.9	37.3 ± 5.7	6.0 ± 0.2
ZEO-treated (21)	3.1 ± 1.3	37.5 ± 7.7*	59.3 ± 7.5	34.2 ± 6.5*	2.7 ± 1.2*	22.9 ± 2.7*	5.0 ± 0.3*

*$P < 0.03$, ZEO-treated *versus* NS-treated animals.

2.3. Statistical Analysis. Data analysis was performed using the IBM SPSS Statistics software, v. 16 (Chicago, USA). Further, Mann-Whitney U-test was used to analyse the histological data. $P < 0.05$ was considered statistically significant.

3. Results

The results showed no significant difference in NS- and ZEO-treated groups regarding the volume density of the epidermis, dermis, and hypodermis of the wounded skin after 12 days (Table 1) (Figure 1). However, the length density of the vessels was reduced by 31% in the ZEO-treated group after this period. The diameters of the large and small vessels (capillaries) were also, respectively, reduced by 38% and 16% in the ZEO-treated rats in comparison to the other group during 12 days. Additionally, volume density of both the dermis and collagen bundles was reduced by 25% in the ZEO-treated rats in comparison to the NS-treated animals after 21 days. Nevertheless, no significant changes were seen in the epidermis and hypodermis of the animals' skin samples in both groups at that time. Length density of the vessels was reduced by 46% in the experimental group. The diameters of the large vessels and capillaries was also reduced, by 39% and 16%, respectively, in the ZEO-treated rats compared to the controlled ones after 21 days. Reduction of the length density and diameter indicates angioinhibitory and vasoconstrictive actions in 12 and 21 days post-wounding.

4. Discussion

This work assessed the impact of one-time direct application of zeolite–bentonite powder to a wounded skin tissue on its healing process. Our findings showed that this compound could affect the healing process through angioinhibitory and vasoconstrictive properties. In addition, this study indicated that application of zeolite–bentonite compound could reduce the volume density of collagen bundles in the healed tissue.

Because of some previously poor experiences regarding the use of haemostatic products, their safety for human tissues remains a constant concern [13]. For instance, QuikClot (Z-Medica, Wallingford, CT, USA) could cause significant exothermic reaction, thermal tissue injury, and necrosis after topical usage (it is claimed that this side effect is considerably resolved in the later generation of this agent called QuikClot ACS+™) [11]. Dry Fibrin Sealant Dressing (DFSD, American Red Cross Holland Laboratory, Rockville, MD) could also transmit viral diseases (particularly hepatitis and human immunodeficiency virus) [12]. Hence, this issue is a detriment to the idealness of haemostatic agents as they should be risk-free and cause no further tissue injury [1–3]. Therefore, assessment of the safety of any newly introduced haemostatic material is necessary. Zeolite–bentonite powder, as a product whose impact on wounded tissues has not been completely examined, is no exception.

Previously, Khoshmohabat et al. performed an experiment to histopathologically evaluate the effects of one-time topical administration of a zeolite–bentonite composition called CoolClot, on the skin wound healing process [3]. In that study, three main and overlapping phases of cutaneous wound healing—including inflammation, proliferation, and maturation—were examined using the scoring system introduced by Abramov and his colleagues (Table 2) [3, 13, 14]. It is noteworthy that Abramov's scoring system was developed to make qualitative histopathological data available for secondary statistical analysis. According to the results of that study, one-time topical usage of Cool-Clot had no significant negative impact on the wound healing process, neither histopathologic nor macroscopic (photographic) [3]. However, our study, having quantitatively evaluated the structural changes of skin using stereological methods, revealed different results from those of the previous histopathologic research. According to our results, one-time topical application of zeolite–bentonite compound could lead to angioinhibitory and vasoconstrictive features that remained even towards the end of the healing process.

Angiogenesis or neovascularization is a critical event occurring during wound repair [15]. Furthermore, newly established blood supply is essential to provide the metabolic demands of the healing tissues. In addition, vasodilatation is a necessary component for angiogenesis. It has been shown that various cell types, such as epidermal cells, macrophages, fibroblasts, and vascular endothelial cells, can stimulate neovascularization by the production of different factors, including transforming growth factor ß (TGFß), nitric oxide (NO), vascular endothelial growth factor (VEGF), and basic fibroblast growth factor (bFGF) [14–17]. Our stereological study indicated that zeolite–bentonite powder could negatively affect angiogenesis and its associated vasodilation. Consequently, it can have a negative impact on the healing process. However, it remains questionable why and by which mechanism zeolite–bentonite compound could affect the aforementioned events.

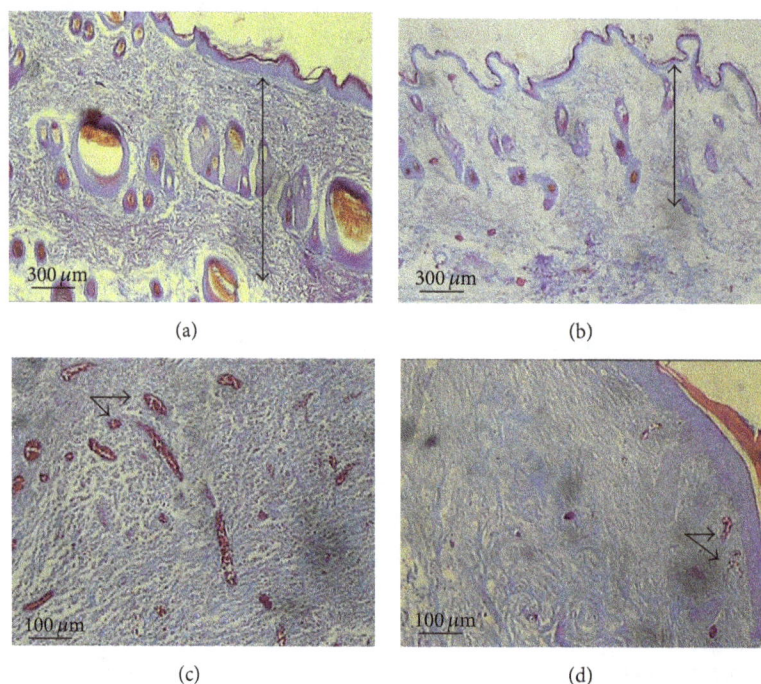

FIGURE 1: The photomicrograph of the rat skin stained with Heidenhain's AZAN trichrome. (a) and (b) images show the wounded skin of the rats 21 days after treatment with NS and ZEO, respectively. The two-head arrows indicate reduction in the dermis size of the ZEO-treated animals. (c) and (d) images display the dermis of the rats 21 days after treatment with normal saline and ZEO, respectively. The arrows indicate reduction in the vessels' density and diameter in the ZEO-exposed rats.

TABLE 2: The Abramov's histological scoring system for wound repair.

Parameter	Score			
	0	1	2	3
Acute inflammation	None	Scant	Moderate	Abundant
Chronic inflammation	None	Scant	Moderate	Abundant
Amount of granulation tissue	None	Scant	Moderate	Abundant
Granulation tissue maturation	Immature	Mild maturation	Moderate maturation	Fully matured
Collagen deposition	None	Scant	Moderate	Abundant
Reepithelialization	None	Partial	Complete but immature or thin	Complete and mature
Neovascularization	None	Up to five vessels per HPF*	6 to 10 vessels per HPF	More than 10 vessels per HPF

*High power field.

Another important point is that the current results of the study show that the volume density of the collagen bundles was significantly less in the healing tissues of the ZEO-treated rats compared to the NS-treated group on Day 21. It is evident that collagen deposition by fibroblasts is essential for the healing process and provides tissue strength, integrity, and structure. However, excessive amounts of collagen deposition will increase the probability of scar formation [16]. According to our findings, it could be claimed that the possibility of scar formation was less in the ZEO-treated animals in comparison to the other group. Yet, it seems necessary to objectively measure the healed tissue strength to opine about the impact of reduction in volume density of collagen on tissue strength.

This work had some limitations that should be considered while interpreting the findings. First, the present study

examined the impact of the topical application of zeolite–bentonite compound on a skin wound model using stereological techniques. Nonetheless, we did not photographically compare wound surface area between NS- and ZEO-treated groups during the study period. In fact, although our findings showed that the zeolite–bentonite powder could have angioinhibitory and vasoconstrictive features, these effects might result in no significant macroscopic difference between the NS- and ZEO-treated groups regarding the wound surface area. This is similar to the result obtained in the experiment by Khoshmohabat et al. Another limitation of the current work was not comparing the impact of zeolite–bentonite powder on wound healing to that of an FDA-approved haemostatic agent to which we had no access. Because of such inaccessibility, we washed the wounds of the control group (NS-treated animals) using only sterile normal saline. Third, we assessed the skin biopsies taken in the middle and late postwounding periods, although it would have been beneficial to examine the skin biopsies of other groups of animals, stereologically, early on (e.g., on Day 4 or 5). However, our limitation in providing male rats was an obstacle to this. Due to the impact of sex hormones on the wound healing process and fluctuation of their levels during the reproductive cycle in female rats, we could not use them in our work.

In conclusion, according to this stereological study, one-time topical usage of zeolite–bentonite haemostatic powder on an animal skin wound could negatively affect the healing process by inhibition of neovascularization and vasoconstriction. In addition, due to the reduction of volume density of collagen bundles after application of zeolite–bentonite compound, the healing tissues had a lesser possibility of scar formation.

Competing Interests

The authors declare that there is no conflict of interests regarding the publication of this article.

Acknowledgments

The authors would like to thank Ms. E. Nadimi for preparing tissue specimens for stereological examination. They are also grateful to Ms. A. Keivanshekouh at the Research Improvement Centre of Shiraz University of Medical Sciences for improving the use of English in the manuscript.

References

[1] A. H. Smith, C. Laird, K. Porter, and M. Bloch, "Haemostatic dressings in prehospital care," *Emergency Medicine Journal*, vol. 30, no. 10, pp. 784–789, 2013.

[2] J. Granville-Chapman, N. Jacobs, and M. J. Midwinter, "Prehospital haemostatic dressings: a systematic review," *Injury*, vol. 42, no. 5, pp. 447–459, 2011.

[3] H. Khoshmohabat, B. Dalfardi, A. Dehghanian, H. R. Rasouli, S. M. J. Mortazavi, and S. Paydar, "The effect of CoolClot hemostatic agent on skin wound healing in rats," *Journal of Surgical Research*, vol. 200, no. 2, pp. 732–737, 2016.

[4] S. M. Mortazavi, A. Atefi, P. Roshan-Shomal, N. Raadpey, and G. Mortazavi, "Development of a novel mineral based haemostatic agent consisting of a combination of bentonite and zeolite minerals," *Journal of Ayub Medical College, Abbottabad : JAMC*, vol. 21, no. 1, pp. 3–7, 2009.

[5] S. Mortazavi, A. Tavasoli, M. Atefi et al., "CoolClot, a novel hemostatic agent for controlling life-threatening arterial bleeding," *World Journal of Emergency Medicine*, vol. 4, pp. 123–127, 2013.

[6] S. Kamp, G. B. E. Jemec, K. Kemp et al., "Application of stereology to dermatological research," *Experimental Dermatology*, vol. 18, no. 12, pp. 1001–1009, 2009.

[7] C. Mühlfeld, J. R. Nyengaard, and T. M. Mayhew, "A review of state-of-the-art stereology for better quantitative 3D morphology in cardiac research," *Cardiovascular Pathology*, vol. 19, no. 2, pp. 65–82, 2010.

[8] C. A. Mandarim-de-Lacerda, "Stereological tools in biomedical research," *Anais da Academia Brasileira de Ciencias*, vol. 75, no. 4, pp. 469–486, 2003.

[9] Y. Garcia, A. Breen, K. Burugapalli, P. Dockery, and A. Pandit, "Stereological methods to assess tissue response for tissue-engineered scaffolds," *Biomaterials*, vol. 28, no. 2, pp. 175–186, 2007.

[10] S. Karbalay-Doust, A. Noorafshan, and S.-M. Pourshahid, "Taxol and taurine protect the renal tissue of rats after unilateral ureteral obstruction: a stereological survey," *Korean Journal of Urology*, vol. 53, no. 5, pp. 360–367, 2012.

[11] F. Arnaud, T. Tomori, W. Carr et al., "Exothermic reaction in zeolite hemostatic dressings: QuikClot ACS and ACS+®," *Annals of Biomedical Engineering*, vol. 36, no. 10, pp. 1708–1713, 2008.

[12] B. Kheirabadi, "Evaluation of topical hemostatic agents for combat wound treatment," *U.S. Army Medical Department Journal*, pp. 25–37, 2011.

[13] Y. Abramov, B. Golden, M. Sullivan et al., "Histologic characterization of vaginal vs. abdominal surgical wound healing in a rabbit model," *Wound Repair and Regeneration*, vol. 15, no. 1, pp. 80–86, 2007.

[14] J. Li, J. Chen, and R. Kirsner, "Pathophysiology of acute wound healing," *Clinics in Dermatology*, vol. 25, no. 1, pp. 9–18, 2007.

[15] M. G. Tonnesen, X. Feng, and R. A. F. Clark, "Angiogenesis in wound healing," *Journal of Investigative Dermatology Symposium Proceedings*, vol. 5, no. 1, pp. 40–46, 2000.

[16] R. F. Diegelmann and M. C. Evans, "Wound healing: an overview of acute, fibrotic and delayed healing," *Frontiers in Bioscience*, vol. 9, pp. 283–289, 2004.

[17] G. Broughton II, J. E. Janis, and C. E. Attinger, "Wound healing: an overview," *Plastic and Reconstructive Surgery*, vol. 117, no. 7S, pp. 1e-S–32e-S, 2006.

5

Adverse Effects of Subchronic Dose of Aspirin on Reproductive Profile of Male Rats

Archana Vyas,[1] Heera Ram,[1] Ashok Purohit,[1] and Rameshwar Jatwa[2]

[1]*Department of Zoology, Jai Narain Vyas University, Jodhpur, Rajasthan 342001, India*
[2]*Molecular Medicine and Toxicology Lab, School of Life Sciences, Devi Ahilya University, Indore, Madhya Pradesh 452001, India*

Correspondence should be addressed to Heera Ram; baradhr@gmail.com

Academic Editor: Massoud Amanlou

Aspirin (acetylsalicylic acid) is widely used for cardiovascular prophylaxis and as anti-inflammatory pharmaceutical. An investigation was carried out to evaluate the influence of subchronic dose of aspirin on reproductive profile of male rats, if any. Experimental animals were divided into three groups: control and aspirin subchronic dose of 12.5 mg/kg for 30 days and 60 days, respectively, while alterations in sperm dynamics, testicular histopathological and planimetric investigations, body and organs weights, lipid profiles, and hematology were performed as per aimed objectives. Subchronic dose of aspirin reduced sperm density, count, and mobility in cauda epididymis and testis; histopathology and developing primary spermatogonial cells (primary spermatogonia, secondary spermatogonia, and mature spermatocyte) count were also significantly decreased in rats. Hematological investigations revealed hemopoietic abnormalities in 60-day-treated animals along with dysfunctions in hepatic and renal functions. The findings of the present study revealed that administration with subchronic dose of aspirin to male rats resulted in altered reproductive profiles and serum biochemistry.

1. Introduction

Aspirin (acetylsalicylic acid) is a nonsteroidal anti-inflammatory drug (NSAID) used in various pathological conditions for its anti-inflammatory, antipyretic, and analgesic benefits [1, 2]. Investigations on aspirin and its underlying mechanism exposed new arena of knowledge, namely, prostaglandin synthesis and platelet inhibition and allowed additional development of efficient antiplatelet agents and anti-inflammatory medications [3]. In the present scenario, with increasing incidence of noncommunicable diseases, aspirin has gained a significant attention not only as an analgesic but also as a cardioprotective agent [4]. On the other hand, reports are there in the literature suggesting morbidity and mortality associated with adverse effects of aspirin. Furthermore, long-term therapeutic use of aspirin is associated with the incidences of gastrointestinal (GI) ulcerations, nephrotoxicity, hepatotoxicity, and even renal cell cancers [5]. The antiplatelet effect of aspirin has been attributed to coronary artery disease, pregnancy complications, and preeclampsia in angiotensin-sensitive primigravida [5–7]. Whereas aspirin treatment causes an increased risk of cerebral microbleeds, tinnitus in children, and Reye's syndrome when given to children or adolescents to treat fever or illnesses, it alters estrogen and progesterone biosynthesis upon chronic administration [8–10].

Interestingly, aspirin-induced inhibition of prostaglandins synthesis resulted in altered cholesterol metabolism and androgen biosynthesis [10]. However, effect of subchronic aspirin administration on male reproductive profile was not well elucidated till date. Therefore, the present study was designed to ravel out the influence of aspirin subchronic dose on male reproductive profile and serum variables of rats.

2. Materials and Methods

2.1. Experimental Animals. Colony bred adult healthy male albino rats weighing 200–235 g were used for present research. All animals were proven fertile and were obtained from the Indian Veterinary Research Institute (IVRI),

Bareilly, India. They were housed in a standard light (14 h light : 10 h dark cycle), controlled room temperature (23 ± 2°C), with the provision of laboratory feed and water ad libitum. The animals were acclimatized for a week before conducting the experiment and care of the laboratory animals was taken as per the guidelines laid down by the Committee for the Purpose of Control and Supervision on Experiments on Animals (CPCSEA), government of India, New Delhi (reg. number: 1646/GO/ERe/S/12/CPCSEA).

2.2. Drug and Dose Regime.
Aspirin (acetylsalicylic acid) tablets (Ecosprin-75®) were purchased from the local registered medical store. Aspirin dose regime was given at low dose of 12.5 mg/kg body weight for 30 and 60 days as per protocol.

2.3. Experimental Design and Preparation of Serum and Tissue Samples.
Twenty-one adult healthy rats were randomly divided into three groups of seven each. While animals of group 1 received vehicle, distilled water served as control and group 2 and 3 animals received aspirin (12.5 mg/kg) by oral gavage for 30 days and 60 days, respectively. On the day of termination, day 31 (group 2) and day 61 (group 3), overnight fasted animals were autopsied after exposing them to mild ether anesthesia. Blood from each animal was collected by cardiac puncture method and serum was isolated and stored at –20°C until assayed for glucose, lipid profiles, and other parameters.

2.4. Estimation of Total Cholesterol.
Total cholesterol concentration in serum was determined by an enzymatic method using commercial available test kit as was routinely done in our laboratory [11, 12]. In brief, cholesterol esters are enzymatically hydrolyzed by cholesterol esterase to cholesterol and free fatty acids. The hydrogen peroxide combines with 4-aminoantipyrine to form a chromophore (quinoneimine dye) which was monitored on a spectrophotometer at 505 nm.

2.5. Triglyceride Assay.
Circulating triglyceride was determined by an enzymatic method using a commercial available triglyceride test kit method. Triglycerides are enzymatically hydrolyzed by lipase to free acids and glycerol. Color reaction is catalyzed by peroxidase; H_2O_2 reacts with 4-aminoantipyrine (4AAP) and 4-chlorophenol to produce a red colored dye [12, 13].

2.6. Fasting Glucose Estimation.
Circulating fasting serum glucose level was measured by a standard method as routinely followed in our laboratory. In brief, glucose is oxidized by glucose oxidase/peroxidase enzyme to yield gluconic acid and hydrogen peroxide. The enzyme peroxidase catalyzes the oxidative coupling of 4-aminoantipyrine with phenol to yield a colored quinoneimine complex. The absorbance is proportional to the concentration of glucose in the sample [14].

2.7. Analysis of Serum Urea.
Urea level in serum was measured by standard diacetyl monoxime method. The enzyme methodology employed as urea is hydrolyzed in the presence of water and urease to produce ammonia and carbon dioxide. The reaction is monitored by measuring the rate of decrease in absorbance at 340 nm as NADH is converted to NAD [15].

2.8. Estimation of Creatinine.
Serum creatinine level was measured by kit method as described earlier. Creatinine reacts with alkaline picrate to produce an orange-yellow color. The absorbance of the orange-yellow color formed is directly proportional to creatinine concentration and is measured on a spectrophotometer at 490–510 nm [16].

2.9. Analysis of SGOT and SGPT Activities.
Measurement of SGOT and SGPT was done by enzymatic methods. In brief, series of reactions involved in the assay for SGOT as the sample catalyzes the transfer of the amino group from L-aspartate to 2-oxoglutarate forming oxaloacetate and L-glutamate. The reaction is monitored by measuring the rate of decrease in absorbance at 340 nm due to the oxidation of NADH to NAD.

Similarly, SGPT catalyzes deamination from alanine to 2-oxoglutarate yielding pyruvate and L-glutamate. Pyruvate is reduced to lactate by LDH present in the reagent with the simultaneous oxidation of NADH to NAD. The reaction is monitored by absorbance at 340 nm on a UV-Vis spectrophotometer [17].

2.10. Quantitative Estimation of Total Protein.
Total serum protein level was estimated by using the method of Lowry et al. [18], as routinely performed in our laboratory. The peptide bonds of protein react with Cu^{+2} ions in alkaline conditions to form a blue-violet ion complex. The color formed is proportional to the protein concentration and is measured at 660 nm on a UV-Vis spectrophotometer [18].

2.11. Hematological Analysis.
Blood samples were collected by direct cardiac puncture method and hematological assessments were performed following standard protocols. The hematological measurements included red blood corpuscles (RBC) count, white blood corpuscle (WBC) count, platelet counts, hemoglobin (Hb) concentration, and hematocrit (HCT) by Wintrobe's methods [12, 19].

2.12. Sperm Dynamics Analysis.
The sperm dynamics analysis was performed following standard method, as routinely done in our laboratory. In brief, the cauda epididymis from each animal was chopped into phosphate buffered saline (0.1 M, pH 7.4) and the following observations were made:

(i) Total number of sperms.

(ii) Total number of motile sperms.

(iii) Normal and abnormal sperm counts.

(iv) Sperms densities in testis and cauda.

The total sperm count was calculated by using Neubauer's haemocytometer. The accuracy of sperm count was increased; the epididymis plasma was diluted with a spermicidal solution, prepared by dissolving 5 g of NaHCO3 and 1 mL of 40% formaldehyde in 100 mL of normal saline.

A twenty times dilution was made by using WBC pipette, which was thoroughly mixed and one drop was added to both sides of Neubauer's haemocytometer. The sperms were allowed to settle down in the haemocytometer by keeping them in a humid chamber for one hour. The sperm count was done in 5 major squares designated as $E1$, $E2$, $E3$, $E4$, and a central $E5$. Each square is 1 mm long, 1 mm wide, and 0.1 mm high. The total volume represented by each major square E is thus 0.1 mm^3 or 10^{-4} mm. The total number of sperms was counted in all the major squares and calculated as follows:

Total no. of sperms/mL plasma

$$= \frac{\text{Total no. of sperms per square } (X)}{\text{Total volume per square } (10^{-4})} \quad (1)$$

$$\times \text{ dilution factor } (20).$$

Similarly, the total number of motile sperms was calculated by using PBGS (phosphate buffered glucose saline) instead of spermicidal solution [20, 21].

2.13. Testicular Histopathological and Planimetric Investigations. After exsanguinations, testis tissues were removed, quickly freed from blood clots, washed thoroughly with phosphate buffered saline (0.1 M, pH 7.4), and used for fixation. Fixed tissues were prepared under paraffin embedding, stained with hematoxylin-eosin (H&E), and examined at 5 μM thick sections. Microscopic observations were made at 100x and 400x magnifications with proper resolution of testicular histoarchitectural alterations. Consequently, planimetric study was performed at 8×4 magnifications for germ cell population dynamics by camera lucida [22].

3. Results

3.1. Effect on Body and Organs Weight. The body weight of the rats was not significantly altered in 30-day- and 60-day-treated groups. Animals in groups 2 and 3 exhibited a significant decrease in the weight of testis and cauda epididymis ($P \leq 0.001$ for both). Similarly, weights of ventral prostate and seminal vesicle of the animals of 30-day and 60-day treatment groups also showed significant decrease ($P \leq 0.001$ for all), whereas there were no significant changes observed in the weights of liver, kidney, and body weights after 30 days or 60 days of treatment, as compared to vehicle treated controls (Table 1).

3.2. Effect on Sperm Dynamics. Analysis of sperm dynamics, namely, total sperm count, total number of motile sperms, sperm density, and abnormal sperm of the cauda epididymis and testis was carried out in the control and animals of 30-day- and 60-day-treated groups.

Aspirin administration for 30 days to rats resulted in significant decrease ($P \leq 0.001$ for all) in sperm dynamics parameters of both groups (Table 2). Total sperm counts in testis and cauda significantly decreased ($P \leq 0.001$ for both) in 30-day- and 60-day-treated group in a gradual manner. Concurrently, the sperm density in cauda and testis was reduced ($P \leq 0.001$ for both) in both the groups who received

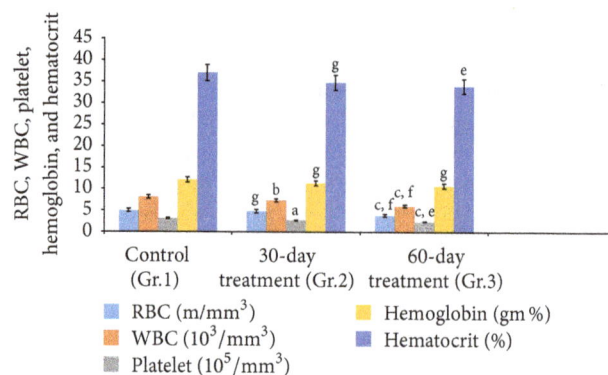

FIGURE 1: Effect of aspirin subchronic dose administration on RBC, WBC, platelets, hemoglobin, and hematocrit of rats. Data are means $\pm$ SEM ($n = 7$). [a]$P \leq 0.05$: [b]$P \leq 0.01$, [c]$P \leq 0.001$ as compared to the respective control values; [e]$P \leq 0.01$ and [f]$P \leq 0.001$ as compared to the respective values of the 30-day-treated groups and [g]nonsignificant.

subchronic dose of aspirin for 30 days and 60 days. Sperm mortality also increased following aspirin treatment for 30 days and 60 days ($P \leq 0.001$ for both) as compared to vehicle control group (Figures 2(a) and 2(b)).

3.3. Serum Biochemistry. The results of serum biochemistry are depicted in Table 3. The concentrations of serum total protein, cholesterol, triglyceride, and glucose were not altered significantly following aspirin administration compared to controls, while serum SGOT and SGPT activities and creatinine and urea levels were increased in both the groups who received subchronic aspirin treatments for 30 and 60 days (Table 2).

3.4. Hematological Study. Aspirin treatments influenced the hematology of the rats. Hematological parameters, namely, Hb (hemoglobin) concentrations, RBC count, WBC count, and HCT (hematocrit) of groups 2 and 3 exhibited significant alterations as compared to controls (Figure 1).

3.5. Testicular Histopathological and Planimetric Investigations. Histoarchitecture of control group testis showed normal testicular architecture with an orderly arrangement of spermatogenic developing cells and interstitial and sertoli cells with connective tissues. The spermatogonia, that is, primary, secondary, and sertoli cells were rested on the basement membrane of the seminiferous tubules. Leydig's cells with large and acidophilic cytoplasm were located in the interstitial tissue among seminiferous tubules (Figures 3(a)-3(b)), while treatment with subchronic dose of aspirin for 30 days or 60 days resulted in varying degrees of abnormalities in testis histology. The primary spermatogonia, secondary spermatogonia, spermatocytes, and Leydig's cells exhibited significant reduction ($P \leq 0.001$ for all) following administration of aspirin for 30 or 60 days (Figures 3(c)-3(d) and Figures 3(e)-3(f)). Concurrently, population of developing spermatogonial cells and fibroblast cells were reduced ($P \leq 0.001$ for all) in aspirin treated groups as compared to vehicle control (Table 3).

TABLE 1: Adverse effects of subchronic dose of aspirin on body and organs weight of male rats.

Treatment groups	Body weight (g)		Testes	Epididymis	Seminal vesicle	Ventral prostate	Heart	Kidney	Liver
	Initial	Final			mg/100 g body weight				g/100 g BW
Control (Gr. 1)	211.3 ± 18.2	227 ± 19.51	1209 ± 72.5	560 ± 15.6	618.6 ± 18.6	279.7 ± 7.4	315.5 ± 16.2	595 ± 25.3	2.6 ± 0.12
30-day-treated group (Gr. 2)	220 ± 20.12^g	228 ± 19.12^g	634 ± 30.16^c	368 ± 13.6^c	273 ± 10.12^c	126 ± 5.76^c	363 ± 11.12^g	608 ± 21.36^g	2.8 ± 0.61^g
60-day-treated group (Gr. 3)	230 ± 22.1^g	237 ± 21.67^g	724 ± 49.79^c	396 ± 16.17^c	319 ± 13.79^c	136 ± 6.12^c	329 ± 12.63^g	642 ± 20.12^g	2.9 ± 0.36^g

Data are means ± SEM ($n = 7$). $^c P \leq 0.001$ compared to the respective control values; ^{g}nonsignificant.

TABLE 2: Adverse effects of subchronic dose of aspirin on testicular cell population dynamics of rats.

Groups	Germinal cell types				Fibroblast	Interstitial cell types		
	Spermatogonia	Primary spermatocyte	Secondary spermatocyte	Spermatids		Immature Leydig's cell	Mature Leydig's cell	Degenerating cell
Vehicle control	26.12 ± 0.76	20.25 ± 0.86	65.16 ± 3.16	160.19 ± 5.16	59.01 ± 1.32	51.33 ± 2.16	73.16 ± 1.06	16.36 ± 1.37
30-day treatment	19.61 ± 1.73^b	12.25 ± 0.62^c	12.16 ± 1.26^c	5.19 ± 0.76^c	55.07 ± 2.31	30.33 ± 3.01^c	32.16 ± 3.05^c	70.16 ± 1.31^c
60-day treatment	5.23 ± 0.36^{c,f}	2.25 ± 0.26^{c,f}	1.56 ± 0.96^{c,f}	2.19 ± 5.16^{c,f}	47.01 ± 2.32^b	21.33 ± 2.67^c	19.01 ± 1.06^{c,f}	81.12 ± 2.16^{c,f}

Data are means ± SEM ($n = 7$). $^b P \leq 0.01$; $^c P \leq 0.001$ compared to the respective control values and $^f P \leq 0.001$ compared to the respective values of the 30-day-treated group.

TABLE 3: Effects of subchronic dose of aspirin on serum total cholesterol, triglyceride, glucose, urea, creatinine, and protein and activities of SGOT and SGPT of male rats.

Groups	Cholesterol (mg/dL)	Glucose (mg/dL)	Triglyceride (mg/dL)	Urea (mg/dL)	Creatinine (mg/dL)	SGOT (U/L)	SGPT (U/L)	Protein (mg/dL)
Control (Gr. 1)	104.1 ± 3.34	97 ± 5	90.21 ± 5.2	21.12 ± 2.16	1.01 ± 0.12	40 ± 3.2	40 ± 2.6	5.52 ± 1.02
30-day-treated group (Gr. 2)	121 ± 7.36^g	103 ± 3.34^g	102.02 ± 2.1^g	30.5 ± 2.76^g	1.65 ± 0.04^a	210 ± 5.26^c	93 ± 2.36^c	7.13 ± 1.63^g
60-day-treated group (Gr. 3)	111 ± 5.23^g	107 ± 4.32^g	97.11 ± 3.1^g	39 ± 1.96^g	1.86 ± 0.043^b	$251 \pm 6.16^{c,f}$	$190 \pm 2.67^{c,f}$	7.87 ± 1.24^g

Data are means $\pm$ SEM ($n = 7$). $^a P \leq 0.05$; $^b P \leq 0.01$; $^c P \leq 0.001$ compared to the respective control values; $^f P \leq 0.001$ compared to the respective values of the 30-day-treated group and ^{g}nonsignificant.

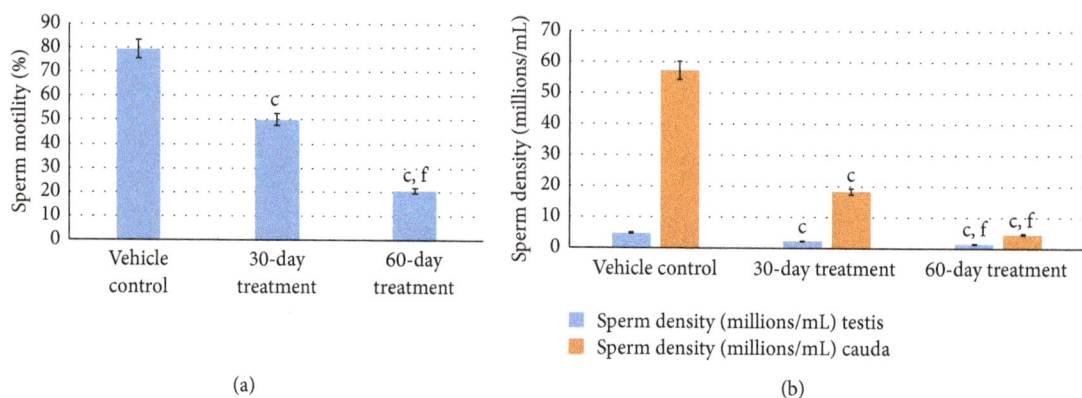

(a)

(b)

FIGURE 2: (a) Effect of aspirin subchronic dose administration on sperm motility of treated rats. Data are means $\pm$ SEM ($n = 7$). $^c P \leq 0.001$ as compared to the respective control values; $^f P \leq 0.001$ as compared to the respective values of the 30-day-treated group. (b) Effects of aspirin subchronic dose administration on sperm density on treated rats. Data are means $\pm$ SEM ($n = 7$). $^c P \leq 0.001$ as compared to the respective control values; $^f P \leq 0.001$ as compared to the respective values of the 30-day-treated group.

4. Discussion

Aspirin is one of most widely used anti-inflammatory drugs with proven cardiovascular benefits [23]. Nonsteroidal anti-inflammatory drugs (NSAIDs) are suggested for analgesic and anti-inflammatory activities to manage oncologic and neurologic diseases in human and veterinary subjects. Despite putting efforts in improving the safety, efficacy, and potency of NSAIDs, adverse effects such as gastrointestinal irritation, renal and hepatic toxicity, interference with hemostasis, and reproductive problems still persist [24]. The findings of the present study clearly reveal that subchronic administration (for 30 or 60 days) of aspirin to male rats caused reproductive abnormalities and liver toxicity. However, treatment with aspirin was found to be safe with reference to organs and body weight, except testis, epididymis, seminal vesicle, and ventral prostate. These alterations might be conducted through indirect involvement of inhibition of androgens biosynthesis [23, 24]. It is well understood that weight, size, and secretary function of testes, epididymis, seminal vesicles, ventral prostate, and vasa differentia are closely regulated by androgens hormones. However, the process of spermatogenesis and the accessory reproductive organs function are dependent on androgen activity [24, 25].

Interestingly, aspirin administration to normal rats resulted in hypercholesterolemia. The increased levels of cholesterol and triglyceride in aspirin treated groups might be due to decreased androgen production, which resulted in accumulation of cholesterol in testes. The impaired sperm dynamics, including spermatogenesis, could be an outcome of aspirin-induced alteration in cholesterol metabolism in testis [26].

Interestingly, subchronic aspirin treatment resulted in reduced sperm count and density; on the other hand, it enhanced sperm motility. Androgens are essential for survival and motility of spermatozoa in the epididymis and cauda region appears to be the most favorable site for the same. Aspirin-induced reduction in sperm dynamics might be an outcome of depressed levels of androgens. Interestingly, subchronic aspirin administration influenced androgen dependent parameters including that of reduced sperm count, motility, and density. The observed reduced sperm activity profile might be an outcome of androgen depletion at target level, particularly in the cauda epididymis, thereby affecting physiological maturation of the sperm [26–28]. In the literature, reports are suggesting that reproductive toxicant which affects sperm motility would in turn influence spermatozoa indirectly through disruption of epididymis epithelial cell function and/or by acting directly on

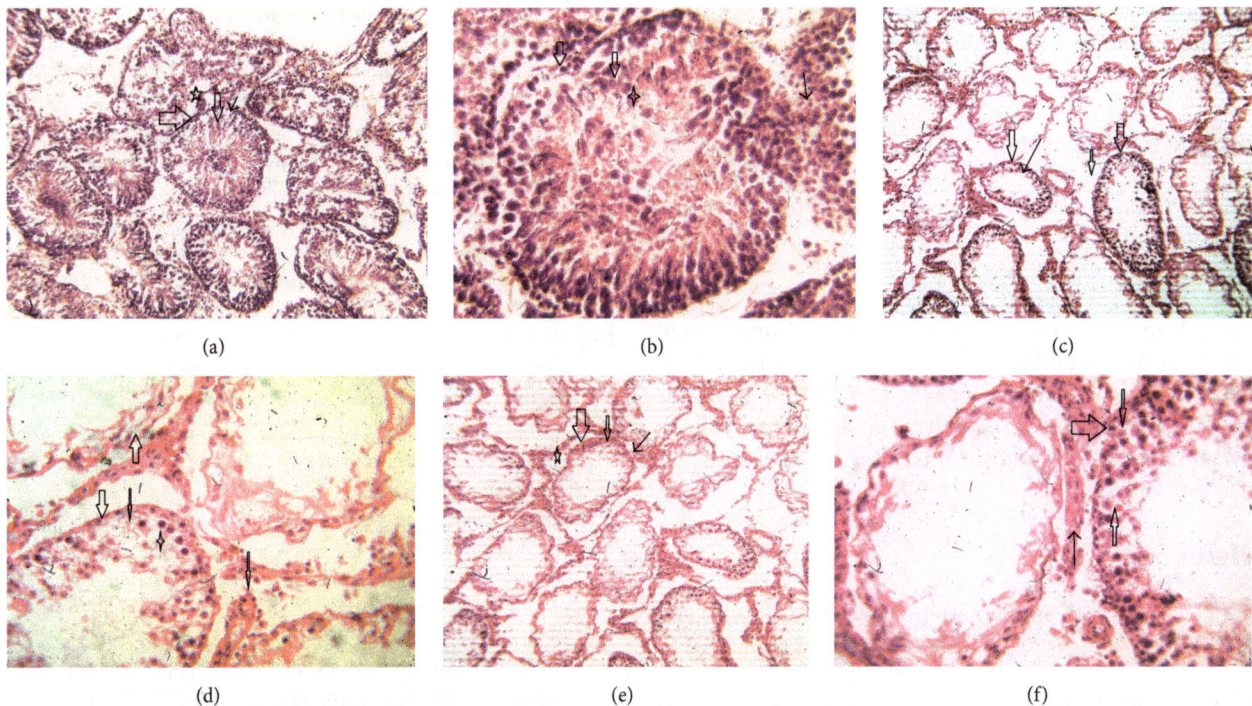

FIGURE 3: (a) Testis histoarchitecture of vehicle control rats (100x HE). Seminiferous tubules consisting of germ epithelium cells, various stages of spermatogonia, and spermatids as normal histoarchitecture of testis (thick arrow). Sertoli cells also exist as supporting and nutritioning cells (→). Interstitial cells or Leydig's cells existing between interseminiferous tubular spaces along with proper framing of connective tissues (star sign). (b) Testis histoarchitecture of vehicle rats (400x HE). At higher magnification, a particular seminiferous showing germ epithelium cells, sertoli cells, and various stages of spermatogonia and spermatids (thick arrow, narrow arrow, and star). (c) Testis histoarchitecture of 30-day-aspirin-subchronic-dose-treated rats (100x HE). The aspirin treatment showing cytological and nuclear degenerative changes in seminiferous tubules (thick arrow) and surrounding tissues as abnormal histoarchitecture (middle sized arrow and thin arrow). (d) Testis histoarchitecture of 30-day-aspirin-subchronic-dose-treated rats (400x HE). A 30-day treatment of aspirin caused abnormal histoarchitecture on particular seminiferous tubule as cytological toxicity by decreased numbers of various stages of spermatogonia (thin arrow). Interstitial cells showing in normal conditions as shown by middle sized arrow. Star showing degenerating stages of spermatogonia. (e) Testis histoarchitecture of 60-day-aspirin-subchronic-dose-treated rats (100x HE). Long-term aspirin treatment caused abnormal histoarchitecture as degenerations and reduced numbers of various stages of spermatogonia (middle sized arrow) and peripheral tissues (star). Thick arrow showing shrinkage in seminiferous tubules. (f) Testis histoarchitecture of 60-day-aspirin-subchronic-dose-treated rats (100x HE). 60-day aspirin treatment caused degenerative changes in particular seminiferous tubule as showing reduced numbers of various stages of spermatogonia (indicated by middle sized arrow), sertoli cells (first middle arrow), and without affecting Leydig's cells (thin arrow).

the spermatozoa by affecting their enzymes [26, 27]. It is speculated that aspirin might have caused reproductive toxicity in male rats through this mechanism, as evidenced by the reduction in androgen dependent parameters.

On the other hand, aspirin treatment for 60 days elevated serum levels of urea, uric acid, creatinine, and the activities of SGOT and SGPT, reflecting the toxic effects on subchronic administration. Adverse effects following aspirin administration in normal rats might be an outcome of NSAIDs induced inhibition of prostaglandin synthesis which leads to renal vasoconstriction and decreased renal perfusion which is responsible for acute renal abnormalities [28–30]. Aspirin-induced liver toxicity is obvious, as liver is the major target organ for drug metabolism and hepatic biotransformation reactions are known to induce apoptosis of hepatocytes [31]. Furthermore, aspirin-induced liver toxicity could be an outcome of idiosyncratic metabolic reaction due to aberrant metabolism of the drug where accumulation of toxic

metabolites in hepatocytes binds to cell proteins and leads to abnormalities [30, 31]. Observations made on total protein levels are in accordance with this fact. The alterations in the level of serum proteins might be an outcome of both hepatic and renal damage, where it causes alteration in a number of enzymes and could also disturb protein synthesis in hepatocytes [31]. Moreover, decreased serum protein levels could be attributed to a reduced hepatic DNA and RNA synthesis which in turn hampered utilization of free amino acids for protein synthesis [32, 33]. In the literature, aspirin-induced hematological disorders are well documented, and the results of the present study are in accordance with this which is suggesting aspirin-induced malfunctions in hemopoiesis of male rats [34, 35].

In conclusion, subchronic administration (for 30 or 60 days) of aspirin resulted in reduced sperm density, count, and mobility in cauda epididymis and testis as well as developing spermatogonial cells count, reflecting the toxic nature in rats. Findings made on the hepatic and renal profiles further reveal toxic nature of the aspirin when administered to rats subchronically.

Competing Interests

The authors declare that they have no competing interests.

Acknowledgments

Financial support from the University Grants Commission, New Delhi, India, under Career Research Award no. F.30-11/2011(SA-II) dated January 16, 2012, to Rameshwar Jatwa is gratefully acknowledged. The authors would like to thank the Polyclinic Center, Government Veterinary Hospital, Jodhpur, Rajasthan, India.

References

[1] V. Fuster and J. M. Sweeny, "Aspirin: historical and contemporary therapeutic overview," *Circulation*, vol. 123, no. 7, pp. 768–779, 2014.

[2] M. K. Nayak, A. Dash, N. Singh, and D. Dash, "Aspirin delimits platelet life span by proteasomal inhibition," *PLoS ONE*, vol. 9, no. 8, pp. e105049–e105058, 2014.

[3] K. O. Oyedeji, A. F. Bolarinwa, and A. K. Adigun, "Effect of aspirin on reproductive functions in male albino rats," *Journal of Pharmacy and Biological Sciences*, vol. 4, no. 7, pp. 49–54, 2013.

[4] S. Halvorsen, F. Andreotti, J. M. Berg et al., "Aspirin therapy in primary cardiovascular disease prevention: a position paper of the European Society of Cardiology working group on Thrombosis," *Journal of American College of Cardiology*, vol. 64, no. 16, pp. 319–327, 2014.

[5] J. Li, Y. Yu, Y. Yang et al., "A 15-day oral dose toxicity study of aspirin eugenol ester in Wistar rats," *Food and Chemical Toxicology*, vol. 50, no. 6, pp. 1980–1985, 2012.

[6] R. G. Schoemaker, P. R. Saxena, and E. A. J. Kalkman, "Low-dose aspirin improves in vivo hemodynamics in conscious, chronically infarcted rats," *Cardiovascular Research*, vol. 37, no. 1, pp. 108–115, 1998.

[7] H. C. S. Wallenburg, J. W. Makovitz, G. A. Dekker, and P. Rotmans, "Low-dose aspirin prevents pregnancy-induced hypertension and pre-eclampsia in angiotensin-sensitive primigravidae," *The Lancet*, vol. 327, no. 8471, pp. 1–3, 1986.

[8] P. Pignatelli, S. Di Santo, F. Barillà, C. Gaudio, and F. Violi, "Multiple anti-atherosclerotic treatments impair aspirin compliance: effects on aspirin resistance," *Journal of Thrombosis and Haemostasis*, vol. 6, no. 10, pp. 1832–1834, 2008.

[9] R. Anthony and M. D. Temple, "Acute and chronic effects of aspirin toxicity and their treatment," *Archives of Internal Medicine*, vol. 141, no. 3, pp. 364–373, 1981.

[10] N. Jain, R. Shrivastava, A. K. Raghuwanshi, and V. K. Shrivastava, "The effect of aspirin on reproductive organs of female albino rat," *International Journal of Pharma Sciences and Research*, vol. 3, no. 8, pp. 2644–2651, 2012.

[11] C. C. Allain, L. S. Poon, C. S. G. Chan, W. Richmond, and P. C. Fu, "Enzymatic determination of total serum cholesterol," *Clinical Chemistry*, vol. 20, no. 4, pp. 470–475, 1974.

[12] H. Ram, R. Jatwa, and A. Purohit, "Antiatherosclerotic and cardioprotective potential of acacia senegal seeds in diet-induced atherosclerosis in rabbits," *Biochemistry Research International*, vol. 2014, Article ID 436848, 6 pages, 2014.

[13] P. Fossati and L. Prencipe, "Serum triglycerides determined colorimetrically with an enzyme that produces hydrogen peroxide," *Clinical Chemistry*, vol. 28, no. 10, pp. 2077–2080, 1982.

[14] R. J. L. Bondar and D. C. Mead, "Evaluation of glucose phosphate dehydrogenase from leuconostoc mesteteroides in hexokinase method for determining in serum," *Clinical Chemistry*, vol. 20, pp. 586–593, 1974.

[15] D. R. Wybenga, J. Di Giorgio, and V. J. Pileggi, "Manual and automated methods for urea nitrogen measurement in whole serum," *Clinical Chemistry*, vol. 17, no. 9, pp. 891–895, 1971.

[16] R. J. Mitchell, "Improved method for specific determination of creatinine in serum and urine," *Clinical Chemistry*, vol. 19, no. 4, pp. 408–410, 1973.

[17] S. Reitman and S. A. Frankel, "A colorimetric method for the determination of serum glutamic oxalacetic and glutamic pyruvic transaminases," *American Journal of Clinical Pathology*, vol. 28, no. 1, pp. 56–63, 1957.

[18] O. H. Lowry, N. J. Rosebrough, A. L. Farr, and R. J. Randall, "Protein measurement with the Folin phenol reagent," *Journal of Biological Chemistry*, vol. 193, no. 1, pp. 265–276, 1951.

[19] M. A. Merchant and D. N. Modi, "Acute and chronic effects of aspirin on hematological parameters and hepatic ferritin expression in mice," *Indian Journal of Pharmacology*, vol. 36, no. 4, pp. 226–231, 2004.

[20] J. Seed, R. E. Chapin, E. D. Clegg et al., "Methods for assessing sperm motility, morphology, and counts in the rat, rabbit, and dog: a consensus report," *Reproductive Toxicology*, vol. 10, no. 3, pp. 237–244, 1996.

[21] M. A. Besley, R. Eliarson, A. J. Gallegosm, K. S. Moghissi, C. A. Paulsen, and M. N. R. Prasad, *Laboratory Manual for the Examination of Human Semen and Semen Cervical Mucus Interaction*, WHO Press Concern, Singapore, 1980.

[22] M. M. Almathkour and E. S. AlSuhaibani, "Protective effect of aspirin on γ radiation-induced sperm malformations in Swiss Albino male mice," *American Journal of Life Sciences*, vol. 2, no. 4, pp. 205–215, 2014.

[23] K. K. Wu, "Aspirin and salicylate: an old remedy with a new twist," *Circulation*, vol. 102, no. 17, pp. 2022–2023, 2000.

[24] E. H. Awtry and J. Loscalzo, "Aspirin," *Circulation*, vol. 101, no. 10, pp. 1206–1218, 2000.

[25] R. H. Aladakatti, B. Sukesh, U. C. Jadaramkunti, and M. B. Hiremath, "Effect of graded doses of nimbolide, a major component of Azadirachta indica leaves, on biochemical and sperm functional parameters in male albino rats," *Journal of Laboratory Animal Science*, vol. 1, pp. 24–31, 2011.

[26] R. S. Bedwal, M. S. Edwards, M. Katoch, A. Bahuguna, and R. Dewan, "Histological and biochemical changes in testis of zinc deficient BALB/c strain of mice," *Indian Journal of Experimental Biology*, vol. 32, no. 4, pp. 243–247, 1994.

[27] N. J. Chinoy, J. M. D'Souza, and P. Padman, "Contraceptive efficacy of *Carica papaya* seed extract in male mice (*Mus musculus*)," *Phytotherapy Research*, vol. 9, no. 1, pp. 30–36, 1995.

[28] A. Purohit and H. M. M. Daradka, "Effect of mild hyperlipidaemia on testicular cell population dynamics in albino rats," *Indian Journal of Experimental Biology*, vol. 37, no. 4, pp. 396–398, 1999.

[29] C. Huerta, J. Castellsague, C. Varas-Lorenzo, and L. A. García Rodríguez, "Nonsteroidal anti-inflammatory drugs and risk of ARF in the general population," *American Journal of Kidney Diseases*, vol. 45, no. 3, pp. 531–539, 2005.

[30] G. R. Matzke, "Nonrenal toxicities of acetaminophen, aspirin, and nonsteroidal anti-inflammatory agents," *American Journal of Kidney Diseases*, vol. 28, no. 1, pp. S63–S70, 1996.

[31] J. S. Aprioku, L. L. Nwidu, and C. N. Amadi, "Evaluation of toxicological profile of ibuprofen in Wistar albino rats," *American Journal of Biomedical Sciences*, vol. 6, no. 1, pp. 32–40, 2014.

[32] H. D. Lewis, J. W. Davis, D. G. Archibald, W. F. Steinkes, T. C. Smitherman, and J. E. Doherty, "Protective effect of aspirin against acute myocardial and death in men with unstable angina," *The New England Journal of Medicine*, vol. 309, pp. 396–404, 1983.

[33] C. Doutremepuich, O. Aguejouf, V. Desplat, and F. X. Eizayaga, "Paradoxical effect of aspirin," *Thrombosis*, vol. 2012, Article ID 676237, 4 pages, 2012.

[34] S. K. Pachathundikandi and E. T. Varghese, "Blood zinc protoporphyrin, serum total protein, and total cholesterol levels in automobile workshop workers in relation to lead toxicity: our experience," *Indian Journal of Clinical Biochemistry*, vol. 21, no. 2, pp. 114–117, 2006.

[35] A. S. El-Sharaky, A. A. Newairy, N. M. Elguindy, and A. A. Elwafa, "Spermatotoxicity, biochemical changes and histological alteration induced by gossypol in testicular and hepatic tissues of male rats," *Food and Chemical Toxicology*, vol. 48, no. 12, pp. 3354–3361, 2010.

6

Xyloglucan Based In Situ Gel of Lidocaine HCl for the Treatment of Periodontosis

Ashlesha P. Pandit, Vaibhav V. Pol, and Vinit S. Kulkarni

Department of Pharmaceutics, JSPM's Rajarshi Shahu College of Pharmacy & Research, Pune-Mumbai Bypass Highway, Tathawade, Pune, Maharashtra 411033, India

Correspondence should be addressed to Ashlesha P. Pandit; panditashleshap@rediffmail.com

Academic Editor: Diego Chiappetta

The present study was aimed at formulating thermoreversible in situ gel of local anesthetic by using xyloglucan based mucoadhesive tamarind seed polysaccharide (TSP) into periodontal pocket. Temperature-sensitive in situ gel of lidocaine hydrochloride (LH) (2% w/v) was formulated by cold method. A full 3^2 factorial design was employed to study the effect of independent variables concentrations of Lutrol F127 and TSP to optimize in situ gel. The dependent variables evaluated were gelation temperature (Y_1) and drug release (Y_2). The results revealed the surface pH of 6.8, similar to the pH of saliva. Viscosity study showed the marked increase in the viscosity of gel at 37°C due to sol-gel conversion. TSP was found to act as good mucoadhesive component to retain gel at the site of application in dental pocket. Gelation of formulation occurred near to body temperature. In vitro study depicted the fast onset of drug action but lasting the release (90%) till 2 h. Formulation F7 was considered as optimized batch, containing 18% Lutrol F127 and 1% tamarind seed polysaccharide. Thus, lidocaine hydrochloride thermoreversible in situ gel offered an alternative to painful injection therapy of anesthesia during dental surgery, with fast onset of anesthetic action lasting throughout the dental procedure.

1. Introduction

Periodontosis is a serious gum infection, which affects the supporting structure of teeth such as gums, periodontal ligaments, alveolar bones, and dental cementum. Periodontosis is caused by the bacteria that stick to the surface of tooth and multiply. Toxins produced by these bacteria in plaque, formed below the gum line, irritate the gums and stimulate an inflammatory response. This results in progressive loss of alveolar bone round the teeth and thus forms the pockets (spaces between the teeth and gums) that become infected [1]. As the disease progresses, the pockets deepen and more gum tissues and bones are destroyed [2]. The number and depth of periodontal pocket vary from patient to patient. The scaling and root planning is the common practice to cure this problem. This scaling procedure needs the application of local and nerve block/infiltration anesthesia by painful needle therapy [3]. An alternative to this therapy of anesthesia is the application of gel [4]. Even though topical anesthetic gels are easy to apply, they possess some drawbacks such as tendency to spread in other areas or lower retention in plaque area, thus causing numbness of lips, tongue, and cheeks and chances of swallowing of the gel. To improve the residence time, in situ gels show promising effect [5]. In situ gel stays at application site due to increased viscosity and mucoadhesiveness and shows fast onset of action. Lutrol is a triblock polymer, consists of polyoxyethylene-polyoxypropylene-polyoxyethylene units, as shown in Figure 1(c), and forms micelles at low concentration and clear thermoreversible gel at a high concentration. The concentrated solution of Lutrol F127 (16–30%) gets transformed from low viscosity transparent solution at 5°C to a solid on heating at body temperature [6]. Formulation which consisted of Lutrol F127 forms a gel in periodontal pocket at a body temperature by modulating the gelation temperature [7]. Gel remains on application site and enhances the residence time in the periodontal pocket. It is used both internally and externally in various products that are designed for animal and human use [8]. The dental gel can be easily rinsed out with water to stop the anesthetic effect after the treatment.

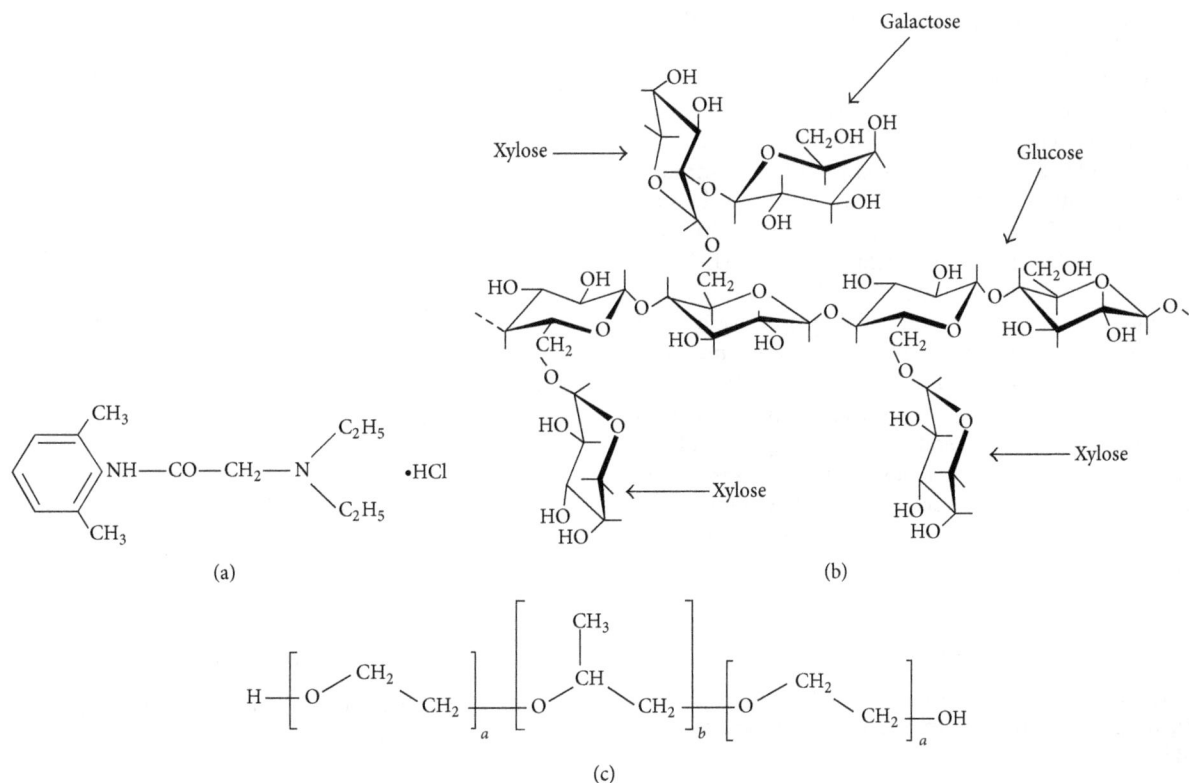

FIGURE 1: Chemical structures of (a) lidocaine hydrochloride, (b) tamarind seed polysaccharide (TSP), and (c) Lutrol F127.

Lidocaine hydrochloride (LH) (Figure 1(a)) is the first amino amide type of local anesthetics and has been in use for many years. In dentistry, it is a drug of choice to temporarily anesthetize the tiny nerve endings located on the surfaces of the oral mucosa. As a local anesthetic, lidocaine is characterized by a rapid onset of action and intermediate duration of efficacy, making it suitable for infiltration and nerve block anesthesia [9]. Lidocaine stabilizes the neuronal membrane by inhibiting the ionic fluxes required for the initiation and conduction of impulses, thereby effecting local anesthetic action.

Tamarind seed polysaccharide (TSP) is a high-molecular-weight, branched polysaccharide and consists of celluloselike backbone that carries xylose and galactoxylose substances, as shown in Figure 1(b) [10]. It is insoluble in organic solvents and dispersible in warm water to form a highly viscous mucilaginous gel with a broad pH tolerance and mucoadhesivity. In addition, it is nontoxic and nonirritant with a haemostatic activity. It is a galactoxyloglucan and possesses properties such as mucomimetic, mucoadhesive, and pseudoplastic properties [11]. TSP has been used for development of bioadhesive drug delivery systems owing to their bioadhesive properties [12]. It has been studied earlier for thermoreversible gelation property [13] and also as mucoadhesive component in mucoadhesive buccal patches for controlled release [14]. TSP is used as mucoadhesive polysaccharide polymer for systemic delivery of rizatriptan benzoate through buccal route, formulated in the form of buccal film [15]. The objective of the present study was to develop thermoreversible in situ gel of local anesthetic LH by using xyloglucan based mucoadhesive polymer TSP for insertion into periodontal pocket to have painless treatment.

2. Materials and Methods

2.1. Materials. LH and Lutrol F127 were generously gifted by Astra Zeneca Pharma Ltd., Mumbai, India, and BASF, Mumbai, India, respectively. Tamarind seeds were purchased from local market. Triethanolamine and benzalkonium chloride were procured from Loba Chemie, Mumbai, India. All chemicals were of analytical grade and were used as received.

2.2. Methods

2.2.1. Isolation of Mucoadhesive Agent from Tamarind Seeds. The seeds of *Tamarindus indica* were washed with water to remove the dirt and adhering material. The seeds were slightly roasted in sand and crushed to remove the outer brownish testa. Soaked seeds in water (24 h) were boiled for 1 h and kept aside for 2 h to liberate sufficient mucilage into water. Mucilage was removed from the marc by squeezing the soaked seeds through the muslin cloth. The mucilage was then isolated with equal quantity of acetone and dried at 50°C, powdered, and passed through sieve number 80 to get uniform size fine powder of TSP. The powder was stored in airtight container at room temperature till further use [16].

2.2.2. Characterization of Isolated TSP. Isolated TSP was characterized for angle of repose, density, and compressibility index. Viscosity of TSP was determined to check the flow of the powder. Accurately weighed, dried, and finely powdered TSP (1 g) was suspended in 75 mL of distilled water for 5 h. Volume was made up to 100 mL to produce the concentration of 1% w/v. The mixture was homogenized by mechanical stirrer for 2 h and viscosity was determined at 500 rpm using spindle 61 and 25°C using a Brookfield viscometer (LVDVE, Brookfield Engineering Ltd., Inc., USA). The swelling index was measured to know the water holding capacity of TSP. Accurately weighed TSP (1 g) was transferred to 100 mL measuring cylinder and initial volume was noted. Distilled water was added and shaken gently. Measuring cylinder was kept aside for 24 h at room temperature. The change in volume occupied by the swelled polymer was noted. Swelling capacity of isolated polymer was expressed in terms of swelling index. Swelling index (SI) was calculated according to the following equation [17]:

$$SI = \frac{S_1 - S_0}{S_0} \times 100, \qquad (1)$$

where S_0 is initial volume of the powder in graduated cylindrical and S_1 is the volume occupied by swollen gum after 24 h.

2.2.3. Design of Experiment. The preliminary study of gel was performed by performing trial and error of batches varying the concentrations of Lutrol F127 (12 to 24%) [7, 8] and TSP (0.5 to 2.0%) [10]. The formulations revealed the effect of two factors, Lutrol F127 and TSP, on the gel formation. A 3^2 factorial design was used to get optimized formulation of the in situ gel. Using the software Design Expert® (version 9.0), two factors were evaluated each at three levels. The concentration of Lutrol F127 (X_1) and TSP (X_2) was selected as independent variables (Table 1). The dependent variables evaluated were gelation temperature (Y_1) and drug release (Y_2).

2.2.4. Formulation of In Situ Gel. Mucoadhesive in situ gel was prepared by cold method described by Schmolka [18]. In situ gel of LH (2%) was prepared using different concentrations of Lutrol F127 and TSP as shown in Table 2. Lutrol F127 and LH were dissolved in cold water by agitation. The temperature of the solution was reduced to 4°C to get the clear dispersion. Mucoadhesive TSP polymer was slowly added to the water with continuous agitation of the solution. The resulting solution was left at 4°C for 24 h to complete the polymer dissolution. Finally, benzalkonium chloride (0.001% w/v) was added as preservative. Formulation was adjusted to neutral pH with required quantity of triethanolamine. Formulations (F1 to F9) were filled in 10 mL vials, capped with rubber plugs, sealed with aluminium caps, and stored in a refrigerator (4–8°C) until further use.

2.2.5. Determination of Clarity and pH. The formulations were visually checked for clarity against white and black background and categorized as follows: very clear (+++),

TABLE 1: Coded levels of factorial design.

Factor	Level		
	(−1)	(0)	(+1)
Concentration of Lutrol F127 (%) (X_1)	14	18	22
Concentration of TSP (%) (X_2)	0.5	1.0	1.5

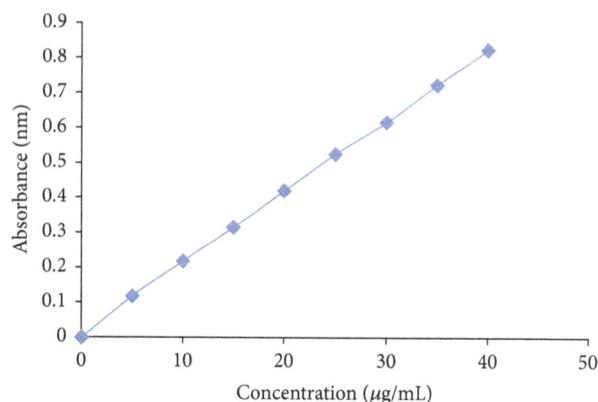

FIGURE 2: Calibration curve of lidocaine hydrochloride.

clear (++), and turbid (+). The pH of each formulation was tested using previously calibrated pH meter (Equiptronics, EQ-610).

2.2.6. Viscosity. The viscosity study of all the formulations (F1 to F9) of the in situgel was determined by the Brookfield viscometer using spindle number 61 (LVDVE, Brookfield Engineering Ltd., Inc., USA). Viscosity of the formulation was noted at two different temperatures, 25°C and 35°C, at 100 rpm shear rate.

2.2.7. Gelation Temperature. Gelation temperature was measured by visual inspection method. 5 mL aliquot of gel was transferred in a test tube and placed in a water bath. With successive increments in temperature of 1°C, the samples were examined visually at which gel formed. Gel was said to have occurred, when the meniscus of the formulation would no longer move, upon tilting through right angle. Each preparation was tested thrice to control the repeatability of the measurement [8].

2.2.8. Drug Content. To get the drug content of gel, the formulation was maintained at 10°C, throughout the test, to remain in the liquid form. 1 mL of liquid was taken in 100 mL volumetric flask; 100 mL pH 6.8 phosphate buffer solution was added to it. Out of this, 4 mL solution was taken out into a 10 mL volumetric flask and volume was adjusted with pH 6.8 phosphate buffer. Absorbance was measured using double beam UV spectrophotometer at 263 nm (UV-1800, Shimadzu, Japan). The amount of drug present was calculated using calibration curve (Figure 2).

TABLE 2: Composition of lidocaine HCl gel formulations.

Ingredient	F1	F2	F3	F4	F5	F6	F7	F8	F9
Lidocaine (%)	2	2	2	2	2	2	2	2	2
Lutrol F127 (%)	14	18	14	22	22	18	18	22	14
TSP (%)	1.0	1.5	1.5	1.5	1.0	0.5	1.0	0.5	0.5
Triethanolamine (mg)	q.s.	q.s.	q.s.	q.s.	q.s.	q.s.	q.s.	q.s.	q.s.
Benzalkonium chloride (%)	0.001	0.001	0.001	0.001	0.001	0.001	0.001	0.001	0.001
Purified water (mL)	10	10	10	10	10	10	10	10	10

2.2.9. Spreadability Test. Spreadability of the in situ gel was performed using a CT3 Texture Analyzer (Brookfield Engineering Lab, Inc., USA) in TPA mode. In this method an analytical probe is depressed into the sample at a defined rate to a desired depth, allowing a predefined necessary period, between the end of the first compression cycle and the beginning of second compression cycle. A cone analytical probe sample holder (TA2/1000) (30 mm diameter, 60°) was completely filled with the gel. The tapered cone was forced down into the sample holder at a defined rate of 1 mm/s and to a defined depth of 10 mm. When a trigger force of 10 g was attained, the probe proceeded to pierce the sample at a test speed of 2 mm/s to a depth of 25 mm. When the specified penetration distance was achieved, the probe departed from the sample at the posttest speed of 2 mm/s. The resulting force-time plot provided hardness, cohesiveness, and adhesiveness. The maximum force attained on the graph was a measure of the firmness of the sample at the specified depth (hardness). The maximum negative force was taken as an indication of the stickiness/cohesiveness of the sample. The work required to deform the gel in down movement of probe indicated cohesiveness. The work necessary to overcome the attractive forces between the surface of the sample and the surface of the probe provided adhesiveness of the sample [19].

2.2.10. Gel Strength. Gel strength is related to the viscosity of the gel. Formulation (50 g) was put in a 100 mL graduated measuring cylinder, which was further placed in thermostatically controlled water bath at 37°C. A calibrated weight of 35 g was slowly placed on the surface of the gel. Time (in seconds) required by the weight to penetrate 5 cm deep into the gel was noted [20]. The diagrammatic sketch of apparatus is as shown in Figure 3.

2.2.11. Mucoadhesive Strength. Mucoadhesive strength of gel F7 was performed using a texture analyzer (CT3 Texture Analyzer, Brookfield Engineering Lab, Inc., USA). A fresh oral gum mucosal tissue of sheep was obtained from local slaughter house, cut (20 × 20 mm), and washed with phosphate buffer pH 6.8. A section of tissue was fixed on the tissue holder, keeping the orifice of the lid open to expose the small section of the tissue. Simulated saliva was placed in the 500 mL beaker and put on the thermostatically controlled heater at 37 ± 0.5°C. Tissue holder was placed in this beaker containing magnetic stirrer and equilibrated for 15 min at physiological temperature. A drop of gel was placed on

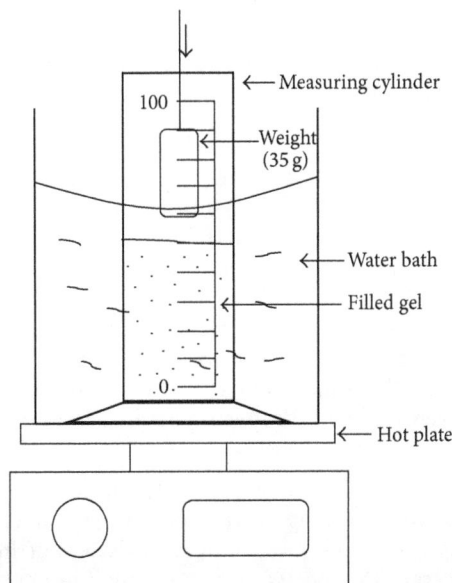

FIGURE 3: Apparatus representing the measurement of gel strength.

the tissue through the opening of the holder. The cylinder probe (TA-5) was lowered at a rate of 0.5 mm/s until it touched the membrane. A contact force of 1 N was maintained for 60 s, and the probe was subsequently withdrawn at a rate of 0.5 mm/s to a distance of 15 mm. The maximum force required to separate the probe from the tissue being maximum detachment force in grams (F_{max}) was noted from TexturePro CT V1.3 Build 14 software and mucoadhesive strength was determined using the following equation:

$$\text{Mucoadhesive strength} \left(\text{dyne/cm}^2\right) = \frac{F_{max} \times g}{A}, \quad (2)$$

where F_{max} is the maximum detachment force in grams, g is acceleration due to gravity, and A is the area of tissue exposed to the gel.

2.2.12. In Vitro Release Studies. In vitro release study of formulations (F1 to F9) was performed using dialysis membrane (Himedia, India). Dialysis membrane consisted of cellophane membrane having an average flat width of 24.26 mm, average diameter of 14.3 mm, and capacity of approximately 1.61 mL/cm, utilized for diffusion. Prior to the diffusion study, the dialysis membrane was soaked overnight in pH 6.8 phosphate buffer solution. Formulation (1 mL) was placed in

TABLE 3: Formulation table.

| Formulation code | Clarity | pH | Viscosity (cps) (±SD) | | Drug content (%) (±SD) | Gelation temperature (°C) (±SD) |
			At 25°C	At 35°C		
F1	Transparent	6.6	233.66 ± 0.57	445.66 ± 6.02	96.5 ± 0.8	37.66 ± 0.3
F2	Transparent	6.8	1422.66 ± 3.5	1634.67 ± 4.16	97.10	35.33
F3	Transparent	6.7	245.0 ± 1	315.33 ± 3.05	95.20	36.66
F4	Transparent	6.6	2760.33 ± 2.51	2957.0 ± 5.67	93.30	20.33
F5	Transparent	6.5	2438.0 ± 8.54	2781.66 ± 4.04	94.60	21.33
F6	Transparent	6.8	934.66 ± 2.08	1322.33 ± 2.51	97.80	35.66
F7	Transparent	6.8	1211.0 ± 10.14	1636.0 ± 5.29	98.10	35.33
F8	Transparent	6.6	2057.33 ± 5.03	2619.33 ± 6.11	94.95	22.66
F9	Transparent	6.7	249.66 ± 222.51	363.67 ± 3.51	96.20	37.66

±SD: Standard Deviation.

the dialysis membrane, cut off in the size of 7 cm length, and sealed on both sides. The dialysis tube was then placed in a glass beaker containing 20 mL of pH 6.8 phosphate buffer solution equilibrated at $37 \pm 0.5°C$ [12]. 1 mL of aliquot was withdrawn after every 10 min till 2 h to get the amount of drug released through the membrane and entered in the phosphate buffer and replaced with same volume of preheated solution to maintain the sink condition. After suitable dilutions, samples were analyzed UV spectrophotometrically at 263 nm.

2.2.13. Ex Vivo Study.

The gel permeated through the oral tissue was performed using ex vivo study. A fresh gum mucosal tissue was carefully removed from the oral cavity of the sheep, obtained from the local slaughter house. The mucosa was stored in the saline solution. The mucosa was cut off in circular shape of 3.5 cm in diameter and fixed in between the donor and the receptor compartment of the Franz diffusion cell, keeping mucosal side up. Prior to study, the mucosa was equilibrated by putting in phosphate buffer pH 6.8 for 1 h. The optimized batch gel formulation (equivalent to 10 mg of LH) was applied evenly on the mucosal membrane. The receptor compartment was filled with 25 mL of pH 6.8 phosphate buffer solution maintained at temperature 37°C. The assembly was put on the magnetic stirrer. At predetermined time periods of 30 min time interval, 1 mL of aliquot was withdrawn from the receptor compartment, replacing the same volume with pH 6.8 phosphate buffer of temperature 37°C, for a period of 2 h. After suitable dilution, samples were analyzed UV spectrophotometrically at 263 nm.

2.2.14. Stability Study.

The optimized batch was packed in amber colour bottle, sealed, kept at 40°C, and maintained at 75% relative humidity in stability chamber (Thermolab, India) for a period of 3 months. Samples withdrawn at 1, 2, and 3 months were characterized for appearance, drug content, and in vitro drug release.

3. Results and Discussion

3.1. Characterization of TSP.

The percentage yield of isolated tamarind seed polysaccharide was 70.3% w/w. The powder obtained was cream in colour with good swelling index (200%) and viscosity (aqueous dispersion of 1% w/v was 8.85 cps). Angle of repose, bulk density, tapped density, and Carr's index revealed good flow properties.

3.2. Design of Experiment.

Experimental trials were performed for nine possible formulations suggested by 3^2 factorial design. Mathematical treatment of the nine possible combinations of batches F1–F9 is shown in Table 2.

3.3. Clarity, pH, Drug Content, and Viscosity.

All formulations (F1 to F9) showed the clear visibility of the gel. The pH of all formulations was found to be in the range of 6.5–6.8, which was similar to the normal pH of mouth saliva (6.8 to 7.4) [2]. Scanning of lidocaine HCl solution in pH 6.8 phosphate buffer solution by UV spectrophotometer showed λ_{max} at 263 nm. At this wavelength the standard curve followed Beer-Lambert's law in the concentration range of 5 to 30 $\mu g/mL$ with $R^2 = 0.9992$. The drug content of all formulations was found to be in the range of 93–99%, thus confirming the uniformity in formulation of the gel (Table 3). As the concentration of the Lutrol F127 (18–22%) and TSP (0.5–1.5) was increased, the viscosity of the gel was also increased. Formulations with the higher concentration of TSP (0.5 to 1.5%) at the same amount of Lutrol F127 (22%) in F8, F5, and F4 showed the increase in viscosity at both temperatures (25°C and 35°C). Formulations consisted of the increased amount of Lutrol F127 (14 to 22%) at the same amount of TSP (1.5%) in F3, F2, and F4 and showed the increase in viscosity (Table 3). Thus, the viscosity of formulations in gel state was found to be proportionate with the increase in concentration of Lutrol F127 and TSP.

3.4. Gelation Temperature.

Gelation temperature range suitable for dental gel is 33–35°C (Table 3), which means a gel should be in liquid form at room temperature and form a gel phase in the buccal cavity. If the gelation temperature of liquid gel is lower than 33°C, gelation occurs at room temperature, leading to difficulty in administering the formulation. If the gelation temperature is higher than 35°C, the gel remains in a liquid form at physiological temperature, resulting in leakage from the periodontal pocket. The gelation temperature of formulations F1 to F9, inspected visually, was found to be within the range of 20 to 37°C. The data presented in Table 3 clearly indicated that the gelation temperature was strongly dependent on the concentration of selected independent variables. An increase in concentration of Lutrol F127 and TSP decreased the gelation temperature. This effect of variables was further supported by the data of design of experiment.

3.4.1. Effect of Formulation Variables on Gelation Temperature.

A mathematical relationship between factors and levels was studied by response surface regression analysis using Design Expert (version 9.0.3.1) software. Equation (3) shows the relationship between the variables and response of gelation temperature (Y_1).

Equation (3), in the form of coded values, is as follows:

$$Y_1 = +35.14 - 8.17X_1 - 0.83X_2 - 0.50X_1X_2$$
$$- 5.79X_1^2 + 0.21X_2^2, \tag{3}$$

where Y_1 is the gelation temperature, X_1 is concentration of Lutrol F127, and X_2 is concentration of TSP.

A negative sign before a factor in polynomial equation (3) indicated that the response has reciprocal effect on both factors. Influence of factors X_1 and X_2 on Y_1 was best fitted to quadratic model and found to be significant with F value of 345.01 ($p < 0.05$). Variables X_1 and X_2 have p value of 0.000404 ($p < 0.05$) and 0.0061. The variables, which have p value less than 0.05, significantly affect the gelation temperature. The predicted R squared value of 0.9828 was in reasonable agreement with the adjusted R squared value of 0.9962. Analysis of variance (ANOVA) was applied to determine the significance and the magnitude of the effects of the variables and their interactions.

As the temperature of Lutrol F127 was increased, the copolymer molecules aggregate to form micelle. This micellization occurs due to the dehydration of hydrophobic propylene oxide blocks. This represents the very first step in the gelling process. The gel formation occurs when the concentration is above the micellar concentration (50%) [21]. This gelation was attributed to the ordered packing of micelles. Interestingly, addition of mucoadhesive polymer (TSP) lowered the gelation temperature of the gel. The viscous nature of TSP may be responsible for lowering the temperature. A micellar association for Lutrol F127 occurs over the temperature range of 10–40°C. Critical micellar temperature is nearer to physiological temperature [7]. These results are in close agreement with the data obtained for in situ gel formulated for periodontal disease using Carbopol 934 P and poloxamer 407 [22].

The regression model obtained was used to generate the counter plots for analyzing interactions of the independent factors. Counter plot shown in Figure 4(a) suggested the correlation between the two variables. Gelation temperature of gel decreased with increase in concentration of Lutrol F127 but showed much less effect on change in concentration of TSP, which was indicated clearly in vertical axis of counter plot. The combined effect of factors X_1 and X_2 can be further elucidated with the help of three-dimensional response surface plot as shown in Figure 4(b). High level of

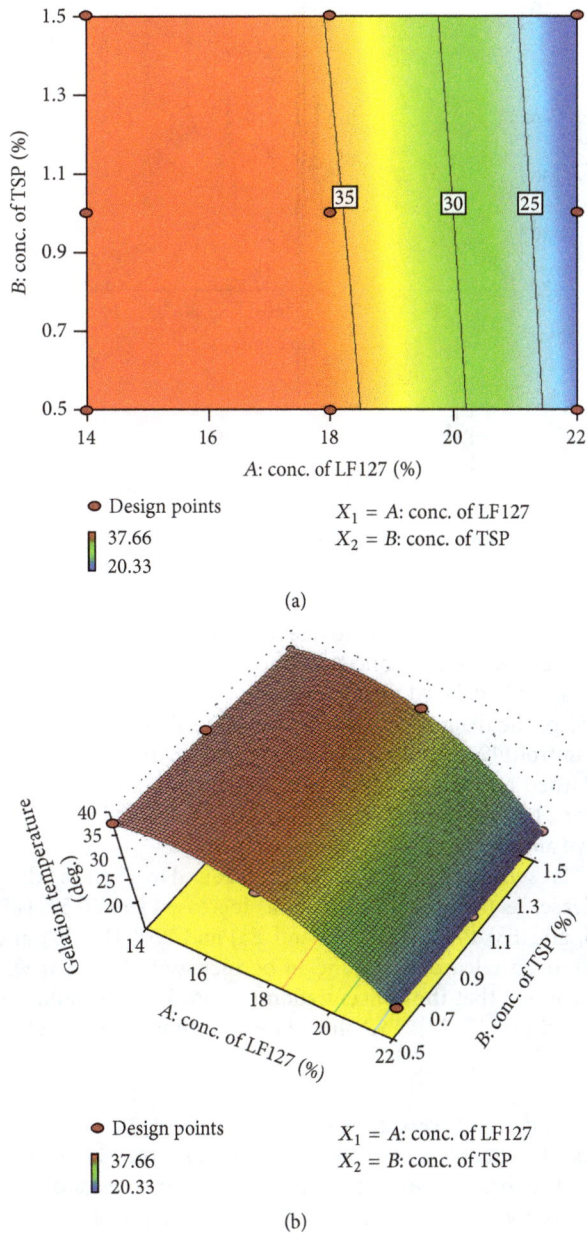

(a)

(b)

FIGURE 4: Counter plot (a) and three-dimensional response surface plot (b) showing the effect of factors on gelation temperature.

factor X_1 showed reduction in gelation temperature and low level showed higher gelation temperature, which indicated that factor X_1 has significant negative effect on gelation temperature of gel. Factor X_2 (TSP) was found to have much less reciprocal effect on gelation temperature. Increase in concentration of TSP lowered the gelation temperature of in situ gel.

3.5. In Vitro Drug Release.

Formulations F1 to F9, subjected to in vitro release study, are represented graphically in Figure 5. Formulations F1, F3, and F9 showed 95% of drug release within 80 min. It was observed that, at less concentration of Lutrol F127 (14%) and higher amount of TSP, the initial rate of

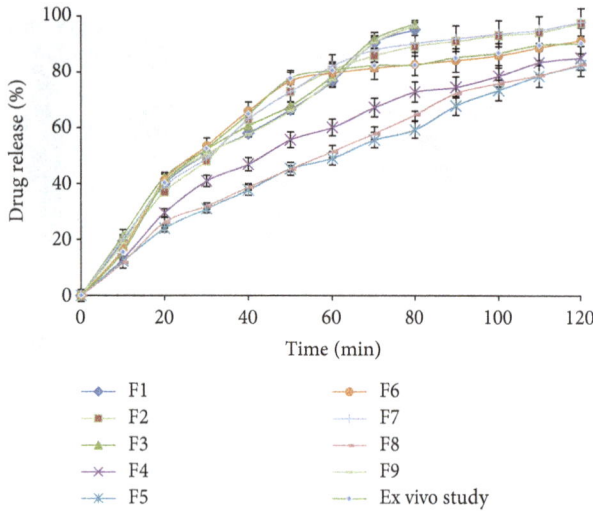

FIGURE 5: Drug release study of in situ gel.

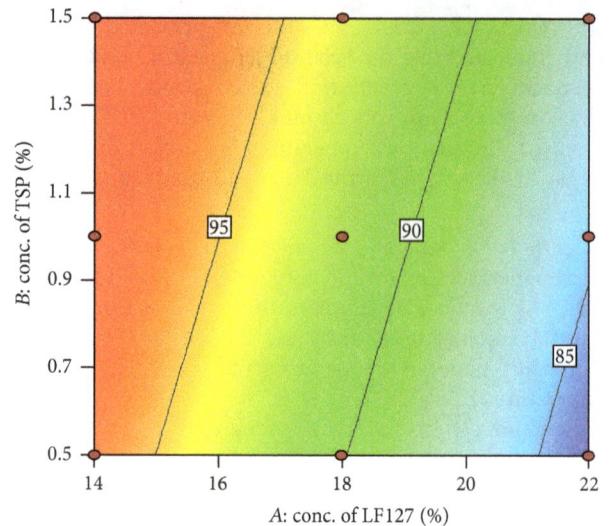

(a)

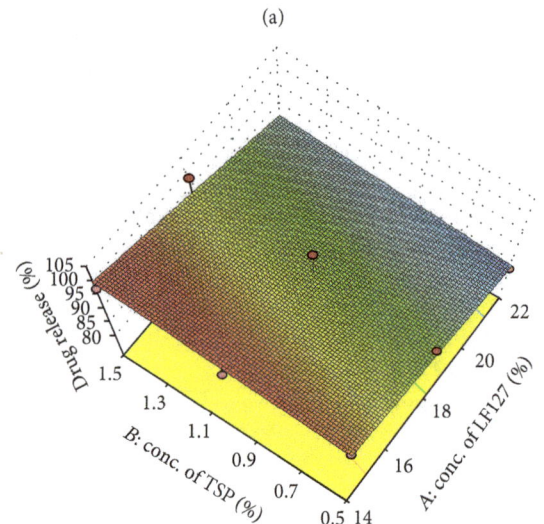

(b) .

FIGURE 6: Counter plot (a) and three-dimensional response surface plot (b) showing the effect of factors on drug release.

drug release was very rapid due to incomplete gel formation. Further, increase in concentration of Lutrol F127 to 18% (F2, F6, and F7) delayed the drug release and released more than 95% of the drug within 2 h. However, further more amount of Lutrol F127 (22%) in F4, F5, and F8, the drug release was retarded and was not released (82%–85%) completely even after 2 h, which is maximal time needed for dental surgery to have anesthetic action.

Presence of TSP in in situ gel was found to affect the drug release. As the amount of TSP was increased from 0.5% (F9, F6, and F8) to 1.0% (F1, F7, and F5) and 1.5% (F3, F2, and F4), drug release was found to be increased. Hence it was concluded that the concentration of Lutrol F127 should not exceed 18% [7, 22]. TSP should be at optimal concentration of 1.0–1.5%.

3.5.1. Effect of Formulation Variables on Drug Release. Analysis of variance was applied to determine the significance and the magnitude of the effects of the variables and their interactions on drug release. The obtained regression model was used to generate the counter plot for analyzing the interactions of the independent variables on dependent variable. Equation (4) shows the polynomial equation in terms of coded levels obtained for drug release:

$$Y_2 = +91.80 - 6.47X_1 + 1.67X_2. \tag{4}$$

The contour plot and three-dimensional analysis showed that drug release was decreased with increase in concentration of Lutrol F127 and increased with increase in concentration of TSP. Figure 6 indicates scale from blue colour to red colour. When colour of response surface shifts from blue towards red it indicates increase in percentage of drug release and vice versa. The same effect was reflected in (4) showing negative sign before X_1 and positive sign before X_2. The variable X_1 showed higher numerical value than X_2, which confirmed the more negative effect of Lutrol F127 compared to the positive effect of TSP on drug release of in situ gel. ANOVA results confirmed the adequacy of the linear model

for drug release (Y_2) and were found to be significant with F value of 9.19 ($p < 0.05$). The predicted R squared value of 0.5491 was in reasonable agreement with the adjusted R squared value of 0.6719.

3.6. Gel Strength. Formulations (F1 to F9) showed good gel strength in the range of 40 to 55 s. Higher gel strength which was related to viscous polymer verified the retaining capacity of gel in the periodontal pocket. F4, F5, and F8 needed more

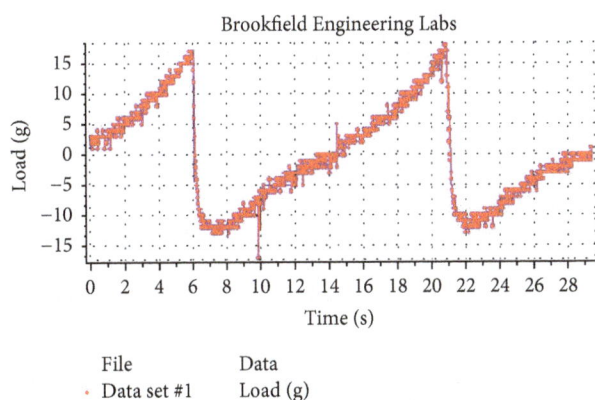

FIGURE 7: Graph of spreadability of gel on texture profile analysis.

time (55 s, 52 s, and 48 s, resp.) to penetrate the weight in it, compared to the other formulations.

3.7. Spreadability Testing.
Spreadability denotes the extent of area to which the gel readily spreads on its application. Hence, it is a property related to the viscosity of mucoadhesive polymer. The greater the viscosity is, the lesser the spreadability is [8] and the more the retention of gel in the dental pocket can be. Texture profile analysis spectra of in situ gel of formulation (F7) showed the hardness of 16.3 g, cohesiveness of 0.81, and adhesiveness of 0.4 mJ (Figure 7). These results expressed the applicability of gels to site of application or adhesivity and indicated the retention time of the gel on the site of application. The more negative value indicated higher adhesivity of the sample. Hardness value confirmed the good firmness of gel and cohesiveness value indicated the better consistency of the gel. As the probe returned to its starting position, the initial lifting of the weight of the sample on the upper surface of the disc produced the negative part of the graph. This indicated the cohesiveness and resistance of the sample to be separated (flow off) from the disc. The maximum negative force on the graph indicated the sample adhesive force.

3.8. Mucoadhesive Strength.
Gel formulation (F7) showed good mucoadhesive strength (1,124 dyne/cm^2) to the sheep mucosa, needed to hold the gel in the dental pocket during surgery, to show therapeutic anesthetic action.

3.9. Ex Vivo Study.
Drug permeation through the oral tissue was performed though the sheep oral mucosa using Franz diffusion cell. The liquid gel was immediately converted to solid gel after putting on the oral mucosa, maintained at 37°C. Initially, faster drug release was observed which was due to the incomplete gel formation. This faster release was actually found to be good to attain faster anesthetic action at the start of dental procedure. As the time progressed, the gelation temperature (35.33°C) was achieved and release rate was slowed down. The gel was retained on the mucosa, which confirmed good mucoadhesion using TSP polymer. The formulation exhibited the good release of LH (98.05%),

as shown in Figure 5. The release was found to be in good correlation with in vitro study (97.5%).

3.10. Stability Study.
Accelerated stability study of an optimized batch of in situ gel (F7) was carried out as per ICH guidelines. There was no significant change in drug content, pH, viscosity, gelation temperature, and drug diffusion for the selected formulation, F7, after 90 days at 40°C ± 0.5/75% ± 5% RH. The drug (92.7%) was diffused through the dialysis membrane within 2 h.

3.11. Optimization of Formulation.
The computer optimization technique by the desirability approach was used to produce the optimum formulation. The process was optimized for the response variables Y_1 and Y_2. The optimized formula was reached by setting maximum percentage of drug release at 2 h and optimal gelation temperature. Formulation F7 was found to be optimized formulation which contained 18% Lutrol F127 and 1% TSP.

4. Conclusion

Lidocaine hydrochloride loaded periodontal temperature-sensitive in situ gel was successfully developed by cold method using xyloglucan based mucoadhesive polymer TSP for insertion into periodontal pocket to have painless treatment. Viscosity study showed the marked increase in the viscosity of gel at 37°C due to sol-gel conversion. Gelation of formulation was observed near to body temperature. In vitro study depicted the rapid onset of drug action, extending till 2 h, to cover period of periodontal treatment. Use of natural, less costly, biodegradable, and easily available mucoadhesive TSP polymer as well as avoidance of needle insertions during scaling and root planning of periodontosis helped achieve patient compliance by ultimately reducing the cost of the treatment. TSP (1%) and Lutrol F127 (18%), in combination, imparted viscous behaviour to gel needed to retain the formulation in periodontal pocket. Thus, lidocaine hydrochloride thermoreversible in situ gel offered an alternative to painful injection therapy of anesthesia during dental surgery, with rapid onset of anesthetic action lasting throughout the dental procedure.

Conflict of Interests

The authors declare that there is no conflict of interests regarding the publication of this paper.

Acknowledgment

The authors thank BASF, Mumbai, India, for providing gift sample of Lutrol F127.

References

[1] M. A. Listgarten, "Nature of periodontal diseases: pathogenic mechanisms," *Journal of Periodontal Research*, vol. 22, no. 3, pp. 172–178, 1987.

[2] S. P. Vyas, V. Sihorkar, and V. Mishra, "Controlled and targeted drug delivery strategies towards intraperiodontal pocket diseases," *Journal of Clinical Pharmacy and Therapeutics*, vol. 25, no. 1, pp. 21–42, 2000.

[3] P. Svensson, J. K. Petersen, and H. Svensson, "Efficacy of a topical anesthetic on pain and unpleasantness during scaling of gingival pockets," *Anesthesia Progress*, vol. 41, no. 2, pp. 35–39, 1994.

[4] S. F. Malamed, P. Sykes, Y. Kubota, H. Matsuura, and M. Lipp, "Local anesthesia: a review," *Anesthesia & Pain Control in Dentistry*, vol. 1, no. 1, pp. 11–24, 1992.

[5] D. J. Estafan, "Invasive and noninvasive dental analgesia techniques," *General Dentistry*, vol. 46, no. 6, pp. 600–603, 1998.

[6] R. C. Nagarwal, A. Srinatha, and J. K. Pandit, "*In situ* forming formulation: development, evaluation, and optimization using 3^3 factorial design," *AAPS PharmSciTech*, vol. 10, no. 3, pp. 977–984, 2009.

[7] J. J. Escobar-Chavez, M. Lopez-Cervantes, A. Naik, and Y. N. Kalia, "Applications of thermoreversible pluronics F-127 gels in pharmaceutical formulations," *Journal of Pharmacy & Pharmaceutical Sciences*, vol. 9, no. 3, pp. 339–358, 2006.

[8] R. J. Majithiya, P. K. Ghosh, M. L. Umrethia, and R. S. R. Murthy, "Thermoreversible-mucoadhesive gel for nasal delivery of sumatriptan," *AAPS PharmSciTech*, vol. 7, no. 3, pp. E80–E86, 2006.

[9] O. E. Ogle and G. Mahjoubi, "Local anesthesia: agents, techniques, and complications," *Dental Clinics of North America*, vol. 56, no. 1, pp. 133–148, 2012.

[10] A. Mishra and A. V. Malhotra, "Tamarind xyloglucan: a polysaccharide with versatile application potential," *Journal of Materials Chemistry*, vol. 19, no. 45, pp. 8528–8536, 2009.

[11] Y. Chandramouli, S. Firoz, A. Vikram, B. Mahitha, B. Rubia Yasmeen, and K. Hemanthpavankumar, "Tamarind seed polysaccharide (TSP)—an adaptable excipient for novel drug delivery systems," *International Journal of Pharmacy Practice & Drug Research*, vol. 2, no. 2, pp. 57–63, 2012.

[12] A. K. Bandyopadhyay and R. Datta, "A new nasal drug delivery system for diazepam using natural mucoadhesive polysaccharide obtained from tamarind seeds," *Saudi Pharmaceutical Journal*, vol. 14, no. 2, pp. 115–119, 2006.

[13] S. Yamanaka, Y. Yuguchi, H. Urakawa, K. Kajiwara, M. Shirakawa, and K. Yamatoya, "Gelation of tamarind seed polysaccharide xyloglucan in the presence of ethanol," *Food Hydrocolloids*, vol. 14, no. 2, pp. 125–128, 2000.

[14] S. Burgalassi, L. Panichi, M. F. Saettone, J. Jacobsen, and M. R. Rassing, "Development and in vitro/in vivo testing of mucoadhesive buccal patches releasing benzydamine and lidocaine," *International Journal of Pharmaceutics*, vol. 133, no. 1-2, pp. 1–7, 1996.

[15] A. M. Avachat, K. N. Gujar, and K. V. Wagh, "Development and evaluation of tamarind seed xyloglucan-based mucoadhesive buccal films of rizatriptan benzoate," *Carbohydrate Polymers*, vol. 91, no. 2, pp. 537–542, 2013.

[16] R. D. Durai, J. Joseph, S. N. Kanchalochana, G. Rajalakshmi, and V. Hari, "Tamarind seed polysaccharide: a promising natural excipient for pharmaceuticals," *International Journal of Green Pharmacy*, vol. 6, no. 4, pp. 270–278, 2012.

[17] P. K. Mukharjee, *Quality Control of Herbal Drugs: An Approach to Evaluation of Botanicals*, Business Horizons Pharmaceutical Publishers, New Delhi, India, 3rd edition, 2008.

[18] I. R. Schmolka, "Artificial skin. I. Preparation and properties of pluronic F-127 gels for treatment of burns," *Journal of Biomedical Materials Research*, vol. 6, no. 6, pp. 571–582, 1972.

[19] V. Pande, S. Patel, V. Patil, and R. Sonawane, "Design expert assisted formulation of topical bioadhesive gel of sertaconazole nitrate," *Advanced Pharmaceutical Bulletin*, vol. 4, no. 2, pp. 121–130, 2014.

[20] H.-G. Choi, J.-H. Jung, J.-M. Ryu, S.-J. Yoon, Y.-K. Oh, and C.-K. Kim, "Development of in situ-gelling and mucoadhesive acetaminophen liquid suppository," *International Journal of Pharmaceutics*, vol. 165, no. 1, pp. 33–44, 1998.

[21] G. Dumortier, J. L. Grossiord, F. Agnely, and J. C. Chaumeil, "A review of poloxamer 407 pharmaceutical and pharmacological characteristics," *Pharmaceutical Research*, vol. 23, no. 12, pp. 2709–2728, 2006.

[22] K. Garala, P. Joshi, M. Shah, A. Ramkishan, and J. Patel, "Formulation and evaluation of periodontal in situ gel," *International Journal of Pharmaceutical Investigation*, vol. 3, no. 1, pp. 29–41, 2013.

7

Immunooncology: Can the Right Chimeric Antigen Receptors T-Cell Design Be Made to Cure All Types of Cancers and Will It Be Covered?

Regina Au

BioMarketing Insight, Boston, MA, USA

Correspondence should be addressed to Regina Au; regina@biomarketinginsight.com

Academic Editor: Imtiaz Ahmad Siddiqui

Immunooncology (IO) is the buzz word today and it has everyone doing IO research. If we look back at the history of cancer treatment, the survival rate was measured in months which, according to oncologists, was a lot back then because the mortality rate in most cancers was 100%. However, most traditional chemotherapies were not well tolerated because they would kill both cancerous and healthy cells, which lead to major side effects such as loss of hair, nausea and vomiting, and risk of infection. Survival was better but not much better depending on the type of cancer and the patient's own genetic and physiological make-up. IO therapies target specific receptors on the cancer cells. However, with more advance technologies, the cost to develop these types of therapies increases significantly because the biology is more complex and it is more difficult to produce. Find out why these therapies are more complex and therefore more expensive. But the enhanced efficacy of these therapies does justify the cost.

1. Introduction

Scientists have tried to solve the targeting problem with IO therapies by utilizing the patient's own immune system to aid in recognizing and killing only cancer cells, rather than healthy cells, and keep the cancer cells at bay. Most recently, Chimeric Antigen Receptors T-cell (CAR-T) therapy is a cellular therapy that appears to be a game changer in cancer treatment. This review will cover (1) types of immunooncology therapies; (2) the different types of functioning T-cells; (3) the roadblocks to cellular therapies; (4) adaptive CAR-T therapy and the design of CAR-T-cells which are important; (5) the efficacy of CAR-T therapy in leukemia; (6) the efficacy of CAR-T in solid tumors; (7) the advantages of CAR-T therapy; (8) the side effect profile; (9) CAR-T therapy will be expensive; (10) CAR-T therapy does justify the cost; and (11) questions still facing the CAR-T field.

2. Types of Immunooncology Therapies

There are two categories of IO: (1) checkpoint therapies and (2) Adoptive Cell Transfer (ACT) therapies.

(1) Checkpoint therapies include cytokine therapy, therapeutic vaccine (dendritic cell vaccines), antibody drug conjugates, and tumor specific T-cell.

Checkpoint therapies currently on the market are Merck & Co.'s pembrolizumab (Keytruda®) [1] and Bristol Myers Squibb's (BMS) nivolumab (Opdivo®) [2] for specific types of cancers that have made significant inroads with some patients being cancer-free. Both Keytruda and Opdivo are human monoclonal antibodies that block the interaction between PD-1 and its ligands, PD-L1 and PD-L2, that inhibits the body's immune response, including antitumor immune response. BMS second monoclonal antibody ipilimumab (Yervoy®) [3] binds to CTLA-4 and blocks the interaction of CTLA-4 with its ligands CD80/CD86 that also inhibits T-cell activation and proliferation.

(2) Adoptive Cell Transfer (ACT) therapies, tumor infiltrating lymphocytes (TILs) from tumor mass that are excised, and gene transfer methods, Chimeric Antigen Receptors (CARs) T-cells and TCR (T-cell receptor) T-cells for blood, are included.

For the purpose of this review, we will focus on CAR-T therapy.

3. The Different Types of Functioning T-Cells

Our body has four basic types of functioning T-cells (Grupp 2014) [4]: (1) naive; (2) terminal effector (Te); (3) effector memory (Em); and (4) central memory (Cm). When there is no new infection present, the levels of naive cells are high and the rest are low. Once a bacteria or virus is introduced, there are high levels of T-Em, low levels of T-Cm, and no naive cells. When the T-cells are killing the bacteria or virus, there are high levels of T-Te and T-Em are low. These terminal effector cells, however, are subject to exhaustion and senescence and then they disappear. When the infection is cured, there are high levels of T-Cm that is activated when there is a reinfection.

4. The Roadblocks to Cellular Therapies

There are a number of roadblocks to cellular therapies [4], some of which scientists have figured out and others they still need to perfect.

Problems

(1) Targeting. CD19+ tumor cell and normal B cell both express CD19 where T-cells cannot recognize the tumor cells, getting T-cells to recognize only the cancer cells and not the normal cells.

Solution. T-cell recognition therapies are needed: CAR or TCR therapies; scientists have been developing these types of therapies and there are a number of CAR-T clinical trials worldwide.

(2) Expansion Ex Vivo. Making CAR-T-cells for each patient is complex and time consuming. We need a process where cells can expand significantly in cell culture or ex vivo.

Solution. We need to incorporate good manufacturing practice (GMP) cell culture approach in order for cells to proliferate significantly.

(3) Expansion in Host. Getting "programmed" T-cells to expand or proliferate significantly in the human body: in order to get an effector T-cell response, cells have to proliferate tremendously from a small number of precursor cells to a large number of effector cells and then convert to a memory response. This requires an enormous amount of T-cells.

Solution. We need to incorporate a significant amount of young T-cells that are not exhausted due to the expansion. This has not been proven yet.

(4) Persistence. We should get "programmed" T-cells to remain in the body for a long-term effect.

Solution. We need to use central memory T-cell (T-Cm) that will recognize the cancer cells for an unlimited period of time. This has not been proven yet.

(5) Effector Cells and Target Ratio. We must create more efficient effector memory T-cells (T-Em) with more cytotoxic T lymphocytes (CTL) activity.

Solution. We need proliferation or expansion of T-Em that will eventually convert into central memory T-cells (T-Cm), and it is the T-Cm cells that will activate and maintain CTL activity, when exposed to a bacteria or virus again. Efficiency and safety need to be demonstrated in Phase I clinical trials, not just safety, in order to demonstrate long-term efficacy in subsequent trials.

5. Adaptive CAR-T Therapy

In ACT, more specifically CAR-T-cells, a CAR gene has two major components: (1) an external receptor that recognizes an antigen binding site on the cancer cells and (2) an internal component or signaling/expression that directs the T-cell to the cancer binding site and is inserted into a T-cell via a retrovirus or lentivirus vector. See Figure 1.

5.1. The Design of CAR-T-Cells Is Important. Scientists have been working on CAR-T-cells for over a decade and developed the first generation of CAR-T back in 1991 for HIV. This first generation of CD4/CD8z (CD4/CD8 T-cells) + CD3 ζ- (zeta) chain (to generate an activation signal in T lymphocytes) and CAR-T for HIV (CD4) using a retrovirus went into clinical trial in 1997; the CAR-T-cells persist now for 10 years (June 2015) [5].

The second generation of CAR-T uses a single chain fragment variable (scFv) or antibody fragment as the external component designed with the internal signaling CD28 or 4-1BB (CD137) + CD3 ζ-chain. Immunologists have found that they needed two (2) signals; signal 1 for activation and signal 2 for survival for T-cell proliferation (Looney 2013 [6], Maude et al. 2015 [7], and Sadelain et al. 2013 [8]). They looked at the power of dual signaling for proliferation or activation of T-cells. In one study, if you are using only signal 1, the anti-CD3 signal was low. If you are using only signal 2, the anti-CD28 signal was absent. Combining anti-CD3 and anti-CD28, the signal had at least a 1,000-fold increase (57K units). Scientists discovered that if you have signal 2 but not signal 1, it has no effect on T-cell. If you have signal 1 but no signal 2, there is inactivation (anergy) or deletion of T-cell (Hanada and Restifo 2013) [9].

The costimulatory properties of second-generation Chimeric Antigen Receptors (CARs) determine the overall potency of adoptive transferred T-cells. But the combination of CD28-4-1BB and CD28-OX40 has demonstrated sustained activation of T-cells in animal models but remains to be evaluated in clinical trials (Almåsbak et al. 2016) [10]. Zhao and colleagues investigated seven (7) different CAR structures of CD28 and/or 4-1BB costimulation. They discovered that using the two signaling domains (CD28 and CD3ζ) configuration and the 4-1BB ligand provided the highest therapeutic efficacy, by providing balanced tumoricidal function and increased T-cell persistence which was accompanied by an elevated CD8/CD4 ratio and decreased exhaustion (Zhao et al. 2015) [11]. The costimulatory signals currently used in third-generation CAR-T-cells are CD28 and 4-1BB or Ox40 + CD3 ζ-chain. Scientists also believe that the microenvironment plays an

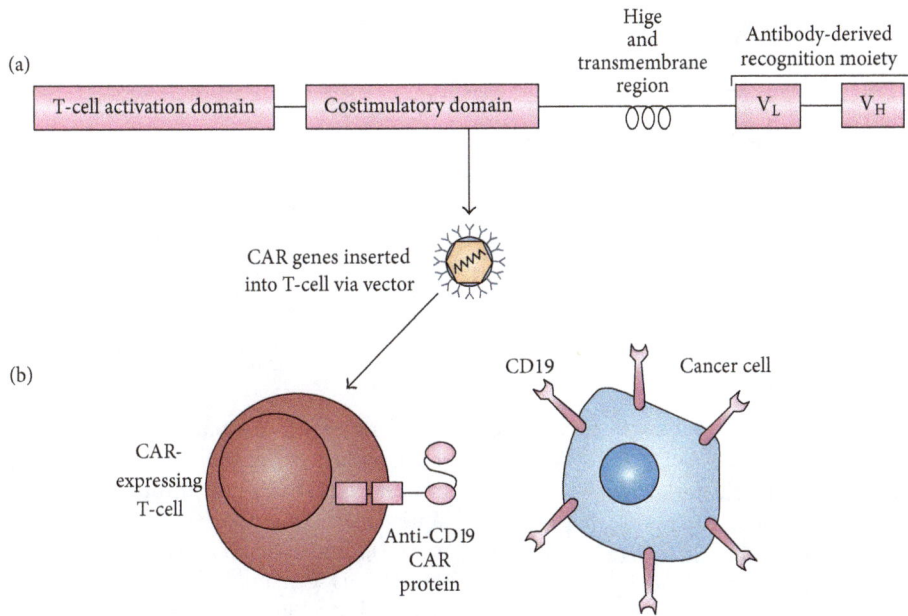

FIGURE 1: An anti-CD19 CAR-expressing T-cell recognizing a CD19+. Reprinted by permission from Macmillan Publishers Ltd. [34].

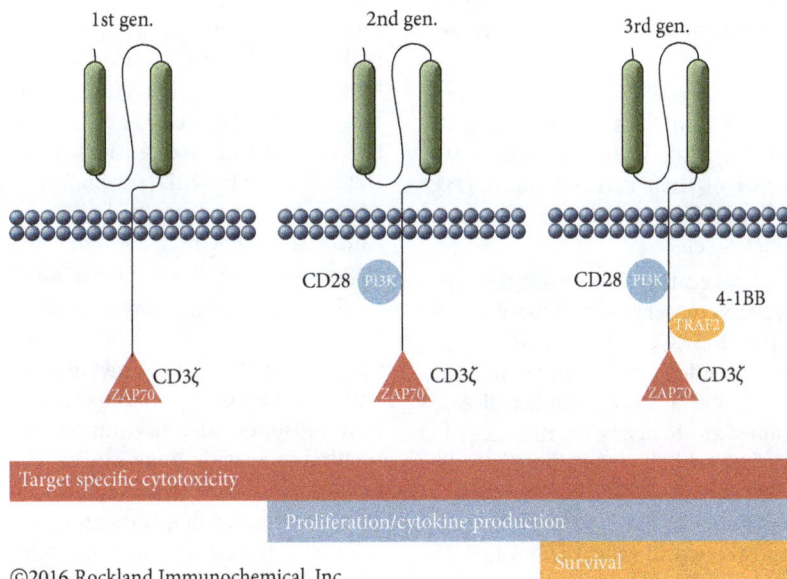

©2016 Rockland Immunochemical, Inc.

FIGURE 2: CAR-T designs. Source: Rockland Immunochemicals, Inc., http://www.rockland-inc.com/car-t-cell-therapy-services.aspx.

important role in the immune system. See Figure 2 (NCI 2014) [12].

To make these cancer-fighting T-cells or CAR-T-cells, T-cells are first collected from the patient and then modified as in Figure 2 to recognize an antigen binding site on the cancer cells. It usually takes 2 and 1/2 to 3 weeks to insert the gene and grow cells. Once this is accomplished the modified T-cells are then infused back into the patient, or autologous therapy.

Once it is infused back into the patient these "programmed" T-cells can multiply and persist for a long time ("living drug"); they are capable of destroying any cells that have the target antigen.

This disruptive technology of modifying T-cells is similar to monoclonal antibody therapy, as it does use a fragment of an antibody, but has more potency and persistence, as living cells that can persist in the body, as opposed to antibodies (proteins) that are active for a limited time.

6. The Efficacy of CAR-T Therapy in Leukemia

In designing CD19 for Leukemia, three (3) different CAR-T therapies were compared from Memorial Sloan Kettering Cancer Center (MSKCC), the National Cancer Institute (NCI), and University of Pennsylvania, (UPenn) [5] (Davila et al. 2012) [13]; see Table 1. Professor Carl June emphasized

TABLE 1: CD-19 designs for leukemia.

	MSKCC	NCI	UPenn
Design	CD28-19-28z	CD28-FMC63-28Z	4-1BB-CD19-BB
Vector	Retrovirus	Retrovirus	Lentivirus
Expression	Approx. 30 days	Approx. 30 days	>4 years
CR in ALL	90%	80%	90%
CR in CLL	0/8		4/14
PR in CLL	0/8		4/14
OOR in CLL	0.00%		57%

CR: complete response, ALL: acute lymphocytic leukemia, CLL: chronic lymphocytic leukemia, PR: partial response, and ORR: overall response rate.

that the design of the CAR-T is very important in addition to which vector you choose.

Viruses can transfer their genetic material to infected cells and then replicate, encapsulate, and package their genome to transfer to other noninfected cells. They were also found to incorporate and transmit genes of cellular origin making them an ideal tool to genetically modify cells [13] (Dufait et al. 2012) [14]. Retrovirus has been the most successful in human gene therapy in correcting genetic disorders. There are two basic types of retroviruses, simple, as in the Moloney mouse leukemia virus (MLV), and complex retroviruses (lentiviruses).

The difference between simple γ-retroviruses and a complex lentiviruses is that simple retrovirus vectors can only transduce cells during mitosis, while lentiviral vectors can transduce cells independently of their division status [14]. This characteristic makes lentiviral vectors ideal for gene therapy for highly differentiated cells.

For Acute Lymphocytic Leukemia (ALL), this is the type of efficacy data that has got everyone very excited about CAR-T therapy [5, 12] (UPenn [15], MSKCC [16], and NCI [17]). Even though the results for Chronic Lymphocytic Leukemia (CLL) were not as successful, it is a more complex disease to tackle and many companies are focusing on this area. In the UPenn study, the lentivirus probably contributed to the longer expression or persistence of CAR-T-cells. Due to these promising results, as of September 16, 2015, 77 CAR-T trials are being conducted around the world (48 in US, 8 in UK, and 20 in China) and China is predicted to outpace the US in clinical trials [5].

Emily Whitehead, the first pediatric patient with ALL treated with CAR-T therapy at the Children's Hospital of Philadelphia (CHOP), was a complete responder in 2012. She remains cancer-free for 4 years so far. When President Obama announced the Precision Medicine Initiative, Emily was invited to the White House in January of 2015 as a successful example of Precision Medicine or Personalized Medicine.

7. The Efficacy of CAR-T in Solid Tumors

CAR-T therapy has been successful combating circulating tumors such as ALL because the tumors are in the vicinity of the CAR-T-cells. However in solid tumors, the CAR-T-cells need a mechanism to hone in onto the cancer cells.

Checkpoint inhibitors or monoclonal antibodies have been used to treat prostate cancer due to its specificity in honing in on the tumor through prostate-specific membrane antigen (PSMA) and prostate stem cell antigen (PSCA). However, significant clinical efficacy has not been demonstrated. Surgery is generally the treatment for localized prostate cancer, but a high percentage of patients have a reoccurrence of tumors that progress to the lymph nodes and bone.

T-cells unlike antibodies have the ability to penetrate inflamed epithelial tissues, clonally expand, and generate memory cells producing a stronger antitumor activity thereby making modified CAR-T-cells directed at PSMA possibly a better treatment option. Hillerdal and Essand [18] and Abate-Daga et al. [19] both showed delayed tumor growth but not cure in mice treated with PSCA CAR-T-cells based on the 1G8 and Ha1-4.117 antibodies, respectively. Interestingly, Abate-Daga first developed a PSCA CAR-T to treat pancreatic cancer since PSCA is a glycoprotein overexpressed in early stages of malignancy in pancreatic cancer.

In prostate cancer that progresses to lymph node and bone metastases, T-cell infiltration is influenced by blood vessel quality and bone metastases have poor vessel quality with dysfunctional junctions [18]. The microenvironment or immunosuppressive environment creates many challenges in treating metastatic bone cancer. There are many factors that may enhance the CAR-T-cell efficacy in the tumor environment including using antiangiogenesis drugs for increased T-cell infiltration, targeting tumor stroma to improve antitumor effect, and depleting Treg as preconditioning, to TGFβ blocking agent to reduce immunosupression and osteolysis [18]. But more studies are needed to confirm these hypotheses.

The first successful clinical trial using CAR-T therapy to treat solid tumors in pancreatic cancer was presented at the American Society of Clinical Oncology (ASCO) Annual Meeting in 2015. Six patients with refractory pancreatic cancers were treated: four patients showed progressive disease and two had stable disease (for 3.7 and 5.3 months) including one patient that resulted in the absence of some metastatic lesions (Castellino 2015) [20]. The investigators, from the University of Pennsylvania in Philadelphia, used specialized CAR-Tmeso (mesothelin + and a costimulatory molecule, 4-1BB) cell which was shown to hone in on the tumor sites of the patients. Mesothelin (MSLN) is a membrane-anchored protein normally seen in mesothelial cells and is overexpressed in all pancreatic cancer tissue according to investigator Gregory L. Beatty, M.D., Ph.D., assistant professor of medicine.

However, solid tumors in pancreatic cancer are uniquely challenging as they may have many different types of markers that have not yet been discovered. Researchers at the Perelman School of Medicine at Penn discovered a novel marker in a patient's tumor that did not possess any of the usual markers but had a specific change in protein glycosylation, a unique pattern of sugars on the cell surface of the protein (Cell Press 2016) [21]. In collaboration with other researchers, they developed a novel CAR-T-cells that expressed a monoclonal antibody called 5E5, which specifically recognizes the Tn glycan on the mucin 1 (MUC1) protein, a sugar modification. This marker is absent on normal cells but abundant on different types of cancer cells [21] (Posey Jr. et al. 2016) [22]. 5E5 modified CAR-T-cells were injected into mice with leukemia and pancreatic cancer that resulted in reduction of tumor growth and increased survival. All six mice with pancreatic cancer were alive at the end of the experiment.

8. The Advantages of CAR-T Therapy

There are a number of advantages to CAR-T therapy [4, 5, 7] (Brentjens 2015) [23]:

(1) It uses human leukocyte antigen (HLA) restricted T-cell receptors, similar to a monoclonal antibody; it has very specific antigen recognition and therefore can have universal application.

(2) It is active in both CD4 and CD8 T-cells.

(3) It can target antigens on proteins, carbohydrates, and glycolipids.

(4) It can rapidly produce tumor specific T-cells with GMP processes in 7–12 days.

(5) It has minimal risk of autoimmunity or Graft versus Host Disease (GvHD).

(6) It is a "living drug" that requires only a single infusion and persists for a unlimited period of time.

(7) It destroys the cancer cell membrane in killing the tumor cell, and therefore, there is no cross reactivity unlike traditional chemotherapy.

(8) CAR scFv or TCR (external) can reprogram specificity of T-cells for tumor target. Specificity is important to avoid toxicity.

(9) CAR signaling domains can reprogram T-cell metabolism. This can enhance survival in tumor microenvironment and effector function.

The metabolism of CAR-T-cells plays an important role in the microenvironment, which had two phases: (1) resting to effector or activation (living off sugar) and then (2) effector to resting or memory cell (living off the mitochondrial) where memory cell will activate should there be a reinfection.

Therefore, choosing the appropriate signals can arm the T-cells better [5]:

(1) CD28 domains: studies show that CD28 costimulation of human peripheral blood T-cells enhances expression of glucose transporters, glucose uptake, and glycolysis (Frauwirth et al., 2002) [24], the "Warburg" effect. After antigen encounter, T-cells shift to a glycolytic metabolism to sustain effector function (Sukumar et al. 2013) [25]. However, induction of high glycolytic activity in $CD8^+$ T-cells severely compromises the ability of $CD8^+$ T-cells to form long-term memory or decreased persistence.

(2) 4-1BB domains enhance mitochondrial biogenesis and are associated with enhanced persistence. 4-1BB enhances primary $CD8^+$ T-cell responses and the maintenance of memory $CD8^+$ T-cells (Zhong et al. 2010) [26] associated with enhanced persistence.

9. The Side Effect Profile

One of the potentially lethal side effects with CAR-T therapy is cytokine release syndrome (CRS) which involves elevated levels of several cytokines including interleukin- (IL-) 6 and interferon γ. Clinical symptoms include fever, hypotension, respiratory insufficiency, and neurological changes such as delirium, global encephalopathy, aphasia, and seizure-like activities/seizure. This particular side effect was not evident in mice models and was presented only when it was infused into humans.

There were several cases of CRS at Children's Hospital of Philadelphia (CHOP) with significantly elevated levels of IL-6 which made the patients extremely ill. After a cytokine blockade failed, one 8 mg/kg dose of an IL-6 receptor antagonist, Tocilizumab, and the IL-6 levels returned to normal (Maude et al. 2015) [4, 7, 12]. IL-6 is a classic feedback loop mechanism possessing a network effect and one needs to interrupt multiple nodes or block the IL-6 mechanism to halt this toxicity.

It was also found that, by measuring the percentage of bone marrow blast (BMB), defined as disease burden, BMB correlates with the severity of CRS in children. Those with no disease burden are characterized as having BMB below 50%, and those with disease burden (yes) have greater than 50% BMB. Those who have a "yes" for disease burden have a greater likelihood and severity of CRS [4, 7]. It is more advantageous to deploy therapy in patients with a low burden of disease resulting in less toxicity. The more the BMB, the more severe the CRS. This could also be applied to adults as they have a mature immune system compared to children, who are still developing their immune system.

Other side effects can include the following [4, 7]:

(1) Macrophage Activation Syndrome (MAS)/Hemophagocytic Lymphohistiocytosis (HLH) depicted by extraordinarily high ferritin levels (16K to 415K ng/mL).

(2) Coagulopathy-elevated D-dimer and low fibrinogen.

(3) Hepatosplenomegaly (HSM) and transaminitis and increased transaminases (AST, ALT) coupled with nonspecific hepatitis.

(4) Moderate marrow hemophagocytosis.

10. CAR-T Therapy Will Be Expensive

People want to live longer with a better quality of life. To achieve this, scientists have gone into uncharted waters in understanding the etiology or mechanism of action of diseases, which is not an easy feat. In order to achieve this, drug development has got longer and longer and, therefore, more and more expensive. On average, according to a 2016 study published by Tuft's Center for the Study of Drug Development, it takes 11 years (range 10–15) to develop a drug from research to approval with a cost of $2.6 billion dollars (DiMasi et al. 2016) [27].

In the past, drug development was mostly focused on small molecule of chemical pathways that were well known, where a chemical reaction will occur in the same manner whether it is the first time or the 10^n time. Then the industry moved into biologics or large molecule where the biology is more complicated, and one cannot predict how a cell is going to react each time. Large molecule drug discovery, therefore, is inherently more expensive and scientists also had to figure out a way to get these large molecules to the right target.

Today, there is IO therapy, which is extremely complex compared to small or large molecule. Scientists understand how our immune system works, but not thoroughly enough to know how the immune system will react when one starts to manipulate the human immune system.

In order to administer CAR-T therapy, scientists had to figure out the following steps to manufacturing this therapy:

(1) Depending on the type of cancer, design a CAR with the best external and internal signals (signal 1 and signal 2).

(2) Design it with the best viral vector to transmit the gene to the T-cell and proliferate.

(3) Get the CAR-T-cells to expand ex vivo in order to infuse it back to the patient.

(4) Get the reprogrammed cells to expand in the host and persist for unlimited amount of time in order for the patient to remain cancer-free.

(5) Collect T-cells from the patient.

(6) Reprogram the patient's T-cell to CAR-T-cells.

(7) Infuse it back into the patient.

(8) It usually takes 2 1/2 to 3 weeks to insert the gene and grow cells.

(9) Average time from screening to implantation into the patient with CAR-Tmeso was 41 days.

All these steps take an extraordinary amount of scientific knowledge, experimentation, and time for each individual. This is truly personalized medicine. CAR-T therapy is uncharted territory and no one knows whether this will work for every individual, even if one is using an individual's own immune system. In the comparison study of SKMCC, NCI, and UPenn for leukemia, the therapy worked well for ALL in a small number of patients, but not very well for CLL. The expression of CAR-T-cells only lasted for 30 days in the SKMCC and NCI which may account for why the response rate was poor for CLL. However, even with an expression rate of greater than 4 years in the UPenn study, the overall response rate was 57% for CLL versus 90% for ALL.

For patients who only achieved a partial response or is nonresponsive to the CAR-T therapy, doctors and scientists have to figure out why the patient did not have a complete response. It may mean going back to the drawing board in designing a different CAR, using a different viral vector, or using a different type of T-cell. This path adds on cost to the CAR-T therapy. Or, they may decide to either add another drug or go with a different class of agents.

In calculating the cost to produce this therapy, because the process described has to be done separately for each individual, it becomes very costly. Manufacturing cost only comes down when there is economy of scale, and with CAR-T therapy, there is no economy of scale since it is personalized to each individual. The cost of this therapy can only be determined by the biotech company that is actually developing the CAR-T therapy.

This is the dilemma. Society wants personalized medicine yet who is going to pay for the cost of personalized medicine? Insurance providers will not pay for CAR-T therapy because it is unproven by regulatory standards right now as well as their standards; the side effect profile is risky even though it can be remedied, and it is very expensive. Today, most insurance companies will only pay for the standard treatments and only when all therapies fail will the insurance company consider adoptive cellular therapy with special circumstances.

11. CAR-T Therapy Does Justify the Cost

If one can use their own immune system to fight cancer, this is ideal and the therapy would be a one dose cure as opposed to traditional treatments including checkpoint inhibitors, where the patient would take the drug/biologic for a specific period of time and hope the cancer is eradicated. Any inhibitor is only viable for a limited period of time compared to programmed T-cells, which could be expressed for an unlimited time period. In non-CAR-T therapy, the cancer could return and the same or different drug/biologic would have to be administered again similar to a maintenance therapy versus a cure, which is less expensive in the long run. And as each episode of a relapse occurs, the odds of survival are diminished significantly because the body gets weaker and the cancer gets smarter in terms of resistance.

But the real answer relies on the payer. The insurance company will not pay for a new therapy unless it is proven that CAR-T therapy works and is a cure, by their standards, not just FDA approval, it is safe, and it saves the insurance company money. But in order to determine this, health economic data must be collected for a determined length of time to demonstrate not only efficacy and safety, but also the fact that the therapy saves the company money compared to standard of care treatment, which many times are generic versions of the drug or biosimilar of a biologic.

If the insurance company will not cover the therapy, then the patient or family will have to pay for it. But most patients and families can not afford it and they will have to rely on the standard treatment and hope for the best.

12. Questions Still Facing the CAR-T Field

The development of CAR-T therapy is at the beginning of its era. There are still many questions facing the CAR field [4, 5]:

(1) Does persistence correlate with outcome?

(2) Is long-term persistence of CAR cells desired?

(3) Which approaches give durable persistence of CAR-Ts?

(4) What is the best vector to introduce the CAR: retroviral, lentiviral, or nonviral vectors?

(5) Which is better: scFv or endodomain construction?

(6) What is the optimal T-cell type and composition of the infused product?

(7) How can checkpoint therapy and CAR-T therapy be combined?

One of the issues that contribute to compromised immune response is T-cell exhaustion and senescence and loss of CD8 and CD4 T-cell function, which occurs with chronic infections and cancer. The addition of a PD1 inhibitor, which is a checkpoint inhibitor, can rescue partially exhausted cell [6] and why scientists should investigate how checkpoint and CAR-T therapies can be used in combination.

In addition to questions facing the CAR field, there are clinical questions such as degree of disease burden and pre- and postinfusion therapy that can affect how well the CAR-T therapy works. Juno Therapeutics' CAR-T trial was halted when three patients died due to neurotoxicity, an adverse event well recognized in cases with CAR-T therapy but mild to moderate in a previous trial (Timmerman 2016) [28]. Juno believes that the deaths may have been related to the type of preconditioning therapy that patients got before receiving their reengineered T-cell infusions. Fludarabine (can cause neurologic affects) [29], a chemotherapy agent, was added to cyclophosphamide as the preconditioning regiment months after the trial started. Scientists believed that the depletion of certain blood cells would create a more favorable environment for the programmed infused T-cells to engraft and start attacking cancer. Later, with the elimination of Fludarabine from their protocol, Juno received the green light to restart the trial.

In order to bring the cost of this complex therapy down, scientists are looking at the possibility of allogenic (donor) therapy in lieu of autogenic therapy. Cellectis, a French biopharmaceutical company, has developed an allogenic CAR-T therapy, "UCAR-T" or universal CAR-T therapy. A pediatric patient with a refractory relapsed ALL was given UCAR-T in the UK after all previous treatment had failed in 2015. According to the CEO of Cellectis, at that time, the patient did not exhibit any adverse effects such as CRS and the UCAR-T-cells were still active after three months (Labiotech 2015) [30]. With these results, in June of 2016, Cellectis announced the enrollment of their first pediatric patient in a Phase 1 clinical trial for acute B lymphoblastic leukemia (B-ALL) at the University College of London (UCL) (Cellectis 2016) [31].

Kite Pharmaceutical is also pursuing the same path by partnering with the University of California Los Angeles (UCLA) for an allogenic T-cell therapies developed by Dr. Gay Crooks at UCLA, a type of artificial cell culture system that would support ex vivo differentiation of T-cells from pluripotent stem cells (Biopharm Drive 2016) [32].

13. Conclusion

It has been established that CAR-T therapy can work thus far as a cure in some patients. But the design of the CAR can be very complex and critical since the choice of costimulatory signals will determine whether or not an immune response is induced (CD28) or inhibited (CTLA 4 and PD1) [6]:

(1) Inadequate costimulation can weaken host defenses leading to infection of cancer.

(2) Inappropriate costimulation can lead to allergy, autoimmunity, and graft rejection.

(3) Inadequate coinhibition leads to autoimmunity or autoinflammatory disease.

(4) Inappropriate coinhibition leads to immunologic exhaustion.

It is a fine balance between the design of the CAR-T-cells, the microenvironment, and clinical influences such as disease burden or pretherapy in order for this therapy to work. Two main areas that warrant further research are the following.

(1) Determining Why Some Patients Only Have a Partial or No Response. T-cell exhaustion, senescence, and loss of CD8 and CD4 T-cell function due to chronic infection; inadequate amount of efficient effector memory T-cells (T-Em) converting to central memory cells which leads to increased cytotoxic T lymphocytes (CTL) activity; and lack of enough central memory cells for persistence are all roadblocks to cellular therapy that could explain why some patients have partial or no response. It could also be another mechanism that researchers will discover upon further research.

(2) Designing a CAR-T Therapy That Is Specific to Each Type of Solid Tumors. The complexity of treating solid tumors is twofold: (1) the T-cells have to hone in onto specific binding sites of the cancer cell and (2) T-cell infiltration can be hindered by poor microenvironment such as poor vessel quality and dysfunctional junction or toxic immunosuppressive environment as in prostate cancer. There are also a number of proteins that are overexpressed in many different types of solid tumors.

For pancreatic cancer, PSCA, Tn glycan on the mucin 1 (MUC1), and mesothelin are all overexpressed. Prostate and pancreatic cancer have the same PSCA that is overexpressed but PSCA is overexpressed in the premalignant stages of pancreatic cancer, and MSLN is overexpressed at later stages according to studies by Abate-Daga et al. [19]. Two different types of protein are overexpressed depending on the stage of the cancer, adding to the complexity in developing the right CAR-T to treat tumors. Castellino and his group [20] were the first to developed CAR-Tmeso cells to treat pancreatic cancer in mice.

Choosing or discovering the right target or targets for each individual in addition to knowing which protein to target at the appropriate stage of the cancer appears crucial in finding successful treatments for cancer. Many companies in the past have tried to use two, sometimes three, immunotherapies for pancreatic cancer, but have not produced favorable results since Gemcitabine (Gemzar) was approved in 1996 for pancreatic cancer. However, Gemzar only works in about 10% of the patients.

Apexian pharmaceuticals is taking a different approach in developing a drug that binds to APE1/Ref-1, a dual protein that is crucial in the development and growth of tumors in pancreatic cancer and is particularly dependent on APE1/Ref-1 [33]. In preliminary studies, it has shown to have activity in different types (breast, prostate, renal, head and neck, and colorectal) of cancers. If this drug comes to fruition, perhaps combination therapy with this drug and CAR-T for partial responders or nonresponders will result in more patients being and remaining cancer-free.

The issue of cost is always a topic at hand as to who is going to pay for these advance therapies. But it is already costing the healthcare system significant amount of money every time a drug does not work on a patient just because the other drugs are cheaper. Each failure adds cost to the system in keeping the patient in the hospital or returning to the emergency room due to complications as the cancer progressing further. A patient also should not have to suffer through failure after failure just because the other drugs are cheaper when one dose of a CAR-T therapy could have cured the patient. These new therapies should be covered by insurance. When allogenic CAR-T-cells are demonstrated to work as well as autogenic CAR-T-cells, the cost of therapy will definitely decrease significantly.

There has been many legislative orders from Obamacare to curb the rising cost of healthcare. But what some may not realize is that as people are living longer, they require more healthcare due to more comorbidities, which automatically increases the cost of healthcare. In order to prevent healthcare cost from spiraling out of control, the whole healthcare system has to change. Until we can change the mindset of everyone to foster preventive care, have patient's take responsibility of their own health, embrace the notion of treating the right patient with the right drug, with the freedom of advance technology being covered by insurance, and foster the expectation that not every disease needs to be treated with a machine gun when a pistol will achieve the same outcome, things will not change.

The advances in technology that scientists have made today are extraordinary, where cancer may be "cured" rather than in "remission." The concept of cure would have been considered fiction 25 years ago. We have the technology. We should be able to use the technology and trust that people will use it appropriately.

Competing Interests

The author declares that there is no conflict of interests regarding the publication of this paper.

References

[1] Keytruda prescribing information, http://www.merck.com/product/usa/pi_circulars/k/keytruda/keytruda_pi.pdf.

[2] Opdivo prescribing information, http://packageinserts.bms.com/pi/pi_opdivo.pdf.

[3] Yervoy prescribing information, http://packageinserts.bms.com/pi/pi_yervoy.pdf.

[4] S. Grupp, "Immunotherapy: CAR-T cells," in *Proceedings of the Society for Adolescent and Young Adult Oncology Conference*, 2014, https://www.youtube.com/watch?v=r9fVKcNOkUE.

[5] C. June, "Cells: from Robert Hooke to Cell Therapy—a 350 year journey," The Royal Society scientific programme, October 2015, https://www.youtube.com/watch?v=GAQ5tCi44II.

[6] J. Looney, *T Cell Activation and Control*, Cleveland Clinic Foundation Center for Continuing Education and the R.J. Fasenmyer Center for Clinical Immunology, 2013, https://www.youtube.com/watch?v=GXVLdbkRkhw.

[7] S. L. Maude, D. T. Teachey, D. L. Porter, and S. A. Grupp, "CD19-targeted chimeric antigen receptor T-cell therapy for acute lymphoblastic leukemia," *Blood*, vol. 125, no. 26, pp. 4017–4023, 2015.

[8] M. Sadelain, R. Brentjens, and I. Rivière, "The basic principles of chimeric antigen receptor design," *Cancer Discovery*, vol. 3, no. 4, pp. 388–398, 2013.

[9] K.-I. Hanada and N. P. Restifo, "Double or nothing on cancer immunotherapy," *Nature Biotechnology*, vol. 31, no. 1, pp. 33–34, 2013.

[10] H. Almåsbak, T. Aarvak, and M. C. Vemuri, "CAR T cell therapy: a game changer in cancer treatment," *Journal of Immunology Research*, vol. 2016, Article ID 5474602, 10 pages, 2016.

[11] Z. Zhao, M. Condomines, S. J. C. van der Stegen et al., "Structural design of engineered costimulation determines tumor rejection kinetics and persistence of CAR T cells," *Cancer Cell*, vol. 28, no. 4, pp. 415–428, 2015.

[12] National Cancer Institute, *CAR T-Cell Therapy: Engineering Patients' Immune Cells to Treat Their Cancers*, 2014, http://www.cancer.gov/about-cancer/treatment/research/car-t-cells.

[13] M. L. Davila, R. Brentjens, X. Wang, I. Rivière, and M. Sadelain, "How do CARs work? Early insights from recent clinical studies targeting CD19," *OncoImmunology*, vol. 1, no. 9, pp. 1577–1583, 2012.

[14] I. Dufait, T. Liechtenstein, A. Lanna et al., "Retroviral and lentiviral vectors for the induction of immunological tolerance," *Scientifica*, vol. 2012, Article ID 694137, 14 pages, 2012.

[15] S. L. Maude, N. Frey, P. A. Shaw et al., "Chimeric antigen receptor T cells for sustained remissions in leukemia," *New England Journal of Medicine*, vol. 371, no. 16, pp. 1507–1517, 2014.

[16] M. L. Davila, I. Riviere, X. Wang et al., "Efficacy and toxicity management of 19-28z CAR T cell therapy in B cell acute lymphoblastic leukemia," *Science Translational Medicine*, vol. 6, no. 224, Article ID 224ra25, 2014.

[17] D. W. Lee, J. N. Kochenderfer, M. Stetler-Stevenson et al., "T cells expressing CD19 chimeric antigen receptors for acute lymphoblastic leukaemia in children and young adults: a phase 1 dose-escalation trial," *The Lancet*, vol. 385, no. 9967, pp. 517–528, 2015.

[18] V. Hillerdal and M. Essand, "Chimeric antigen receptor-engineered T cells for the treatment of metastatic prostate cancer," *BioDrugs*, vol. 29, no. 2, pp. 75–89, 2015.

[19] D. Abate-Daga, K. H. Lagisetty, E. Tran et al., "A novel chimeric antigen receptor against prostate stem cell antigen mediates tumor destruction in a humanized mouse model of pancreatic cancer," *Human Gene Therapy*, vol. 25, no. 12, pp. 1003–1012, 2014.

[20] A. Castellino, First Success with CAR T-Cells in a Solid Tumor, Medscape Medical News, June 2015, http://www.medscape.com/viewarticle/846702.

[21] Cell Press, 'CAR T cell therapy can now target solid tumors: Mouse study', ScienceDaily, June 2016, https://www.science-daily.com/releases/2016/06/160621132523.htm.

[22] A. D. Posey Jr., R. D. Schwab, A. C. Boesteanu et al., "Engineered CAR T cells targeting the cancer-associated Tn-glycoform of the membrane mucin MUC1 control adenocarcinoma," *Immunity*, vol. 44, no. 6, pp. 1444–1454, 2016.

[23] R. Brentjens, "Immunological approaches: CARS to armored CARS—T cell treatment of cancer," in *Proceedings of the Lymphoma and Myeloma Conference*, New York, NY, USA, October 2015, https://www.youtube.com/watch?v=-e1UPNQD3qI.

[24] K. A. Frauwirth, J. L. Riley, M. H. Harris et al., "The CD28 signaling pathway regulates glucose metabolism," *Immunity*, vol. 16, no. 6, pp. 769–777, 2002.

[25] M. Sukumar, J. Liu, Y. Ji et al., "Inhibiting glycolytic metabolism enhances CD8$^+$ T cell memory and antitumor function," *The Journal of Clinical Investigation*, vol. 123, no. 10, pp. 4479–4488, 2013.

[26] X.-S. Zhong, M. Matsushita, J. Plotkin, I. Riviere, and M. Sadelain, "Chimeric antigen receptors combining 4-1BB and CD28 signaling domains augment PI3kinase/AKT/Bcl-X$_L$ activation and CD8$^+$ T cell–mediated tumor eradication," *Molecular Therapy*, vol. 18, no. 2, pp. 413–420, 2010.

[27] J. A. DiMasi, H. G. Grabowski, and R. W. Hansen, "Innovation in the pharmaceutical industry: new estimates of R&D costs," *Journal of Health Economics*, vol. 47, pp. 20–33, 2016.

[28] L. Timmerman, Juno Therapeutics' Lead Drug Trial Halted as Patients Die From Neurotoxicity, Timmerman Report, July 2016, http://www.forbes.com/sites/luketimmerman/2016/07/07/juno-therapeutics-lead-drug-goes-on-clinical-hold-after-two-patients-die/#1d3692d25f59.

[29] FDA Labeling, "Fludara prescribing information," 2003, http://www.fda.gov/ohrms/dockets/ac/04/briefing/2004-4067b1_15_fludarabine%20label.pdf.

[30] Labiotech, 2015. Cellectis' CEO: "I'm just trying to be realistic, CAR-T is not THE miracle cure for Cancer", Cellectis Interview with LaBiotech, http://labiotech.eu/cellectis-interview-car-t-is-not-the-cure-of-cancer/.

[31] Cellectis News, 2016. Cellectis Announces First Patient Treated in Phase 1 Trial of UCART19 in Pediatric Acute B Lymphoblastic Leukemia (B-ALL), Cellectis News Release, June 2016, http://www.cellectis.com/en/content/cellectis-announces-first-patient-treated-phase-1-trial-ucart19-pediatric-acute-b-0.

[32] Biopharma Drive, "Kite eyes off-the-shelf T-cell therapies with UCLA research deal," Biopharma Drive News, July 2016, http://www.biopharmadive.com/news/Kite-Pharma-UCLA-tcell–allogeneic/423263/.

[33] F. Vinluan, Led by Former Lilly Exec, Apexian Out to Tackle Pancreatic Cancer, Xconomy, November 2016, http://www.xconomy.com/indiana/2016/11/16/led-by-former-lilly-exec-apexian-out-to-tackle-pancreatic-cancer/?single_page=true.

[34] J. N. Kochenderfer and S. A. Rosenberg, "Treating B-cell cancer with T cells expressing anti-CD19 chimeric antigen receptors," *Nature Reviews Clinical Oncology*, vol. 10, pp. 267–276, 2013.

8

Methanolic Extract of Dill Leaves Inhibits AGEs Formation and Shows Potential Hepatoprotective Effects in CCl$_4$ Induced Liver Toxicity in Rat

Ebrahim Abbasi Oshaghi,[1] Iraj Khodadadi,[1] Fatemeh Mirzaei,[2] Mozafar Khazaei,[3] Heidar Tavilani,[1] and Mohammad Taghi Goodarzi[1,4]

[1]Department of Clinical Biochemistry, School of Medicine, Hamadan University of Medical Sciences, Hamadan, Iran
[2]Student Research Committee, Kermanshah University of Medical Sciences, Kermanshah, Iran
[3]Fertility and Infertility Research Center, Kermanshah University of Medical Sciences, Kermanshah, Iran
[4]Research Center for Molecular Medicine, Hamadan University of Medical Sciences, Hamadan, Iran

Correspondence should be addressed to Mohammad Taghi Goodarzi; mtgoodarzi@yahoo.com

Academic Editor: István Zupkó

The research was aimed at evaluating the antiglycation, antioxidant, and hepatoprotective properties of methanolic extract of *Anethum graveolens* (dill). The antioxidant properties, photochemical characteristics, and antiglycation effects of dill extract were measured. Carbon tetrachloride-induced hepatotoxic rats were used to show the hepatoprotective activity of dill leaves. Different concentration of dill extract (0.032, 0.065, 0.125, 0.25, 0.5, and 1 mg/mL) showed potential antioxidant ability. The extract of dill leaves significantly reduced AGEs formation and also fructosamine and protein carbonyl levels in rats' liver. Thiol groups' oxidation, amyloid cross-β, and protein fragmentation ($P < 0.001$) significantly reduced in treated rats. Liver damage markers significantly reduced in dill-treated animals ($P < 0.05$). Dill with potential antioxidant, antiglycation, and hepatoprotective effects can be suggested for treatment of diabetes complications.

1. Introduction

Free radicals are involved in many chronic and acute disorders such as diabetes, cancer, cardiovascular disease, immunosuppression, and neurological problems [1]. The detrimental effects of the free radicals can be blocked by natural antioxidants [2]. Numerous kinds of herbal medicine have studied for their antioxidant and antiradical properties [3]. *Anethum graveolens* L. (dill) belongs to Apiaceae family and grows mostly in Europe, Mediterranean region, and Asia [4]. Dill is used for various purposes in many countries and traditionally used for medicinal purpose such as digestive disorders, reduction of the bad breath, and stimulation of lactation and also known as a lipid lowering, anticancer, antimicrobial, antidiabetic, antigastric irritation, anti-inflammatory, and antioxidant agent [4, 5]. Administration of dill in human and animal models had antioxidant activity and normalized blood glucose and lipid profile [4–9]. Dill also showed potential antidiabetic activity [10]. The exact antidiabetic mechanism of dill has not been recognized until now. The previous reports have not investigated all of the antioxidant indices of *Anethum graveolens*, neither its antiglycation effects. Furthermore, variance in cultivating area and the method of extraction cause different antioxidant ability [3]. Consequently, this study was planned to assess the antiglycation and oxidant scavenging as well as hepatoprotective effects of dill cultivated in Hamadan (west of Iran).

2. Materials and Methods

2.1. Extraction of Plant Materials and Phytochemical Screening. *Anethum graveolens* was prepared from Hamadan (west of Iran) and identified by our colleague in the Buali-Sina

University, Hamadan, Iran. For preparation of methanolic extract, dill leaves powder was dried and crushed. Dried dill powder (100 g) was mixed with 300 mL of methanol at room temperature for 48 hours. The prepared solution was filtered and subsequently concentrated and evaporated to dryness in vacuum. The extract was kept in dark vials at $-20°C$ until analysis [11].

2.2. Phytochemical Screening.

Phytochemical screening was performed according to Salmanian et al. [12] and Abbasi Oshaghi et al. [13] method. Total phenolic content of methanolic extract was determined using Folin-Ciocalteu reaction. Briefly, one milligram of methanolic extract was dissolved in the reaction solution (3.8 mL of deionized water + 2 mL of 2% Na_2CO_3 + 100 μL of 50% Folin-Ciocalteu). The prepared mixture was incubated at room temperature for 30 min and the absorbance of the sample was determined at 750 nm. Flavonoids content of dill was determined by using $AlCl_3$ assay. Briefly 500 μL of the dill extract (1 mg/mL in methanol) was mixed with the reaction solution (1.5 mL of 95% alcohol + 100 μL of 10% $AlCl_3$ + 100 μL of 1 M potassium acetate + 2.8 mL of deionized water). After 40 min of incubation at room temperature the absorbance of the samples was measured at 415 nm. Total flavonols content of dill was determined by adding of 1 mg/mL dill extract to the reaction solution (200 μL of 20 mg/mL $AlCl_3$) + 6 mL sodium acetate solution (50 mg/mL). After 2.5 hours of incubation at room temperature the absorbance of the prepared solution was measured at 440 nm. The results were calculated per mg equivalents of gallic acid (for phenolic) and quercetin (for flavonoids and flavonols) per gram of each extract.

2.3. Antioxidant Activity.

To measure the antioxidant activity of prepared dill extract different tests were carried out including ferric reducing antioxidant power (FRAP), DPPH radical scavenging, superoxide anion and hydrogen peroxide scavenging, metal chelating, reducing power, and nitric oxide scavenging activity, according to the previously published methods [12].

2.4. Glycation of BSA and Fructosamine.

Glycated BSA was prepared using treatment of BSA with different concentration of fructose (200 and 500 mM) at different time periods (1, 2, 3, and 4 weeks) [14]. Aminoguanidine (AG) a known antiglycation agent was used as a positive control. After dialysis in PBS, glycated BSA formation was determined using a fluorometry method at an excitation wavelength of 440 nm and emission wavelength of 460 nm (spectrofluorometer, Jasco FP-6200) [14]. Nitroblue tetrazolium (NBT) reaction was used to measure the fructosamine level [15].

2.5. Thiol Group and Protein Carbonyl Content.

The free thiol and carbonyl contents in glycated BSA were determined according to Adisakwattana et al.'s report [14].

2.6. Protein Aggregation and Fragmentation.

Amyloid cross-β structure, which is recognized as an indicator of protein aggregation, was determined using Congo red dye [14]. The fragmentation of protein was estimated and shown using SDS-PAGE [14].

2.7. In Vivo Studies

2.7.1. Hepatoprotective Activity.

Male Wistar rats weighing 210–220 g were divided randomly into four groups (n = 6): (1) normal rats that received 30% CCl_4 in olive oil (1 mL/kg body wt i.p) every 72 hours for a period of 10 days (hepatotoxic group); (2) CCl_4 hepatotoxic induced rats that received 100 mg/kg dill extract for 10 days; (3) CCl_4 induced hepatotoxic rats that received 300 mg/kg dill extract for 10 days; (4) normal rats that received distilled water (1 mL/kg body wt) orally for 10 days [16]. After that, the animals were anesthetized and blood was collected from their heart. All of biochemical assays were performed using commercial kits (Pars Azmun, Iran) [5]. All procedures were approved by ethics committee of Hamadan University of Medical Science, Hamadan, Iran.

2.7.2. Histopathological Examination.

The pieces of rats' liver were excised and then fixed in 10% formalin solution and processed by standard way. Liver sections with thickness of 5 μm were stained with haematoxylin and eosin (H&E). The stained slides were evaluated under a light microscope.

2.8. Statistical Analysis.

Data are expressed as means $\pm$ SEM of three duplicate measurements and then analyzed by SPSS package (version 16, SPSS, Inc). One way analysis of variance (ANOVA) followed by Tukey test was used to analyze the results. The P values less than 0.05 were regarded as statically significant.

3. Results

3.1. In Vitro Antioxidant Study.

Dill extract showed strong DPPH radical scavenging activity in a dose dependent manner with IC50 of 0.064 mg/mL. Dill extract also had potential FRAP value and reducing power ability (Figure 1). Dill showed potential super oxide anion-, hydrogen peroxide- and NO-scavenging activity and metal chelating with IC_{50} of 0.110, 0.125 mg/mL, 0.064, and 0.056 mg/mL, respectively (Figure 1). The total phenols, flavonoids, flavonols, alkaloid, anthocyanin, tannins, and saponin contents were 176 $\pm$ 5.2, 130$\pm$4.4, 121$\pm$3.8, 88$\pm$5.1, 46$\pm$2.9, 66$\pm$3.7, and 45$\pm$3.2 mg/g of extract, respectively.

In vitro antiglycation study of dill extract at different concentration significantly declined AGEs formation at 1, 2, 3, and 4 weeks of incubation. Dill also significantly declined fructosamine levels (Table 1) and carbonyl content (Table 2) and also inhibited thiol groups oxidation (Table 2), amyloid cross-β structure, and protein fragmentation rate (Figure 2).

In the in vivo study the serum levels of LDH, ALP, AST, ALT, γ-GT, total bilirubin, direct bilirubin, triglycerides, total cholesterol, and liver weight were significantly increased, whereas total protein, albumin, and body weight significantly reduced in CCl_4 group. These values normalized in the animals which were pretreated with dill extract ($P < 0.05$ for all factors) (Table 3).

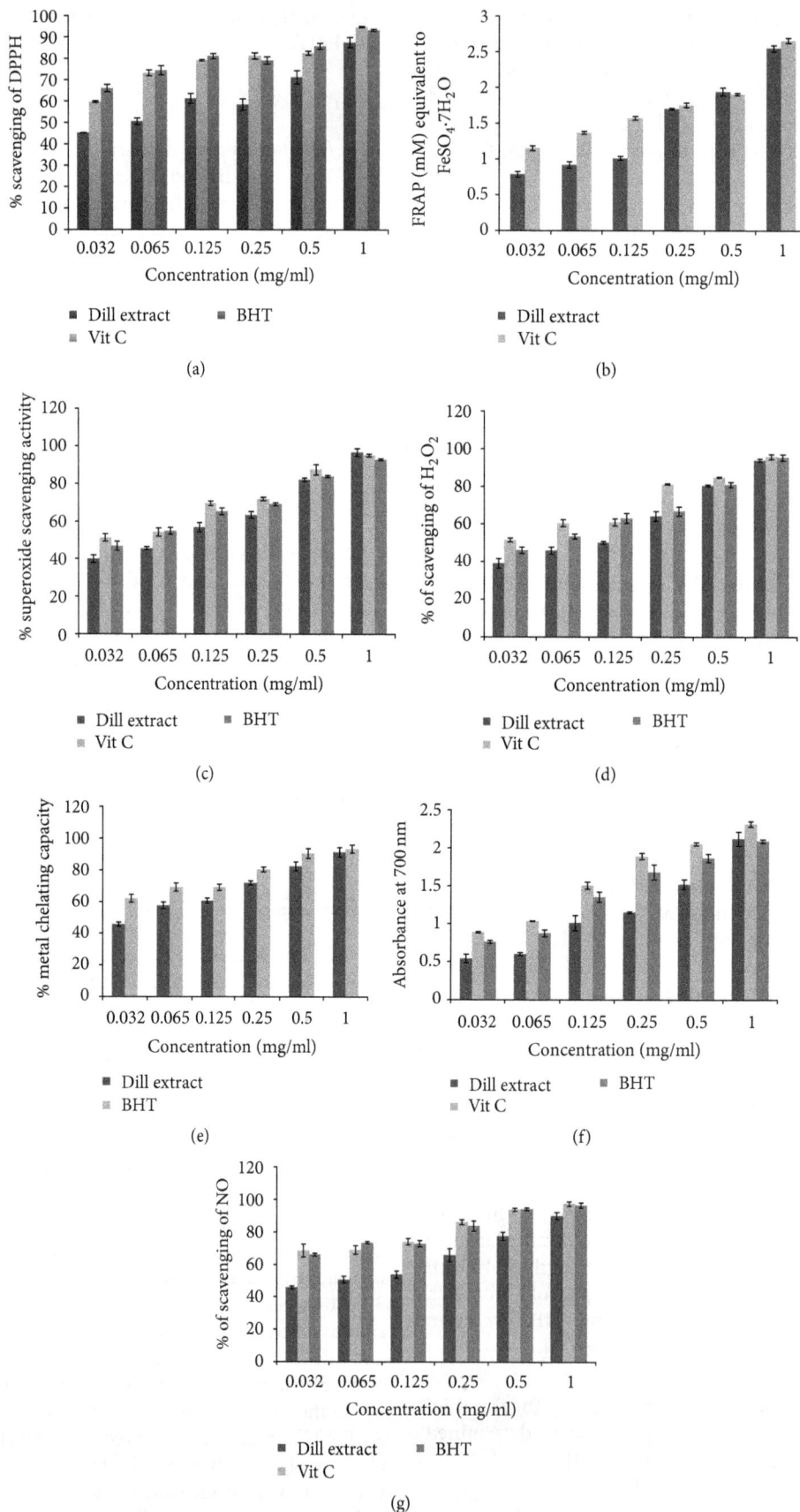

FIGURE 1: Antioxidant and antiradical activity of dill extract. Values are the average of triplicate experiments and presented as mean ± SEM. (a) DPPH radical scavenging activity. (b) FRAP assays. (c) Superoxide radical scavenging activity. (d) Hydrogen peroxide radical scavenging activity. (e) Metal chelating activity. (f) Reducing power activity. (g) Nitric oxide scavenging activity.

(a)

(b)

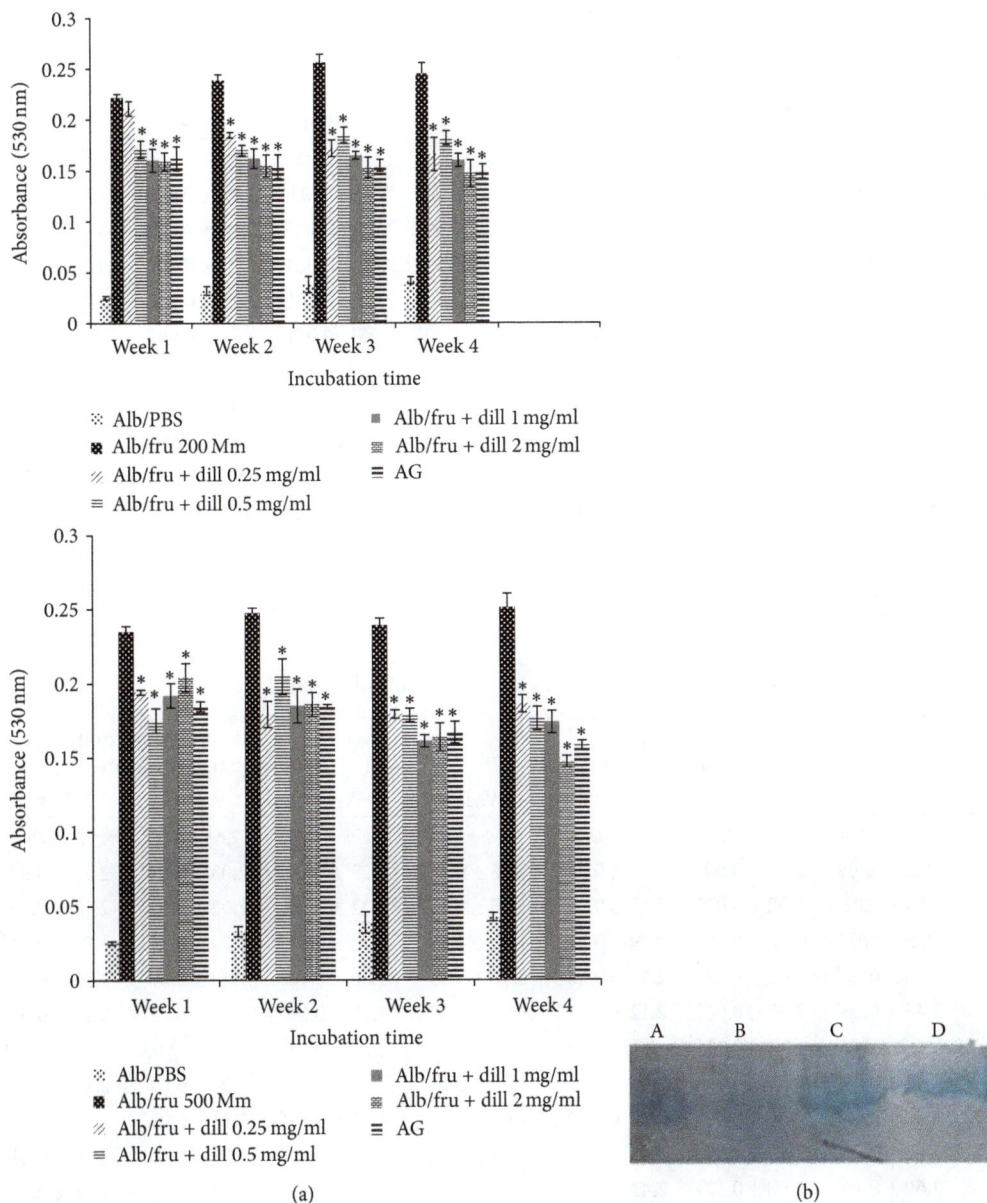

FIGURE 2: (a) The effect of dill extract on the level of protein aggregation. Data are represented as mean ± SEM ($n = 3$); $^*P < 0.001$ compared with BSA/fructose at the same incubation time. AG: aminoguanidine. Data are represented as mean ± SEM ($n = 3$); $^*P < 0.001$ compared with BSA/fructose at the same incubation time. (b) Protein fragmentation in BSA incubated with 200 mM fructose in the presence of Cu^{+2} ion, aminoguanidine, and dill extract for 7 days, detected by SDS-PAGE. Protein fragmentation inhibited by aminoguanidine (lane C) and dill extract (lane D) compared with BSA/fructose. A lane: 10 mg/mL BSA, B lane: 10 mg/mL BSA + 200 mM fructose, C lane: 10 mg/mL BSA + 200 mM fructose + aminoguanidine, and D lane: 10 mg/mL BSA + 200 mM fructose + dill extract.

3.2. Histopathological Change in Liver. The microscopic analysis revealed varying degree of cellular damage from normal to severe in different treated groups (Figure 3). Liver histology in control group showed regular structure including well-organized cells sinusoidal lining and clear central vein. The CCl_4-treated group illustrated the entire damage of hepatocytes, destruction of normal euchromatic nucleus, degeneration of central vein, fat accumulation, and foam cell formation. Also, in CCl_4-treated group, centrilobular necrosis in most cases, various size vacuoles, and mild fibrosis were

observed. These histopathological changes were repaired near to normal structure in the CCl_4-treated animals that received 100 mg/kg and 300 mg/kg dill extract. The restoration of these changes in 300 mg/kg was more than that of CCl_4-treated animals that received 100 mg/kg dill extract.

4. Discussion

In this study extract of dill leaves showed high amount of phenolic and flavonoid. Lisiewska et al. [17] found that the

TABLE 1: The effect of dill extract on AGE and fructosamine formation.

Experimental groups	AGE formation (arbitrary unit)				Fructosamine levels (mmol/mg protein)			
	Week 1	Week 2	Week 3	Week 4	Week 1	Week 2	Week 3	Week 4
BSA/Fru 500 mM	95.22 ± 6.64	100.93 ± 7.35	128.15 ± 6.37	141.09 ± 13.1	3.46 ± 0.070	3.36 ± 0.06	3.64 ± 0.066	3.95 ± 0.063
+Dill 0.25 mg/ml	38.87 ± 4.56*	40.08 ± 7.15*	44.91 ± 6.32*	56.76 ± 8.03*	3.37 ± 0.036	2.95 ± 0.055*	3.03 ± 0.028*	3.43 ± 0.005*
+Dill 0.5 mg/ml	36.49 ± 6.81*	39.78 ± 6.31*	47.94 ± 7.28*	54.65 ± 4.49*	2.68 ± 0.105*	2.86 ± 0.066*	3.04 ± 0.063*	3.39 ± 0.008*
+Dill 1 mg/ml	28.51 ± 4.20*	36.87 ± 5.35*	35.32 ± 6.19*	44.46 ± 7.33*	2.62 ± 0.061*	2.71 ± 0.089*	2.83 ± 0.014*	3.19 ± 0.020*
+Dill 2 mg/ml	23.73 ± 3.01*	31.64 ± 4.40*	41.63 ± 2.98*	47.07 ± 3.45*	2.70 ± 0.105*	2.75 ± 0.080*	2.64 ± 0.008*	2.97 ± 0.026*
+AG 2 mg/ml	37.23 ± 5.51*	45.56 ± 4.35*	49.45 ± 4.02*	55.82 ± 2.90*	2.65 ± 0.081*	2.74 ± 0.043*	2.54 ± 0.139*	2.81 ± 0.010*
BSA/Fru 200 mM	98.07 ± 4.74	109.77 ± 8.30	133.54 ± 9.14	151.46 ± 5.41	2.33 ± 0.05	2.54 ± 0.01	2.77 ± 0.08	2.95 ± 0.02
+Dill 0.25 mg/ml	44.43 ± 5.96*	49.63 ± 5.61*	53.80 ± 6.85*	70.32 ± 8.73*	2.36 ± 0.07	2.03 ± 0.05*	2.10 ± 0.02*	2.50 ± 0.01*
+Dill 0.5 mg/ml	37.05 ± 5.62*	45.01 ± 4.28*	50.83 ± 5.58*	64.54 ± 5.30*	1.71 ± 0.09*	1.94 ± 0.06*	2.11 ± 0.06*	2.46 ± 0.01*
+Dill 1 mg/ml	33.40 ± 6.06*	47.10 ± 5.54*	42.21 ± 4.15*	50.02 ± 4.44*	1.72 ± 0.06*	1.79 ± 0.08*	1.90 ± 0.01*	2.26 ± 0.02*
+Dill 2 mg/ml	32.95 ± 5.28*	41.21 ± 5.50*	45.70 ± 5.47*	43.29 ± 5.22*	1.80 ± 0.10*	1.83 ± 0.08*	1.71 ± 0.01*	2.04 ± 0.02*
+AG 2 mg/ml	51.22 ± 4.91*	53.63 ± 5.55*	52.05 ± 5.22*	59.94 ± 4.10*	1.76 ± 0.08*	2.20 ± 0.06*	2.09 ± 0.04*	2.29 ± 0.01*
BSA/PBS	20.73 ± 2.43*	20.00 ± 2.21*	26.97 ± 5.69*	29.20 ± 4.52*	0.15 ± 0.01*	0.16 ± 0.01*	0.17 ± 0.01*	0.20 ± 0.01*

*$P < 0.01$ when compared to BSA/fructose at the same incubation time.

TABLE 2: The effect of dill extract on the thioland carbonyl group.

Experimental groups	Thiol group (nmol/mg protein)				Carbonyl group (nmol/mg protein)			
	Week 1	Week 2	Week 3	Week 4	Week 1	Week 2	Week 3	Week 4
BSA/Fru 500 mM	2.24 ± 0.01	1.69 ± 0.08	1.35 ± 0.02	0.84 ± 0.05	2.55 ± 0.06	2.68 ± 0.12	3.21 ± 0.06	3.39 ± 0.10
+Dill 0.25 mg/ml	2.29 ± 0.08	2.14 ± 0.09*	1.98 ± 0.03*	1.56 ± 0.06*	2.22 ± 0.11*	2.03 ± 0.05*	2.12 ± 0.03*	2.53 ± 0.02*
+Dill 0.5 mg/ml	2.54 ± 0.02*	2.32 ± 0.02*	2.17 ± 0.09*	1.76 ± 0.07*	2.22 ± 0.09*	2.02 ± 0.06*	2.11 ± 0.05*	2.52 ± 0.01*
+Dill 1 mg/ml	2.4 ± 0.07*	2.48 ± 0.06*	2.39 ± 0.07*	1.41 ± 0.03*	1.72 ± 0.05*	1.79 ± 0.08*	1.92 ± 0.01*	2.29 ± 0.02*
+Dill 2 mg/ml	2.76 ± 0.02*	2.62 ± 0.02*	2.34 ± 0.05*	2.40 ± 0.09*	1.80 ± 0.10*	1.83 ± 0.07*	1.73 ± 0.01*	2.07 ± 0.02*
+AG 2 mg/ml	2.47 ± 0.06*	2.35 ± 0.01*	2.12 ± 0.04*	1.79 ± 0.09*	1.97 ± 0.09*	2.03 ± 0.02*	2.14 ± 0.01*	2.37 ± 0.09*
BSA/Fru 200 mM	1.99 ± 0.05	1.7 ± 0.05	1.52 ± 0.14	0.90 ± 0.05	2.26 ± 0.01	2.57 ± 0.03	2.58 ± 0.10	3.32 ± 0.02
+Dill 0.25 mg/ml	2.37 ± 0.04*	2.20 ± 0.05*	2.09 ± 0.05*	1.75 ± 0.01*	2.27 ± 0.05	2.08 ± 0.04*	2.13 ± 0.06*	2.90 ± 0.03*
+Dill 0.5 mg/ml	2.48 ± 0.07*	2.36 ± 0.09*	2.16 ± 0.07*	1.67 ± 0.10*	1.72 ± 0.03*	1.93 ± 0.01*	2.20 ± 0.05*	2.99 ± 0.02*
+Dill 1 mg/ml	2.66 ± 0.03*	2.49 ± 0.09*	2.48 ± 0.03*	1.54 ± 0.02*	1.73 ± 0.05*	1.75 ± 0.06*	2.06 ± 0.01*	2.71 ± 0.07*
+Dill 2 mg/ml	2.60 ± 0.14*	2.50 ± 0.12*	2.42 ± 0.06*	2.31 ± 0.04*	1.81 ± 0.09*	1.79 ± 0.03*	1.78 ± 0.04*	2.65 ± 0.09*
+AG 2 mg/ml	2.55 ± 0.07*	2.35 ± 0.01*	2.25 ± 0.13*	1.87 ± 0.01*	1.63 ± 0.07*	2.06 ± 0.01*	2.12 ± 0.10*	2.38 ± 0.04*
BSA/PBS	2.73 ± 0.06*	2.63 ± 0.07*	2.53 ± 0.04*	2.51 ± 0.09*	0.21 ± 0.05*	0.25 ± 0.06*	0.23 ± 0.01*	0.24 ± 0.02*

*$P < 0.01$ when compared to BSA/fructose at the same incubation time.

higher leaves of plant have higher amount of phenolics; the stem of dill has the lowest amount of phenolics. These components are able to inhibit lipid peroxidation and have useful effect in mutagenesis, carcinogenesis, atherogenesis, and thrombosis [12]. The hypolipidemic, antidiabetic, and hepatoprotective properties of the dill may be attributed to the high levels of flavonoids, which have been established to have antioxidant activity. The antioxidant properties of these agents are mostly because of their redox activities, which allow them to have different activity such as hydrogen donors, reducing metabolites, reactive oxygen species quenchers, and metal chelating. In this study relatively high amount of alkaloids was found in dill extract. Agrawal et al. [18] reported that alkaloids have potential antioxidant and hypoglycemic effect

in diabetic animals. Anthocyanins also have many biological properties, including anticarcinogenic, antioxidant, and anti-inflammatory activities. Setorki et al. [19] reported that dill had moderate level of anthocyanins. Tannins also are found in dill and many researches showed their useful properties in management of diabetes complications by inhibition of oxidative stress and AGEs formation. Santos et al. [20] showed that administration of tannins markedly declined glucose and lipid levels in diabetic animals. Nakagawa and Yokozawa [21] reported that tannin inhibited AGEs formation. Saponins also were found in the dill extract and have numerous pharmacological properties such as motivation of insulin and C-peptide secretion, antioxidant activity, inhibition of AGEs formation, and also declining of diabetic

TABLE 3: The effect of dill extract on biochemical factors.

Biochemical factors	CCl$_4$-treated	Dill (100 mg/kg) + CCl$_4$	Dill (300 mg/kg) + CCl$_4$	Normal group
LDH (U/l)	196.50 ± 2.29	132.33 ± 2.02*	113.83 ± 4.7*	103.00 ± 5.5*
ALP (U/l)	230.17 ± 6.17	181.67 ± 3.50*	145.67 ± 5.11*	154.00 ± 0.54*
AST (U/l)	273.83 ± 8.47	203.33 ± 4.43*	109.00 ± 3.34*	98.17 ± 3.79*
ALT (U/l)	239.00 ± 5.31	104.50 ± 2.02*	78.50 ± 7.48*	54.33 ± 2.69*
γ-GT (U/l)	5.45 ± 0.611	3.23 ± 0.24#	2.88 ± 0.36#	1.32 ± 0.12*
Total bilirubin (mg/dl)	3.01 ± 0.14	1.78 ± 0.12*	1.49 ± 0.08*	0.85 ± 0.04*
Direct bilirubin (mg/dl)	1.01 ± 0.08	0.89 ± 0.20¥	0.51 ± 0.04#	0.30 ± 0.03*
Total protein (mg/dl)	5.47 ± 0.30	6.00 ± 0.24	6.25 ± 0.11#	6.46 ± 0.08#
Albumin (mg/dl)	2.96 ± 0.14	3.36 ± 0.07¥	3.49 ± 0.09#	3.52 ± 0.07#
Triglyceride (mg/dl)	121.83 ± 5.26	111.50 ± 4.37	99.67 ± 6.69¥	84.16 ± 1.83*
Total cholesterol (mg/dl)	110.83 ± 2.78	88.16 ± 7.10¥	71.16 ± 6.10#	75.16 ± 7.56#
Body weight (g)	195.67 ± 4.54	224.00 ± 1.93*	220.50 ± 1.82*	223.33 ± 1.34*
Liver weight (g)	4.17 ± 0.11	3.37 ± 0.10#	3.42 ± 0.14#	3.34 ± 0.18#

Data are represented as mean ± SEM (n = 6); $^\text{¥}P$ < 0.05, $^\#P$ < 0.01, and $^*P$ < 0.001 compared with CCl$_4$-treated rats.

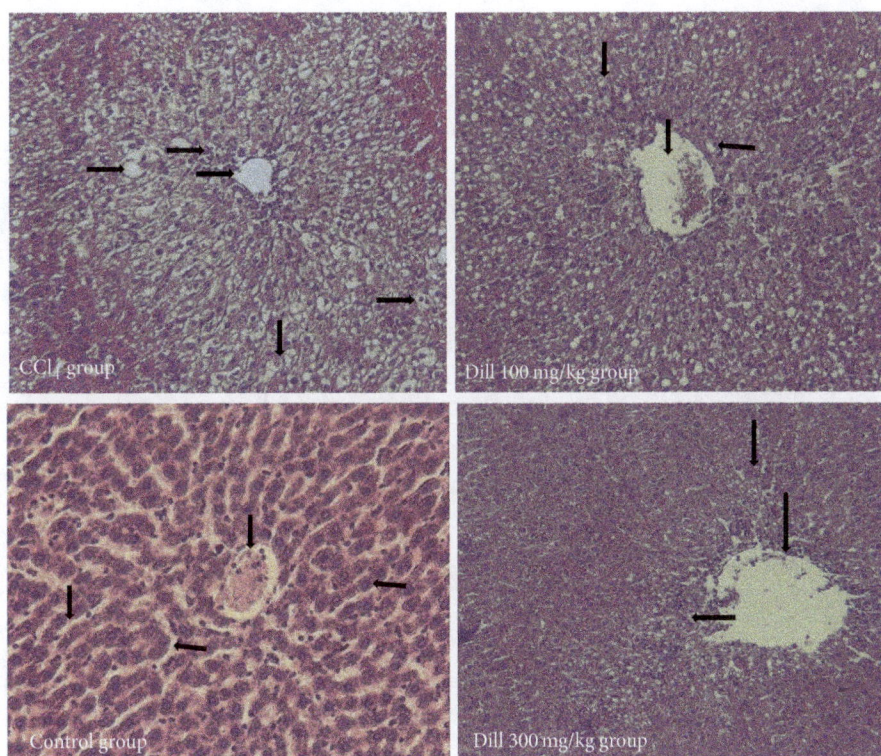

FIGURE 3: Histopathological changes in the liver of different treated animals. Histology of liver in normal group showed regular structure, while CCl$_4$-treated animals show the entire damage of hepatocytes. In dill-treated animals liver damage was restored.

nephropathy [22]. It has been reported that saponins rise permeability of the intestinal mucosal cells and increase the various nutrient absorption. Consequently, these components increased the phenolics absorption. Furthermore, these components possess antioxidant activity that involves effectiveness of the phenolics to protect against CCl$_4$ induced hepatotoxicity [23]. Shyu et al. [3] reported high amounts of

flavonoids, phenols, and proanthocyanidins in the ethanolic extract of *Anethum graveolens* flower.

Our results showed potential antioxidant activity for dill in different tests. The stable free radical of DPPH and FRAP value generally are used to evaluate plant antioxidant ability by working as hydrogen donors or free radical scavengers [12]. Bahramikia et al. [1] reported that water extract fraction of dill had significant DPPH scavenging activity. Superoxide anion involves the development of other ROS including hydroxyl radical, singlet oxygen, and hydrogen peroxide (H_2O_2), which stimulates oxidation of proteins, lipids, and DNA. Studies showed that antioxidant effects of some flavonoids are efficient, predominantly by O_2^- scavenging activity [12, 24]. Among the different species of metal ions, iron (II) is known as the strong prooxidant [12]. Iron chelating activity of dill extract is similar to ascorbic acid and BHT [24]. The reducing power of the agents could serve as a remarkable indicator of their antioxidant activity; therefore, the effectiveness of certain antioxidant agents is famous to be related to high reducing power activity. The reducing power of dill maybe related to its ability to donate hydrogen [24]. NO is a reactive compound which reacts with oxygen and leads to formation of oxidized form of nitrogen [24]. Dill showed potential NO scavenging activity in a dose dependent manner.

Fructose and its metabolites are supposed to be important precursors of AGEs formation in the intracellular condition [25]. Consumption of aminoguanidine (AG) has sufficient effects on diabetic complications; however, it has some harmful side effects such as hepatotoxicity and drug resistance [14]. Therefore, administration of natural products with antiradical and antioxidant effects and low side effects makes them good candidates in treatment of diabetes complications. The dill ability to reduce AGEs formation might contribute to its antioxidant activity [26]. In agreement with Bahramikia et al. [1] studies, we showed that dill has potential antioxidant activity. The metal chelating activity has been shown to be one of the major mechanisms for antiglycation property [25]. In this study, dill extract at different concentration significantly showed iron chelating activity. Presence of tannins in dill extract plays a critical role in treatment of diabetes complications through inhibition of oxidative stress and AGEs formation [20]. Nakagawa and Yokozawa [21] showed that green tea contains high amounts of tannins which significantly inhibits AGE formation. The other mechanism suggested for antiglycation activity is a break of the cross-linking constitution in the AGEs, reducing the carbonyl groups, Amadori products, or Schiff's bases and also reduction of the late-stage Amadori products [26]. Declining of fructosamine levels has beneficial approach to delay vascular complications of diabetes [25]. Our findings indicate dill extract significantly reduced fructosamine levels.

Some studies reported that administration of aqueous extract of dill declined fasting blood glucose in animal models. Mobasseri et al. [8] showed dill normalized lipid profiles and insulin sensitivity in diabetic patients. We previously showed that administration of dill in diabetic animals led to normalized blood glucose, lipid profile, and antioxidant capacity [26, 27]. Rashid Lamir et al. [9] also established that aerobic training with usage of dill significantly increased HDL-C levels and declined blood glucose and LDL/HDL ratio in diabetic women.

Increasing of carbonyl content and declining of free thiol groups are directly reflected to oxidation of protein [26]. Our study showed that dill extract markedly reduced protein carbonyl content and also increased thiol groups.

Aggregation of protein causes amyloid cross-β structure formation which can be determined via reaction with Congo red dye. Dill extracts markedly inhibited protein aggregation. The aggregated protein is able to produce amyloid cross-β structure and subsequently change stability of protein and its structure [28]. Fragmentation of BSA in the presence of fructose and Cu^{2+} was reduced significantly by dill extract. Incubation of glycated BSA with Cu^{2+} is accompanied by the decline of protein-bound glucose, showing that fragmentation of protein occurred at the expense of BSA-bound glucose [29]. Sakai et al. [29] showed that incubation of protein with fructose and Cu^{2+} markedly increased BSA fragmentation, while AG inhibited this process.

The administration of methanol extract of dill protects the liver from induced damage by CCl_4 as manifested by improvement of biochemical factors. The hepatoprotective mechanism of dill is unclear but may be related to presence of many phytoconstituents and lipid peroxidation inhibitors. The hepatotoxicity induced by CCl_4 is correlated to production of $^\bullet CCl_3$, an active metabolite; this is displayed by marked increase in the serum liver enzymes such as AST, ALT, and ALP [23]. In this study the biochemical factor that was measured for liver function was AST, ALT, LDH, GGT, bilirubin, albumin, and total protein. Serum transferases (ALT and AST) are accepted as sensitive markers, strongly related to liver toxicity and damage [27]. Thuppia et al. [30] showed that ethanolic extract of dill has a hepatoprotective activity by declining the AST and ALT levels on acetaminophen-induced hepatic damage in rats. In this study treating the rats with dill extracts especially at the dose of 300 mg/kg did cause significant reduction on both ALT and AST levels. Actually, this extract normalized liver function test in CCl_4 induced liver toxicity. The existence of high amount of phenolic and flavonoid in dill extract elucidates its free radical scavenging properties and probably its in vivo effect on liver function [23].

Liver is known as the main source of serum protein synthesis especially albumin [23]. We showed significant reduction in total protein and albumin by CCl_4, which is consequently revealed the decline in protein synthesis in the liver through necrosis. While, in our experiments, treatment of rat with dill at the dose of 100 and 300 mg/kg normalized these factors. Our results are also reinforced by Rabeh and Aboraya [31] who reported that *Anethum graveolens* or fennel oil and their mixtures have a significant hepatoprotective effect against CCl_4 induced liver toxicity. They showed that treatment of hepatotoxic rats by dill oil markedly reduced ALT, AST, ALP, and blood lipids and also increased total protein and albumin. Oral uptake of dill at doses of 100 and 300 mg/kg significantly decreased the triglycerides and total cholesterol levels. Reduction at dose of 300 mg/kg was more significant. Our result was in agreement with Yazdanparast and Bahramikia [32], Koppula and Choi [6], Thuppia et al. [30], Hajhashemi and Abbasi [33], Madani et al. [5], and other studies [34] as formerly stated that dill significantly reduced blood lipids and liver enzymes.

Histological analysis (Figure 3) also was correlated with biochemical factors. Histological analysis of hepatotoxic liver with CCl_4 displays major morphological changes.

Nevertheless, in rats treated with dill extract at the doses of 100 and 300 mg/kg, the severity of liver damage was reduced significantly, indicating its potential hepatoprotective properties. Our data were similar to the findings of Thuppia et al. [30], Rabeh and Aboraya [31], and Tamilarasi et al. [35] and also our previous results [36] that showed dill oil, dill ethanolic extract, crude powder of dill, and dill tablet have potential antioxidant and hepatoprotective effects on in rats.

5. Conclusion

Extract of dill leaves showed potential antioxidant, antiglycation, and hepatoprotective activities. According to the findings dill can be suggested as a good candidate for healing of diabetes complication and liver toxicity.

Competing Interests

The authors have no competing interests.

Acknowledgments

The authors would like to thank Hamadan University of Medical Sciences (Hamadan, Iran) for financial support.

References

[1] S. Bahramikia and R. Yazdanparast, "Antioxidant and free radical scavenging activities of different fractions of Anethum graveolens leaves using in vitro models," *Pharmacologyonline*, vol. 2, pp. 219–233, 2008.

[2] A. Mohammadi, F. Mirzaei, M. Jamshidi et al., "The in vivo biochemical and oxidative changes by ethanol and opium consumption in Syrian hamsters," *International Journal of Biology*, vol. 5, no. 4, p. 14, 2013.

[3] Y.-S. Shyu, J.-T. Lin, Y.-T. Chang, C.-J. Chiang, and D.-J. Yang, "Evaluation of antioxidant ability of ethanolic extract from dill (Anethum graveolens L.) flower," *Food Chemistry*, vol. 115, no. 2, pp. 515–521, 2009.

[4] S. Jana and G. Shekhawat, "Anethum graveolens: an indian traditional medicinal herb and spice," *Pharmacognosy Reviews*, vol. 4, no. 8, pp. 179–184, 2010.

[5] H. Madani, N. A. Mahmoodabady, and A. Vahdati, "Effects of hydroalchoholic extract of Anethum graveolens (Dill) on plasma glucose an lipid levels in diabetes induced rats," *Iranian Journal of Diabetes and Lipid Disorders*, vol. 5, no. 2, pp. 109–116, 2005.

[6] S. Koppula and D. K. Choi, "Anethum graveolens linn (Umbelliferae) extract attenuates stress-induced urinary biochemical changes and improves cognition in scopolamine-induced amnesic rats," *Tropical Journal of Pharmaceutical Research*, vol. 10, no. 1, pp. 47–54, 2011.

[7] N. Mishra, "Haematological and hypoglycemic potential Anethum graveolens seeds extract in normal and diabetic Swiss albino mice," *Veterinary World*, vol. 6, no. 8, pp. 502–507, 2013.

[8] M. Mobasseri, L. Payahoo, A. Ostadrahimi, Y. K. Bishak, M. A. Jafarabadi, and S. Mahluji, "Anethum graveolens supplementation improves insulin sensitivity and lipid abnormality in type 2 diabetic patients," *Pharmaceutical Sciences*, vol. 20, no. 2, pp. 40–45, 2014.

[9] A. Rashid Lamir, S. Gholamian, S. A. A. Hashemi Javaheri, and M. Dastani, "The effect of 4-weeks aerobic training according with the usage of Anethum graveolens on blood sugar and lipoproteins profile of diabetic women," *Annals of Biological Research*, vol. 3, no. 9, pp. 4313–4319, 2012.

[10] S. Panda, "The effect of Anethum graveolens L. (dill) on corticosteroid induced diabetes mellitus: involvement of thyroid hormones," *Phytotherapy Research*, vol. 22, no. 12, pp. 1695–1697, 2008.

[11] A. Mohammadi, F. Mirzaei, M. Moradi et al., "Effect of flaxseed on serum lipid profile and expression of NPC1L1, ABCG5 and ABCG8 genes in the intestine of diabetic rat," *Avicenna Journal of Medical Biochemistry*, vol. 1, no. 1, pp. 1–6, 2013.

[12] S. Salmanian, A. R. Sadeghi Mahoonak, M. Alami, and M. Ghorbani, "Phenolic content, antiradical, antioxidant, and antibacterial properties of hawthorn (Crataegus elbursensis) seed and pulp extract," *Journal of Agricultural Science and Technology*, vol. 16, no. 2, pp. 343–354, 2014.

[13] E. Abbasi Oshaghi, I. Khodadadi, M. Saidijam et al., "Lipid lowering effects of hydroalcoholic extract of Anethum graveolens L. and dill tablet in high cholesterol fed hamsters," *Cholesterol*, vol. 2015, Article ID 958560, 7 pages, 2015.

[14] S. Adisakwattana, T. Thilavech, and C. Chusak, "Mesona Chinensis Benth extract prevents AGE formation and protein oxidation against fructose-induced protein glycation in vitro," *BMC Complementary and Alternative Medicine*, vol. 14, no. 1, article 130, 2014.

[15] E. A. Oshaghi, I. Khodadadi, H. Tavilani, and M. T. Goodarzi, "Aqueous extract of Anethum graveolens L. has potential antioxidant and antiglycation effects," *Iranian Journal of Medical Sciences*, vol. 41, no. 4, pp. 328–333, 2016.

[16] E. Oshaghi, I. Khodadadi, H. Tavilani, and M. Goodarzi, "Effect of dill tablet (Anethum graveolens L) on antioxidant status and biochemical factors on carbon tetrachloride-induced liver damage on rat," *International Journal of Applied and Basic Medical Research*, vol. 6, no. 2, pp. 111–114, 2016.

[17] Z. Lisiewska, W. Kmiecik, and A. Korus, "Content of vitamin C, carotenoids, chlorophylls and polyphenols in green parts of dill (Anethum graveolens L.) depending on plant height," *Journal of Food Composition and Analysis*, vol. 19, no. 2-3, pp. 134–140, 2006.

[18] R. Agrawal, N. K. Sethiya, and S. H. Mishra, "Antidiabetic activity of alkaloids of Aerva lanata roots on streptozotocin-nicotinamide induced type-II diabetes in rats," *Pharmaceutical Biology*, vol. 51, no. 5, pp. 635–642, 2013.

[19] M. Setorki, M. Rafieian-Kopaei, A. Merikhi et al., "Suppressive impact of anethum graveolens consumption on biochemical risk factors of atherosclerosis in hypercholesterolemic rabbits," *International Journal of Preventive Medicine*, vol. 4, no. 8, pp. 889–895, 2013.

[20] D. T. Santos, J. Q. Albarelli, M. M. Beppu, and M. A. A. Meireles, "Stabilization of anthocyanin extract from jabuticaba skins by encapsulation using supercritical CO_2 as solvent," *Food Research International*, vol. 50, no. 2, pp. 617–624, 2013.

[21] T. Nakagawa and T. Yokozawa, "Direct scavenging of nitric oxide and superoxide by green tea," *Food and Chemical Toxicology*, vol. 40, no. 12, pp. 1745–1750, 2002.

[22] X. Yin, Y. Zhang, H. Wu et al., "Protective effects of Astragalus saponin I on early stage of diabetic nephropathy in rats," *Journal of Pharmacological Sciences*, vol. 95, no. 2, pp. 256–266, 2004.

[23] N. G. Shehab, E. Abu-Gharbieh, and F. A. Bayoumi, "Impact of phenolic composition on hepatoprotective and antioxidant

effects of four desert medicinal plants," *BMC Complementary and Alternative Medicine*, vol. 15, no. 1, article no. 401, 2015.

[24] I. Erdogan Orhan, F. S. Senol, N. Ozturk, S. A. Celik, A. Pulur, and Y. Kan, "Phytochemical contents and enzyme inhibitory and antioxidant properties of Anethum graveolens L. (dill) samples cultivated under organic and conventional agricultural conditions," *Food and Chemical Toxicology*, vol. 59, pp. 96–103, 2013.

[25] E. Selvin, A. M. Rawlings, M. Grams et al., "Fructosamine and glycated albumin for risk stratification and prediction of incident diabetes and microvascular complications: a prospective cohort analysis of the Atherosclerosis Risk in Communities (ARIC) study," *The Lancet Diabetes & Endocrinology*, vol. 2, no. 4, pp. 279–288, 2014.

[26] R. Nagai, D. B. Murray, T. O. Metz, and J. W. Baynes, "Chelation: a fundamental mechanism of action of AGE inhibitors, AGE breakers, and other inhibitors of diabetes complications," *Diabetes*, vol. 61, no. 3, pp. 549–559, 2012.

[27] H. Javad, H.-Z. Seyed-Mostafa, O. Farhad et al., "Hepatoprotective effects of hydroalcoholic extract of *Allium hirtifolium* (Persian shallot) in diabetic rats," *Journal of Basic and Clinical Physiology and Pharmacology*, vol. 23, no. 2, pp. 83–87, 2012.

[28] L. Marzban, K. Park, and C. B. Verchere, "Islet amyloid polypeptide and type 2 diabetes," *Experimental Gerontology*, vol. 38, no. 4, pp. 347–351, 2003.

[29] M. Sakai, M. Oimomi, and M. Kasuga, "Experimental studies on the role of fructose in the development of diabetic complications," *Kobe Journal of Medical Sciences*, vol. 48, no. 5-6, pp. 125–136, 2002.

[30] A. Thuppia, R. Jitvaropas, S. Saenthaweesuk, N. Somparn, and J. Kaulpiboon, "Hepatoprotective effect of the ethanolic extract of Anethum graveolens L. on paracetamol-induced hepatic damage in rats," *Planta Medica*, vol. 77, no. 12, p. PF18, 2011.

[31] N. M. Rabeh and A. O. Aboraya, "Hepatoprotective effect of dill (*Anethum graveolens* L.) and Fennel (*foeniculum vulgare*) oil on hepatotoxic rats," *Pakistan Journal of Nutrition*, vol. 13, no. 6, pp. 303–309, 2014.

[32] R. Yazdanparast and S. Bahramikia, "Evaluation of the effect of Anethum graveolens L. crude extracts on serum lipids and lipoproteins profiles in hypercholesterolaemic rats," *DARU Journal of Pharmaceutical Sciences*, vol. 16, no. 2, pp. 88–94, 2008.

[33] V. Hajhashemi and N. Abbasi, "Hypolipidemic activity of Anethum graveolens in rats," *Phytotherapy Research*, vol. 22, no. 3, pp. 372–375, 2008.

[34] M. T. Goodarzi, I. Khodadadi, H. Tavilani, and E. Abbasi Oshaghi, "The role of *Anethum graveolens* L. (Dill) in the management of diabetes," *Journal of Tropical Medicine*, vol. 2016, Article ID 1098916, 11 pages, 2016.

[35] R. Tamilarasi, D. Sivanesan, and P. Kanimozhi, "Hepatoprotective and antioxidant efficacy of Anethum graveolens Linn in carbon tetrachloride induced hepatotoxicity in Albino rats," *Journal of Chemical and Pharmaceutical Research*, vol. 4, no. 4, pp. 1885–1888, 2012.

[36] E. Abbasi Oshaghi, H. Tavilani, I. Khodadadi, and M. T. Goodarzi, "Dill tablet: a potential antioxidant and anti-diabetic medicine," *Asian Pacific Journal of Tropical Biomedicine*, vol. 5, no. 9, pp. 720–727, 2015.

9

Physicochemical and Antimicrobial Properties of Cocoa Pod Husk Pectin Intended as a Versatile Pharmaceutical Excipient and Nutraceutical

Ofosua Adi-Dako,[1,2] Kwabena Ofori-Kwakye,[1] Samuel Frimpong Manso,[2] Mariam EL Boakye-Gyasi,[1] Clement Sasu,[2] and Mike Pobee[2]

[1]*Department of Pharmaceutics, Faculty of Pharmacy and Pharmaceutical Sciences, College of Health Sciences, Kwame Nkrumah University of Science and Technology (KNUST), Kumasi, Ghana*
[2]*School of Pharmacy, University of Ghana, Legon, Ghana*

Correspondence should be addressed to Kwabena Ofori-Kwakye; koforikwakye@yahoo.com

Academic Editor: Pornsak Sriamornsak

The physicochemical and antimicrobial properties of cocoa pod husk (CPH) pectin intended as a versatile pharmaceutical excipient and nutraceutical were studied. Properties investigated include pH, moisture content, ash values, swelling index, viscosity, degree of esterification (DE), flow properties, SEM, FTIR, NMR, and elemental content. Antimicrobial screening and determination of MICs against test microorganisms were undertaken using agar diffusion and broth dilution methods, respectively. CPH pectin had a DE of 26.8% and exhibited good physicochemical properties. Pectin had good microbiological quality and exhibited pseudoplastic, shear thinning behaviour, and high swelling capacity in aqueous media. The DE, FTIR, and NMR results were similar to those of previous studies and supported highly acetylated low methoxy pectin. CPH pectin was found to be a rich source of minerals and has potential as a nutraceutical. Pectin showed dose-dependent moderate activity against gram positive and gram negative microorganisms but weak activity against *Listeria* spp. and *A. niger*. The MICs of pectin ranged from 0.5 to 4.0 mg/mL, with the highest activity against *E. coli* and *S. aureus* (MIC: 0.5–1.0 mg/mL) and the lowest activity against *A. niger* (MIC: 2.0–4.0 mg/mL). The study has demonstrated that CPH pectin possesses the requisite properties for use as a nutraceutical and functional pharmaceutical excipient.

1. Introduction

Cocoa or *Theobroma cacao* L. (family: Sterculiaceae) is an important agricultural and economic crop which grows in several tropical areas such as West Africa, South America, and Central America [1, 2]. Cocoa beans are the primary economic part of the cocoa fruit and are the main ingredients in the manufacture of chocolate. In West Africa, cocoa is extensively cultivated in many countries, with Cote d'Ivoire and Ghana being the first and second largest producers of cocoa beans in the world, respectively. In Ghana, cocoa cultivation offers employment to about 800,000 farm families and generates about $2 billion annually in foreign exchange, and it is a major contributor to the gross domestic product [3].

The recovery of cocoa beans from the cocoa fruit generates large amounts of waste in the form of cocoa pod shells

or cocoa pod husks (CPHs) estimated at 52–76% of the cocoa fruit [4–6]. In fact, a ton of dry cocoa beans produced generates approximately ten tons of CPH [7, 8] and the waste generally remains underexploited [1, 5]. After harvesting the beans, CPHs are traditionally left as undesirable waste to rot in the cocoa farms and plantations, constituting an environmental menace and presenting a challenging waste management problem. With the increasing demand for cocoa beans to satisfy the increasing demand for chocolates, it is anticipated that the production of CPH will continue to increase in the years ahead. Decomposing CPH waste, apart from producing foul odours in the cocoa farms and plantations, is a carrier of botanical diseases such as black pod rot [5, 7–9].

An economical and environmentally friendly way of dealing with the CPH waste menace is to process them into pectins which are natural polymers containing linear chains of (1, 4)-linked α-d-galacturonic acid residues, with methyl esters of uronic acid [10]. The composition of pectin is influenced by the botanical source, method of extraction, and environmental factors [11]. For instance, pectin extracted from citrus has less neutral sugars and smaller molecular size compared to pectin from apples [12]. Pectins are versatile naturally occurring polysaccharides with wide and innovative applications in the pharmaceutical, cosmetic, and food industries. In the pharmaceutical industry, pectins are employed as excipients in the manufacture of emulsions, suspensions, matrix tablets, film-coated tablets, compression coated tablets, extended release dosage forms, and colonic delivery dosage forms [13–16].

Various techniques and solvent systems such as water, citric acid, hydrochloric acid, and nitric acid have been employed in the recovery and extraction of pectins from CPH with varying levels of success, with respect to yield and quality of pectin extracted [1, 4, 17–20]. The uses of water and citric acid in the extraction process are, however, more appealing because of their safety and environmental friendliness.

Although considerable research has been devoted to the development of pectin from commercial sources, such as apple pomace and citrus peel, with versatile functional properties in pharmaceutical applications, little attention has been paid to the pharmaceutical applications of CPH pectin. The objective of the present study was to evaluate the physicochemical properties, elemental composition, and antimicrobial properties of CPH extracted with water and citric acid. It is envisaged that results from this study would help in determining the suitability or otherwise of CPH pectin as a potential functional pharmaceutical excipient and nutraceutical.

2. Materials and Methods

2.1. Materials. Sodium hydroxide (UK), gelatin and lead acetate (France), ferric chloride (India), hydrochloric acid and Mayer's reagent (England), and Dragendorff's reagent and Marquis reagent (England) were purchased. Mannitol salt agar, MacConkey agar, Bismuth sulphite agar, Cetrimide agar, Sabouraud dextrose agar, nutrient agar, potato dextrose agar, and nutrient broth were obtained from Oxoid (England). Ciprofloxacin powder (batch number AV 4008, Maxheal Labs Pvt. Ltd., India), Amoksiklav powder (Amoxicillin + clavulanic acid) (Lot EN 2737, Lek Pharmaceuticals, Slovenia), and Nystatin (100,000 IU/drop, Egyptian Pharmaceutical Industries, Egypt) were used. All other chemicals used were of analytical grade.

Two typed cultures, *Staphylococcus aureus* NCTC7972 and *Escherichia coli* NCTC5933, and seven clinical strains, *Bacillus subtilis* KBTH2014, *Pseudomonas aeruginosa* KBTH2014, *Salmonella typhi* NMIMR 2014, *Shigella* spp. NMIMR2014, *Enterococcus* spp. NMIMR2014, *Listeria* spp. NMIMR2014, and *Aspergillus niger* NMIMR2014, were used as test microorganisms.

2.2. Collection and Extraction of CPH Pectin. Ripe mature cocoa pods were harvested from *Theobroma cacao* L. in an experimental plantation of the Cocoa Research Institute of Ghana (CRIG), Tafo, Ghana. The pulp and seeds were removed, and the fresh whole pod husks were peeled to avoid the pigmentation of the skin which may cause longer and more extensive extraction [8, 21, 22]. The peeled husks were minced and prepared for extraction. Pectin was extracted from fresh CPHs according to a previously outlined procedure [1, 23] with minor modifications. Fresh CPHs were minced with a mechanical blender. Hot aqueous and hot aqueous citric acid (4% w/v) extraction of the fresh peeled minced husks (1.05 g/mL) were carried out in a water bath at 50°C. The extract was precipitated with ethanol and filtered twice with two-fold linen cloth. The extract was treated with twice its volume of ethanol and washed thrice to remove impurities. Extraction was repeated to exhaustion and the extract was dried under vacuum. The hot water soluble and hot aqueous citric acid soluble extracts were separately freeze-dried in a freeze dryer (Model 7670520, Labconco, USA) at 0–120 mBar and −41°C and the pectin yield was determined. The freeze-dried pectin samples were stored in aluminium foils in a desiccant at −4°C until used.

2.3. Identification Test and Phytochemical Screening of Pectin. One milliliter of 2 N NaOH was added to 5 mL of 1 in 100 solutions of the CPH extract and was allowed to stand at room temperature for 15 minutes. The gel from the preceding test was acidified with 3 N HCl, shaken vigorously, and boiled [24]. Phytochemical screening [25] of CPH pectin was undertaken to determine the presence or otherwise of major phytoconstituents such as tannins, alkaloids, and saponins. Five hundred milligrams of powdered hot water soluble CPH pectin was boiled in 25 mL of water for 5 min. The solution was cooled and filtered and the volume adjusted to 25 mL and used for the phytochemical screening. In the test for tannins, 1 mL portions of the pectin solution were, respectively, added: (a) 10 mL of water and 5 drops of 1% lead acetate solution, (b) a few drops of 1% gelatin solution, and (c) a few drops of 5% ferric chloride solution. The formation of a white precipitate in (a) and (b) and a dark green or deep blue precipitate in (c) indicated the presence of tannins. To test for alkaloids, a few drops of Marquis reagent, Mayer's reagent, and Dragendorff's reagent were separately added to 2 mL portions of the pectin solution. The observation of a colour change (Marquis) and the formation of cream coloured precipitate (Mayer's) and reddish brown precipitate (Dragendorff's) indicated the presence of alkaloids. In the test for saponins, 5 mL of the pectin solution in a test tube was shaken vigorously for 5 min and the formation of stable foam lasting at least 15 min indicated the presence of saponins.

2.4. Physicochemical Properties of CPH Pectin. The moisture content was determined by weighing 1 g of CPH pectin into each of three petri dishes and dried in an oven at 105°C to constant weight. The moisture content was determined as the ratio of the weight of moisture loss to weight of sample expressed as a percentage. The pH of 1% w/v solution of hot water soluble pectin and citric acid soluble pectin samples was determined with a calibrated pH meter. The total ash content and insoluble ash residue were determined according to the British Pharmacopoeia method [26]. One gram of pectin sample was weighed and ignited in a furnace at 450°C. The ash obtained was weighed and boiled in 25 mL of 2 M HCl for 5 minutes. The insoluble matter was filtered and washed with hot water and ignited. The subsequent weight was then determined. The swelling index of the pectin sample was determined according to a WHO method [27]. One gram of the sample was weighed into a 25 mL measuring cylinder and the volume occupied was noted (V_1). Twenty-five milliliters of distilled water was added to the sample and shaken intermittently for 1 hour. The sample was allowed to stand for 3 hours and the volume occupied was noted (V_2). The swelling capacity was calculated as follows: swelling capacity $= (V_2/V_1) \times 100$. The degree of esterification (DE) was determined using the acid-base titration method of the Food Chemicals Codex [28].

In the determination of the bulk and tapped densities, 3 g of pectin powder was weighed into a 10 mL measuring cylinder and the volume occupied was noted. The sample was tapped till the powder was consolidated and the volume after tapping was noted. The bulk and tapped densities, as well as the Hausner ratio and compressibility index, were calculated as follows:

$$\text{Tapped density} = \frac{\text{weight of pectin}}{\text{tapped volume}},$$

$$\text{Bulk density} = \frac{\text{weight of pectin}}{\text{bulk volume}},$$

$$\text{Hausner ratio} = \frac{\text{tapped density}}{\text{bulk density}}, \qquad (1)$$

Carr's compressibility index

$$= \frac{(\text{tapped density} - \text{bulk density})}{(\text{tapped density})} \times 100.$$

The angle of repose was determined by weighing 10 g of pectin powder into a funnel clamped to a stand with its tip 10 cm from a plane paper surface. The powder was allowed to flow freely onto the paper surface. The height of the cone formed after complete flow and the radius of the cone were used to calculate the angle of repose (θ). Consider $\tan\theta = H/R$, $\theta = \tan^{-1}(H/R)$, where H is the height of the heap and R is the radius of the heap. The viscosity of 5% w/v aqueous solution of cocoa pectin was determined at room temperature (25°C) after heating to 33°C, using a Brookfield viscometer (LVT). Determinations were made using spindle 61, by varying the shear rate. Readings on the dial of the viscometer were multiplied by the conversion factor and the results were recorded.

2.5. Scanning Electron Microscopy (SEM) Studies.
Specimens of hot water soluble pectin and citric acid soluble pectin were prepared for SEM analysis with a thin coating of colloidal carbon for electron conductivity. The morphological features of the samples were studied with a scanning electron microscope (Hitachi S3200N, Japan), using EDAX Genesis. All imaging was viewed under conventional high-vacuum mode and secondary electron scintillator detection mode.

2.6. FTIR, NMR, and Elemental Analysis.
A sample of hot water soluble pectin and citric acid soluble pectin was analysed for main functional groups using Bruker Alpha Fourier transform infrared spectrophotometer (Germany) operating on Platinum-ATR to obtain FTIR spectra at 400–4000 cm^{-1}. Specimens of hot water soluble and citric acid soluble pectin were prepared for NMR analysis using a Varian 500 NMR spectrometer (USA). The ^{13}C NMR spectra of the hot water soluble pectin and citric acid soluble pectin extracts in D_2O were obtained at 25°C and 50°C, respectively. Chemical shifts were expressed in δ (ppm) relative to acetone for hot water soluble pectin (δ 30.16) and citric acid soluble pectin (δ 29.65). The results were analysed by MestReNova NMR. In the elemental analysis, pellets of hot water soluble pectin were prepared and irradiated with an energy dispersive X-ray fluorescence spectrometer (Spectro X-Lab 2000, Kleve, Germany). Peaks shown by the spectrometer indicated the presence of particular elements, while the area under the peaks was an indication of the quantity of elements present.

2.7. Evaluation of Microbiological Quality of CPH Pectin.
Profiling of possible microbial contaminants from cocoa pectin was undertaken [26] and the microbial load (total aerobic viable count) of pectin per the plate viable count was determined. Dilutions of pectin sample (1 : 10) were done serially to a sample dilution of 10^8. One mL aliquot of each dilution was transferred aseptically into 20 mL of molten nutrient agar and the plates were allowed to set. The plates were inverted and incubated for up to 48 hours and pure colony forming colonial (cfu) counts were estimated. The presence of the following pathogenic microbes, E. coli, S. aureus, Salmonella spp., P. aeruginosa, and yeasts and moulds in pectin was evaluated. A 1 : 10 dilution of pectin in sterile water was introduced into the primary medium which was nutrient broth. 1 mL of grown culture of the test organism was introduced into the appropriate culture medium in the molten state at 42°C and stabilised at 28°C. The seeded culture media were incubated at 37°C, with an incubation time of 24–72 hours.

2.8. Antimicrobial Screening of CPH Pectin by Agar Diffusion.
Four concentrations (1.25, 2.5, 5.0, and 10.0 mg/mL) of hot water soluble CPH pectin and standard antibacterial agents, Amoksiklav and ciprofloxacin, as well as the antifungal Nystatin, were used to assess their comparative antimicrobial activities by agar diffusion method [26]. Twenty (20) mL aliquots of molten nutrient agar (antibacterial test) and potato dextrose agar (antifungal test) were melted at 42°C and stabilised at 28°C and aseptically seeded with 0.1 mL of 24 h broth cultures of the appropriate test organisms, poured into sterile petri dishes, and allowed to solidify in a laminar flow chamber. A 10 mm diameter cork borer was used to create four ditches in the set agars. Alternate holes were filled with the exact volumes of aqueous solution of the extracts. Positive and negative test controls were set up alongside the test extract. All plates were left in the chamber for an hour to allow for diffusion. The nutrient agar seeded plates were inverted and incubated at 37°C for 18 hours, while the dextrose agar seeded plates were incubated at room temperature (25°C) for

72 hours. Zones of growth inhibitions due to the activity of the extract and the commercial antimicrobial agents were measured after the incubation periods and recorded.

2.9. Determination of Minimum Inhibitory Concentration (MIC). The MIC of hot water soluble CPH pectin was determined using the broth dilution technique. Graded concentrations of pectin (0.125, 0.25, 0.5, 1.0, 2.0, 4.0., and 8.0 mg/mL) in nutrient broth and potato dextrose liquid medium were compared to those of Amoksiklav, ciprofloxacin, and Nystatin. A set of seven double strength nutrient broth tubes were arranged from a prepared stock solution of 50 mg/mL pectin test sample. Volumes of the stock solution required to produce the respective concentrations with the double strength nutrient broth were calculated and added aseptically to the broth by means of sterile syringes in a laminar flow chamber. The volumes of sterile distilled water required to make the broth tubes single strength were also calculated for and added to the broth tubes aseptically. Finally, 0.1 mL inoculum of a 24 h test microbial culture was inoculated into the broth to complete the procedure. Uniform mixing was ensured and the tubes were incubated at 37°C for 24 h. The tubes were observed for growth (turbidity) after the incubation period and MICs for pectin and the standard antimicrobial agents were determined.

3. Results and Discussions

3.1. Extraction, Identification, and Phytochemical Constituents of CPH Pectin. The extraction yield obtained from CPHs was $23.30 \pm 2.00\%$ and $10.50 \pm 0.04\%$ (on dry weight basis) for hot water soluble pectin and citric acid soluble pectin, respectively. Previous reports indicate that pectin was extracted from dried residue pod husk flour [1, 29]. However, in the current study, extraction was undertaken using fresh CPHs and repeated to exhaustion to optimize the yield [17] which is sometimes affected by drying and associated enzymatic activity [30, 31]. It has been reported that the major part of hot water soluble polysaccharides of CPHs is pectin [32]. Aqueous extraction of pectin has advantages over extraction with mineral acids as there is no production of corrosive effluents [29]. Citric acid is a natural, safe food additive and more attractive to use than other strong mineral acids used in the extraction of commercial pectins, which could adversely affect the environment [1]. The extractive yield of cocoa pectin is known to vary depending on the extraction conditions employed and recent studies have shown yields as low as 2% and as high as 20% [4, 18, 19, 22, 29]. Identification test carried out on the extracted samples yielded colourless gelatinous precipitates indicating the possible presence of pectin in the two extracts.

Phytochemical screening of CPH yielded polyphenols such as tannins, alkaloids, and saponins. Phenolic compounds of cacao include catechins, epicatechins, anthocyanins, proanthocyanidins, phenolic acids, condensed tannins, other flavonoids, and some minor compounds [33–35]. Polyphenolic compounds usually accumulate in the outer parts of plants, such as shells, skins, and husks [36]. Previous reports have shown that CPH flour is a source

TABLE 1: Some physicochemical properties of hot water soluble CPH pectin.

Parameter	Value
Yield on extraction (%)	23.3 ± 2.00
	$10.5 \pm 0.04^{*}$
Moisture content (%)	0.19 ± 0.06
Ash value (%)	1.0
pH (1% w/v @ 25°C)	6.73 ± 0.06
	$3.43 \pm 0.06^{*}$
Swelling index	
0.1 M HCl	357.3 ± 4.6
Phosphate buffer pH 6.8	274.7 ± 4.6
Distilled water	360.0 ± 0.0
Degree of esterification (%)	26.8 ± 2.5
Precompression properties	
Bulk density (g/mL)	1.881
Tapped density (g/mL)	2.200
Hausner ratio	1.17
Compressibility index (%)	14.58
Angle of repose (°)	37.97

*Citric acid soluble pectin.

of functional compounds such as phenolics, pectins, and fibre which possess good health benefits [29]. Polyphenols offer protection against coronary heart disease, cancer, and neurodegenerative disorders due to their antioxidant and free radical scavenging properties [37].

3.2. Physicochemical Properties of CPH Pectin. Table 1 presents some physicochemical properties of cocoa pectin. The pH of a 1% w/v hot water soluble pectin and citric acid soluble pectin was 6.7 and 3.4, respectively. Thus, pH of the aqueous soluble pectin was near neutral, while the high acidity of the citric acid soluble pectin is likely due to the use of citric acid in the extraction process. The moisture content of pectin was very low (0.2%). This is likely to protect the powdered samples from microbial attack and also to improve the mechanical properties of the powders. The level of purity of pectin sample can be determined by its ash value. This value is indicative of the level of adulteration or handling of the sample. The acid insoluble ash value is an index of mineral or extraneous matter present in a sample. High ash values for cocoa pectin in contrast to pectin from other sources have been reported and generally range between 6.7 and 9.8% [18, 22, 29]. However, these varied values could have been affected by the mode of extraction of the sample [18]. In the present study, the acid insoluble ash value of cocoa pectin was 1.0%, in accordance with official specification [24].

The swelling characteristics of cocoa pectin in various media were investigated. The swelling index of cocoa pectin was 274.7 in 0.1 N HCl, 357.3 in phosphate buffer pH 6.8, and 360 in water. Cocoa pectin can swell to varying extents depending on the pH, ionic strength, and presence of salts in the medium. The swelling behaviour of CPH pectin shows that it can function as a binder or matrix agent in controlled release formulations. This is because swelling is an important mechanism in diffusion controlled release in drug delivery [38]. The degree of esterification (DE) of CPH pectin was 26.8%, indicating that it is a low methoxy pectin. This observation is in agreement with earlier reports [1, 29]. The DE determines the behaviour of pectin and influences its mechanism of gelation. Low methoxy pectins have a DE of 20–40%, while high methoxy pectins have a DE of 60–75%. Low methoxy pectins require a controlled amount of calcium or divalent cations to achieve gelation, while high methoxy pectins undergo gelation in the presence of sugar [39].

The precompression parameters of cocoa pectin powder studied were the angle of repose, bulk density, tapped density, Hausner ratio, and Carr's compressibility. The ease of flow of powders is of paramount importance in tablets and capsules formulation as free flowing powders ensure reproducible filling of tablet dies and capsule dosators, thereby improving weight uniformity and consistency in physical properties. Hausner ratio is related to interparticle friction in a powder and values close to 1.2 are indicative of less cohesive and free flowing powder while values greater than 1.6 are powders which are cohesive and have poor flow properties. In terms of flowability, powders with compressibility index of 5–15% are regarded as excellent, 12–16% good, 18–21% fair, and >40% extremely poor. A high angle of repose is indicative of a cohesive powder, while a low angle of repose connotes a noncohesive powder. In general, powders with angles of repose >50° have unsatisfactory flow properties, whereas minimum angles close to 25° have very good flow properties [40]. In the current study, cocoa pectin powder had Hausner ratio of 1.17, compressibility index of 14.58%, and angle of repose of ~38°. These values are indicative of a powder which is less cohesive and has good flow properties.

The rheograms of 5% w/v hot water soluble cocoa pectin at 25°C and 33°C showed a non-Newtonian, pseudoplastic, shear thinning behaviour (Figure 1). This is similar to earlier reports of other pectin solutions and polysaccharide pharmaceutical excipients [1, 29]. Increasing the temperature of the sample from 25°C to 33°C did not have any marked effect on viscosity of the pectin sample ($p > 0.05$, Student's t-test p value of 0.59). Although further investigation is necessary, the pseudoplastic behaviour of cocoa pectin is advantageous in its use as a pharmaceutical excipient.

The scanning electron micrographs of hot water soluble pectin and hot citric acid soluble pectin are shown in Figure 2. The surface characteristics of the samples depict irregular shapes, nonuniform sizes, and rough surfaces. Drug release from a dosage form is affected by the surface characteristics of the excipients used. A rough surface will entrap drug particles in the pores and crevices, resulting in retarded drug release. Hot water soluble and hot citric acid soluble pectin would be able to sustain drug release due to the rough surface exhibited [41]. Both powders contained large to fine particle sizes. Fine particles have a tendency of filling the voids between the larger ones and help to reduce the bulkiness of the powder. Also, the dissolution rate of polysaccharide powders tends to increase with the reduction in particle size [42, 43].

Figure 3 shows the FTIR spectra of CPH pectin extracted with different solvents. The two spectra are identical and

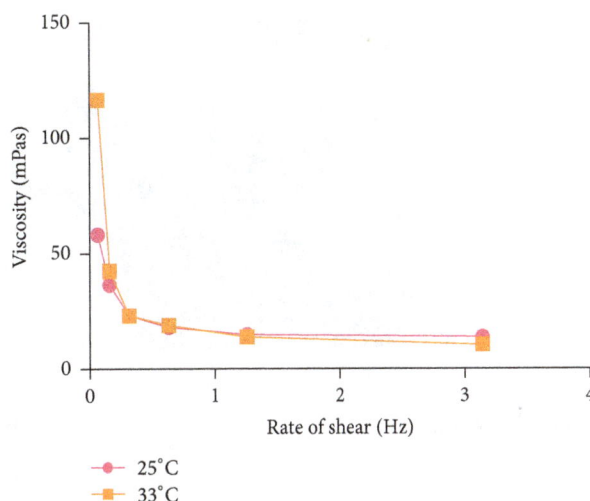

FIGURE 1: Viscosity profiles of 5% w/v hot water soluble pectin.

showed similar functional groups. Data obtained is indicative of –OH stretching absorption bond. Alcohols show a conspicuous –OH stretching absorption bond at 3000–3700 cm^{-1}, which could be narrow or broad depending on whether it is free or involved in hydrogen bonding. The band observed between 2800 and 3100 cm^{-1} is typical of sp3-C–H stretch. Moreover, there was a prominent band between 1000 cm^{-1} and 1200 cm^{-1} which was indicative of a typical C–O stretch such as a glycosidic linkage. The band appearing at 1716 cm^{-1} was typical of a carbonyl group and another band at 1596 cm^{-1} suggests a carboxylate, a salt of a free acid. Furthermore, the band at 2360 cm^{-1} suggests an S–H or C–S bond.

The ^{3}C NMR spectrum of hot water pectin is shown in Figure 4. Chemical shifts were expressed in δ (ppm) relative to acetone (δ 30.16). Chemical shifts due to anomeric carbons were identified in the range δ 95.82–101.4. Signals at δ 101.4 and δ 97.98 were assigned to C-1 of esterified and nonesterified units of α-galacturonic acids, respectively. Previous work showed these signal shifts at δ 100 and 99.3 [1] and δ 100.1 and 99.4 [19], respectively. This is also similar to earlier reports of signals of C-1 of low methoxy pectins in the range δ 101.03–101.43 [44] and of anomeric carbon of α-linkage [45]. Signals observed in the region, δ 170.78, 173.95, 179.87, and 185.44, were assigned to carbonyl groups of the esterified and nonesterified units [46, 47]. C-6 methylated carbonyl signal shifts were identified at δ 170.78 and carboxylic acid signals were identified at δ 173.95. Previous report showed similar high frequency C-6 signals at δ 170.6 and 173.4, respectively [19]. Signals at δ 17.59 were attributed to methyl carbons of rhamnose residues [44]. Signals attributed to C-2, 3, 4, and 5 in the galacturonic acid units were found in the range δ 66.76–80.59. C-4 signal shifts of galacturonic acid units were identified at δ 70.14–71.38 and δ 80.59. Previous work showed signals in the range δ 70-71, with substituted residues with C-4 shifts at δ 77–79, indicating (1, 4) glycosidic linkages in the homogalacturonan region [47]. In the anomeric region, C-1 rhamnose shift was detected at δ 95.82, with the methyl carbon at δ 16.63. Chemical shifts at δ 19.93 were assigned

(a)   (b)

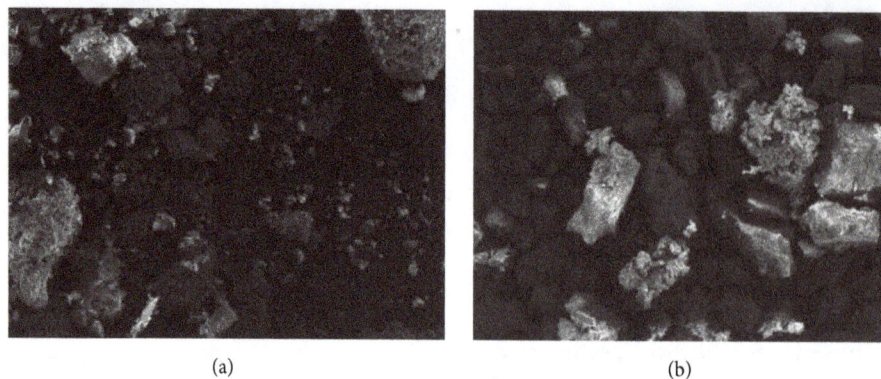

FIGURE 2: Scanning electron micrographs of (a) hot water soluble pectin (mag ×20) and (b) citric acid soluble pectin (mag ×20).

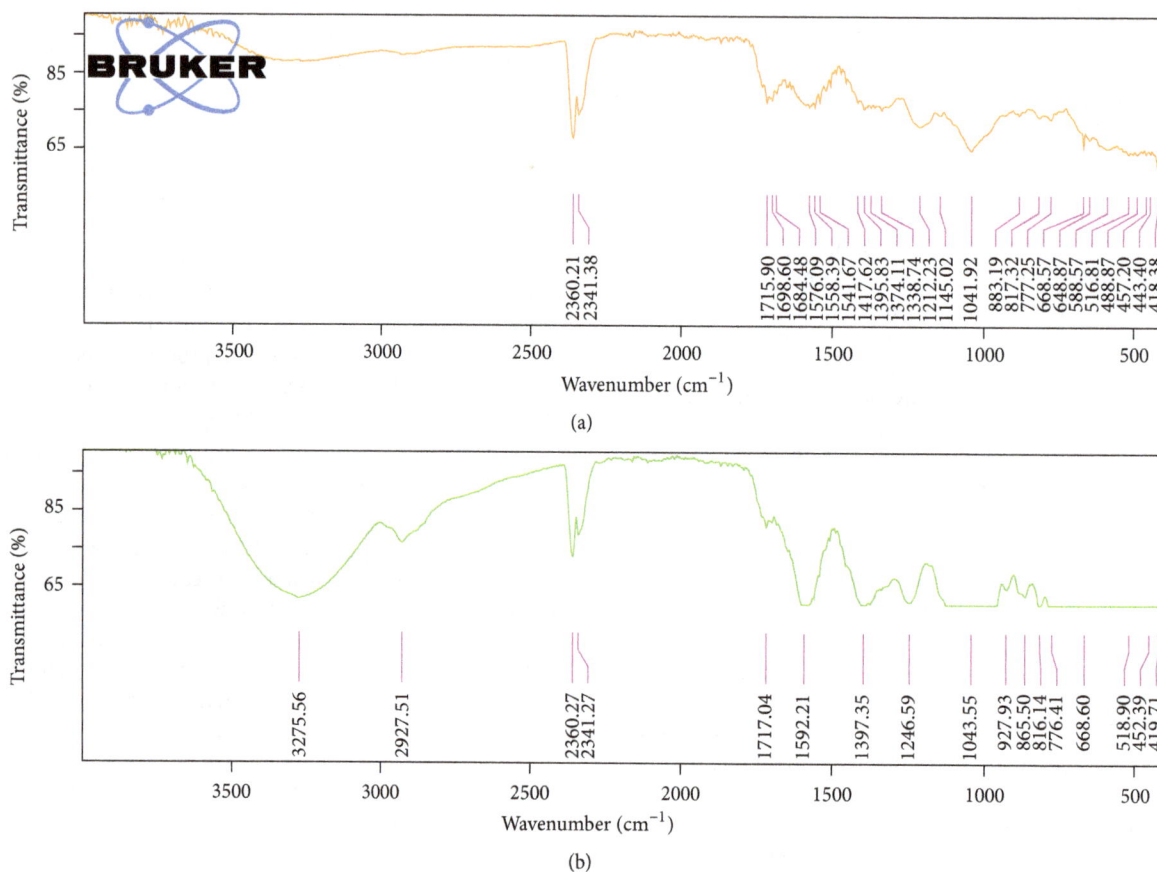

(a)

(b)

FIGURE 3: FTIR spectra of (a) citric acid soluble pectin and (b) hot water soluble pectin.

to methyl groups from the acetyl group [1, 47]. Signals at δ 215.29 were attributed to a carbonyl group from the aldehyde or ketone of the reducing sugar. The data above supports the structure of a highly acetylated low methoxy pectin.

Figure 5 shows the ^{13}C NMR spectrum of citric acid soluble pectin. Chemical shifts of citric acid soluble pectin were expressed in δ (ppm) relative to acetone (δ 29.65). Signal shifts attributed to carbons from citric acid were seen at δ 39.80. Signals at δ 101.4 and δ 97.98 were assigned to C-1 of esterified and nonesterified units of galacturonic acids. Previous work showed these signal shifts at δ 100 and 99.3,

respectively, from methyl ester carbonyl carbons of esterified and nonesterified units from a homogalacturonan [1]. Signal shifts of δ 97.26 were attributed to C-1 rhamnose units with the methyl group at δ 16.62 [46]. Previous reports identified signals at δ 98.5 and 16.6, respectively [1, 19]. Methyl carbons of acetyl groups were seen at a signal shift of δ 19.66. Earlier reports showed the signal at δ 20.5 with C-6 carbonyl carbon of the acetyl group at δ 174.51 [47]. The C-1 signal shifts of δ 102.67 were assigned to C-1 of the anomeric region of substituted and nonsubstituted galacturonic acid units, further supporting β-linkage [45]. Previous reports showed signals at

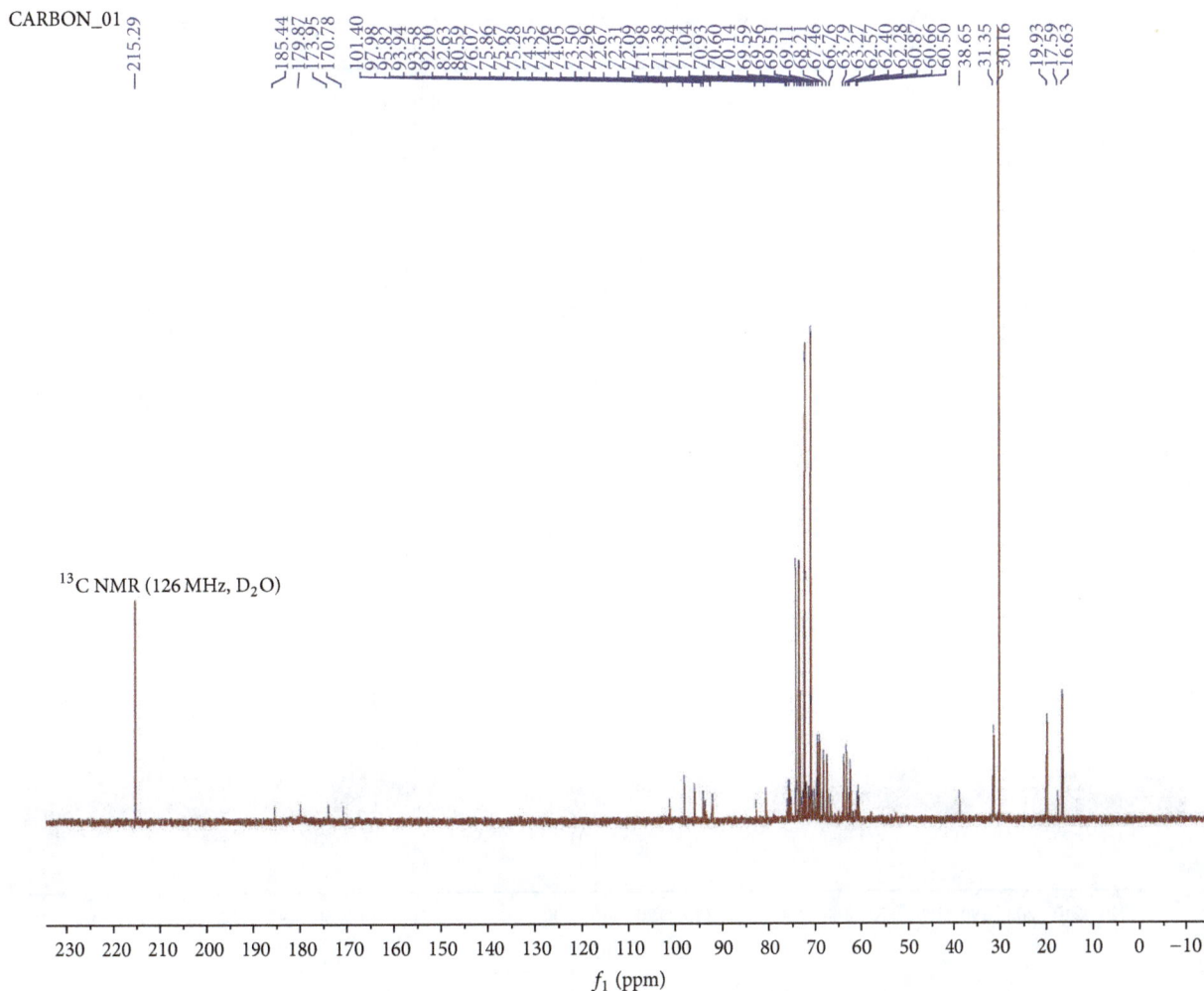

FIGURE 4: ^{13}C NMR spectrum of hot aqueous extract of pectin at 25°C in D$_2$O.

δ 103.3 and δ 102.4, of β 1, 4-D galacturonic acid units. Aromatic carbon signal shifts were observed at δ 151.76 indicating the presence of phenolics [1]. The NMR data shows the presence of highly acetylated pectins with low methoxy groups [1]. The two pectin extracts basically had the same chemical structure which is in accordance with published reports [1, 19].

Results of the elemental analysis of hot water soluble CPH pectin are shown in Table 2. Some major elements or macrominerals identified were sodium, magnesium, calcium, iron, potassium, phosphorus, and sulphur. For the major elements, K was the predominant element (2.269%) followed by Mg (0.219%), P (0.096%), and S (0.094%). Minor elements or microminerals found in cocoa pectin include chromium, copper, zinc, and cobalt. The highest concentration of the minor elements was Cu (10.90%) followed by Zn (8.30%) and Ni (3.70%). Minerals are inorganic substances usually in trace amounts required for the normal functioning of the body. They are involved in bones and teeth development and regulation of metabolic processes of the body by acting as cofactors for enzymes and as catalysts for cell reactions.

TABLE 2: Elemental content of hot water soluble CPH pectin.

Type of element	Content (%)
Macroelements	
Na	>0.038
Mg	0.219
P	0.096
S	0.094
K	2.269
Ca	0.011
Fe	0.024
Microelements	
Cr	<0.0006
Co	<1.90
Ni	3.70
Cu	10.90
Zn	8.30
Ga	0.70
Mo	<0.9

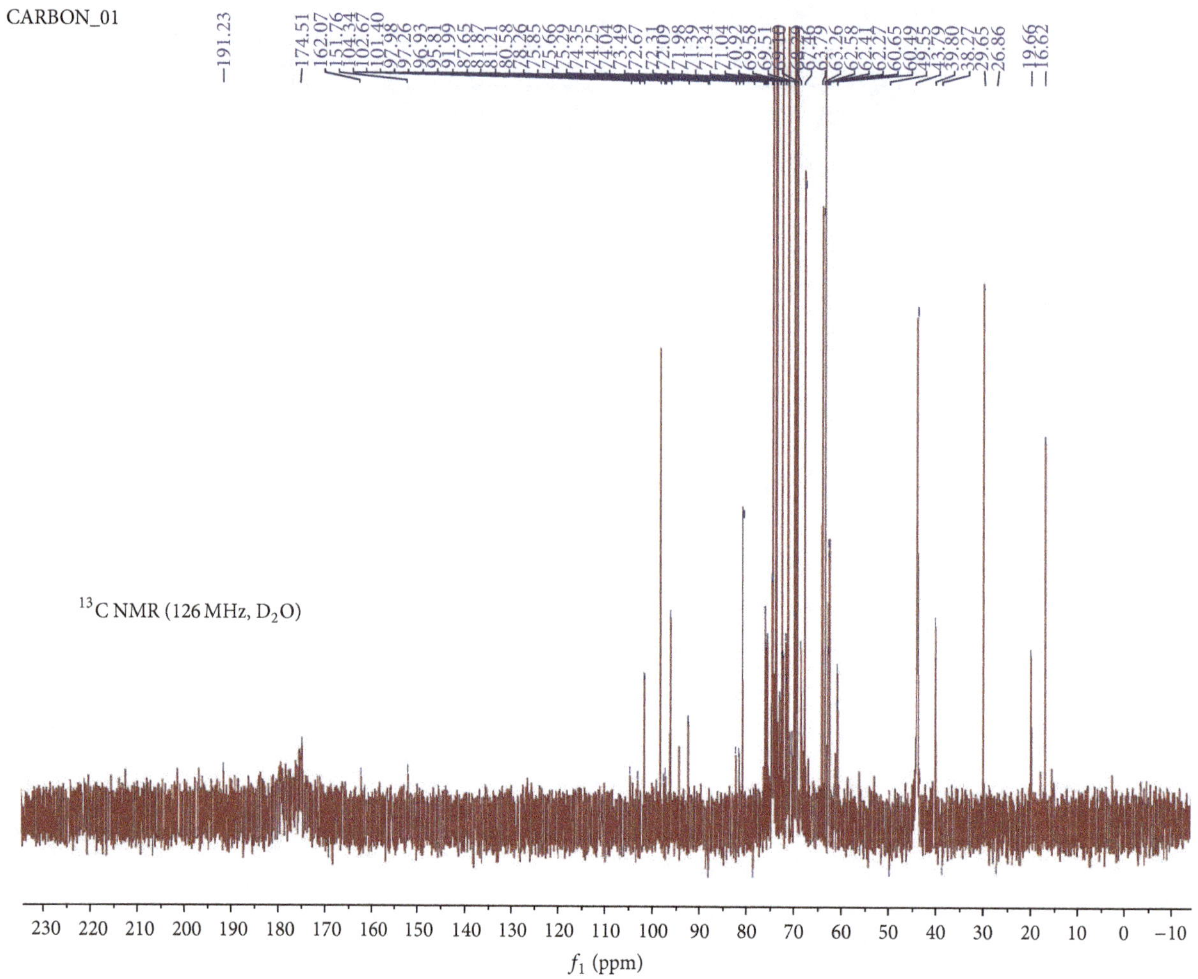

CARBON_01

^{13}C NMR (126 MHz, D$_2$O)

FIGURE 5: ^{13}C NMR spectrum of citric acid soluble pectin at 50°C in D$_2$O.

Previous reports show that CPH flour also contained a variety of minerals. The qualitative components are similar to those reported in previous studies [5]. In one study, a predominance of K was observed, followed by Ca and Mg, with intermediate proportions of Na, Fe, Mn, and Zn and minor amounts of Cu and Se [29]. Another study reported Ca and K as the major elements [18], while an African cocoa pod husk was found to contain K (3.18%), Ca (0.32%), and P (0.15%) as the major elements [48]. The minerals content of CPH pectin affects both the viscosity and the swelling capacity of the polymer in aqueous media.

The wide range of macro- and microminerals found in cocoa pectin shows the potential of this natural polymer to provide medical or health benefits users. Cocoa pectin is therefore a potential plant-based nutraceutical. There is a growing interest in the use of plant-derived bioactive compounds in foods as "multifunctional food additives" due to their additional nutritional and therapeutic effects [49, 50]. Other plant-based bioactive materials with demonstrable nutraceutical properties include citrus fruits, modified citrus pectin, and apple pectin [51–54]. Plant polysaccharides such as cocoa pectin are generally nontoxic, chemically stable, readily available and renewable, and a rich source of macro- and micronutrients. These polysaccharides are under extensive investigation as potential excipients for the formulation of solid and liquid dosage forms and also as a nutraceutical.

3.3. Microbial Quality and Antimicrobial Properties of CPH Pectin.

In general, microbial contaminants may be grouped into harmful, objectionable, and opportunistic organisms. Harmful organisms are toxins-producing, disease causing organisms such as *S. typhi*, *E. coli*, *P. aeruginosa*, and *S. aureus*. Objectionable organisms can cause disease or may interrupt the function of the agent leading to the deterioration of the product. These include *Salmonella* species (proteolytic types) and fungi (mycotoxin producing types), *Pseudomonas* spp., and *Candida albicans*. Organisms are said to be opportunistic if they produce disease or infection under special environmental conditions. Harmful organisms are excluded from all pharmaceutical products and excipients. With regard to the CPH pectin sample tested, no harmful microorganisms were identified (Table 3) and the total microbial count was within the specified limit; hence, it passed the microbial quality test [26].

The antimicrobial activity of CPH pectin against selected microbial strains is presented in Table 4. The activity of CPH pectin against test microbial strains indicated by the zones

TABLE 3: Microbial quality of hot water soluble CPH pectin.

Test protocol	Results	Inference
Total aerobic viable count of sample (BP 2007 specification: $\leq 1 \times 10^5$ cfu/mL)	1.2×10^1 cfu/mL	Passed
Test for *Escherichia coli*, MCA/37°C/48 h (BP 2007 specification: nil)	None detected	Passed
Test for *Staphylococcus aureus*, MSA/37°C/48 h (BP 2007 specification: nil)	None detected	Passed
Test for *Salmonella* spp., BSA/37°C/48 h (BP 2007 specification: nil)	None detected	Passed
Test for *Pseudomonas aeruginosa*, CA/37°C/48 h (BP 2007 specification: nil)	None detected	Passed
Test for *yeasts and moulds*, SDA/25°C/5 days (BP 2007 specification: $\leq 1.0 \times 10^4$ cfu/mL)	None detected	Passed

MCA = MacConkey agar; MSA = Mannitol salt agar; BSA = Bismuth sulphite agar; CA = Cetrimide agar; SDA = Sabouraud dextrose agar.

TABLE 4: Antimicrobial properties of hot water soluble CPH pectin and standard antimicrobial agents against test organisms.

Organisms	Mean zones of inhibition (mm)			
	10 mg/mL	5 mg/mL	2.5 mg/mL	1.25 mg/mL
Gram negative bacteria				
	26.0 ± 0.5	25.0 ± 1.0	22.5 ± 0.5	20.0 ± 0.0
Escherichia coli	$35.0 \pm 0.0^{a*}$	$32.0 \pm 1.0^{a*}$	$30.9 \pm 0.1^{a*}$	$29.0 \pm 0.0^{a*}$
	$37.0 \pm 1.0^{a***}$	$34.9 \pm 0.9^{a***}$	$30.0 \pm 1.0^{a***}$	$26.9 \pm 0.9^{a***}$
	24.0 ± 0.5	23.2 ± 0.2	22.0 ± 0.0	19.4 ± 0.6
Pseudomonas aeruginosa	$36.9 \pm 0.1^{a*}$	$35.0 \pm 1.0^{a*}$	$30.0 \pm 1.0^{a*}$	$27.8 \pm 0.8^{a*}$
	$38.9 \pm 0.8^{a***}$	$37.8 \pm 0.8^{a***}$	$32.0 \pm 0.0^{a***}$	$30.0 \pm 0.0^{a***}$
Salmonella typhi	25.0 ± 1.0	23.2 ± 0.2	20.5 ± 0.5	18.0 ± 0.0
Shigella spp.	22.0 ± 0.0	20.3 ± 0.8	18.0 ± 0.0	16.0 ± 0.0
Gram positive bacteria				
	24.0 ± 0.0	22.5 ± 0.5	19.6 ± 0.6	17.0 ± 0.0
Staphylococcus aureus	$33.9 \pm 0.1^{b*}$	$27.3 \pm 0.6^{b*}$	$25.0 \pm 0.0^{b*}$	$22.0 \pm 1.0^{b*}$
	$36.0 \pm 0.0^{a***}$	$33.9 \pm 0.9^{a***}$	$29.9 \pm 0.1^{a***}$	$24.7 \pm 0.6^{a***}$
	24.0 ± 0.0	22.5 ± 0.5	20.0 ± 0.5	17.0 ± 0.0
Bacillus subtilis	$36.0 \pm 0.0^{a*}$	$30.9 \pm 0.2^{a*}$	$28.0 \pm 1.0^{a*}$	$25.0 \pm 1.0^{a*}$
	$38.0 \pm 0.0^{a***}$	$33.0 \pm 1.0^{a***}$	$24.9 \pm 0.9^{b***}$	$20.1 \pm 0.9^{b***}$
Enterococcus spp.	18.0 ± 0.5	16.0 ± 0.0	15.0 ± 0.0	12.7 ± 0.3
Listeria spp.	15.0 ± 0.0	13.0 ± 0.0	12.0 ± 0.0	ND
Fungus				
	18.0 ± 0.7	16.3 ± 0.4	15.0 ± 0.0	ND
Aspergillus niger	$20.3 \pm 0.4^{b***}$	$18.5 \pm 0.0^{b***}$	$17.0 \pm 0.0^{b***}$	$15.1 \pm 0.1^{***}$

*Amoksiklav; **ciprofloxacin; ***Nystatin; ND = not determined; ᵃstatistically different from pectin ($p < 0.05$); ᵇnot statistically different from pectin ($p > 0.05$).

of growth inhibitions was interpreted as follows: ≥ 30 mm, exceptionally active; 25–30 mm, active; 20–25 mm, moderately active; 15–20 mm, slightly active; <15 mm, peripheral/weak activity [55]. CPH pectin showed dose-dependent moderate antibacterial activity in concentrations of 1.25–10 mg/mL against *S. aureus*, *P. aeruginosa*, *B. subtilis*, *E. coli*, *Salmonella typhi*, and *Shigella* spp. and slight activity against *Enterococcus* spp. and *Aspergillus niger*. It however showed weak activity against *Listeria* spp. in concentrations up to 10 mg/mL. On the other hand, Amoksiklav and ciprofloxacin showed active and exceptionally active activity, respectively.

Generally, CPH pectin exhibited better activity against gram negative than gram positive bacteria.

Table 5 presents a comparative analysis of the MICs of CPH pectin and three standard antimicrobial agents on selected bacteria and fungus strains. For the three gram positive bacteria tested, cocoa pectin had the lowest MIC hence the highest activity against *E. coli*, while the MICs of ciprofloxacin were generally lower than that of cocoa pectin against the test organisms. The MIC of cocoa pectin was lower for *S. aureus* than *B. subtilis*; hence, pectin is more active against *S. aureus*. Also, the MICs of Amoksiklav were

TABLE 5: Minimum inhibitory concentrations (MICs) of CPH pectin and standard antimicrobial agents against test organisms.

Organisms	MIC (mg/mL)			
	CPH pectin	Amoksiklav	Ciprofloxacin	Nystatin
Gram negative bacteria				
Escherichia coli	0.5–1.0	ND	0.125–0.250	ND
Pseudomonas aeruginosa	1.0–2.0	ND	0.500–1.000	ND
Salmonella typhi	1.0–2.0	ND	0.250–0.500	ND
Gram positive bacteria				
Staphylococcus aureus	0.5–1.0	0.25–0.50	ND	ND
Bacillus subtilis	1.0–2.0	0.50–1.00	ND	ND
Fungus				
Aspergillus niger	2.0–4.0	ND	ND	0.5–1.0

ND = not determined.

lower than that of pectin against the gram positive bacteria tested. The MIC of cocoa pectin against *A. niger* was four times higher than that of Nystatin, the standard antifungal product. The study has demonstrated that cocoa pectin has some activity against all the tested microorganisms. However, the antimicrobial activity was generally lower than that of the three standard antimicrobial agents compared.

The antimicrobial activity of CPH extract was assessed recently against *S. aureus*, *S. epidermidis*, *B. subtilis* (gram positive), *P. aeruginosa*, *K. pneumoniae*, and *S. cholerae* [55]. The researchers found the extract to be ineffective up to 10 mg/mL against the gram positive bacteria tested, but it showed activity against *P. aeruginosa*, *S. choleraesuis*, and *S. epidermidis*. The strongest antibacterial activity was shown against *S. choleraesuis* (MIC: 1.0 mg/mL) and *S. epidermidis* (MIC: 2.5 mg/mL) and the bioactive fractions of the extract were found to be phenols, steroids, or terpenes [56]. The antimicrobial properties of cocoa phenolics against some food bacterial pathogens and certain cariogenic bacteria have also been reported [57]. In that study, the activity of cocoa phenolics was directly correlated with the ability of the chemical substances to penetrate the bacterial cell wall [33, 57]. In view of the antibacterial properties observed, cocoa pectin has the potential to be developed as an antimicrobial agent for extended release natural products and in food preservation [58].

4. Conclusion

It can be concluded from the study that cocoa pectin has the requisite microbial quality and physicochemical parameters to be employed as a multifunctional excipient in the pharmaceutical, food, and allied industries. The elemental content analysis showed the presence of a broad range of micro- and macronutrients in cocoa pectin, making it a potentially useful health promotion polymer. Cocoa pectin showed moderate activity against selected gram positive and gram negative bacteria and could be useful as a preservation agent in pharmaceutical formulations and food products. The study has demonstrated the enormous potential of cocoa pectin as a pharmaceutical excipient, a nutraceutical agent, and an antibacterial agent.

Competing Interests

The authors declare that there is no conflict of interests regarding the publication of this paper.

Acknowledgments

The authors gratefully acknowledge the University of Ghana Office of Research, Innovation and Development (ORID) for providing a Faculty Development Grant to OAD in support of this study. Special thanks are also due to Dr. Jeremy Takrama of the Cocoa Research Institute of Ghana (CRIG), Tafo, Ghana, for his technical assistance.

References

[1] L. C. Vriesmann, R. F. Teófilo, and C. Lúcia de Oliveira Petkowicz, "Extraction and characterization of pectin from cacao pod husks (*Theobroma cacao* L.) with citric acid," *LWT— Food Science and Technology*, vol. 49, no. 1, pp. 108–116, 2012.

[2] D. Sailaja, P. Srilakshmi, K. Puneeth, and C. Ramya Krishna, "Estimation of protein content and phytochemicals studies in cocoa fruit outer covering," *International Journal of Plant, Animal and Environmental Sciences*, vol. 5, no. 1, pp. 111–115, 2015.

[3] Ghana Cocobod, "Maintaining the standard for Ghana's premium quality cocoa," October 2015, https://www.cocobod.gh/home_section.php?sec=1.

[4] S.-Y. Chan and W.-S. Choo, "Effect of extraction conditions on the yield and chemical properties of pectin from cocoa husks," *Food Chemistry*, vol. 141, no. 4, pp. 3752–3758, 2013.

[5] A. Donkoh, C. C. Atuahene, B. N. Wilson, and D. Adomako, "Chemical composition of cocoa pod husk and its effect on growth and food efficiency in broiler chicks," *Animal Feed Science and Technology*, vol. 35, no. 1-2, pp. 161–169, 1991.

[6] O. A. Fagbenro, "Results of preliminary studies on the utilization of cocoa-pod husks in fish production in South-west Nigeria," *Biological Wastes*, vol. 25, no. 3, pp. 233–237, 1988.

[7] Z. Kalvatchev, D. Garzaro, and F. G. Cedezo, "*Theobroma cacao* L.: un nuevoenfoque para nutrición y salud," *Agroalimentaria*, vol. 6, pp. 23–25, 1998.

[8] A. Figueira, J. Janick, and J. N. BeMiller, "Partial characterization of cacao pod and stem gums," *Carbohydrate Polymers*, vol. 24, no. 2, pp. 133–138, 1994.

[9] H. Barazarte, E. Sangronis, and E. Unai, "Cocoa (Theobroma cacao L.) hulls: a posible commercial source of pectins," *Archivos Latinoamericanos de Nutricion*, vol. 58, no. 1, pp. 64–70, 2008.

[10] S. Sungthongjeen, T. Pitaksuteepong, A. Somsiri, and P. Sriamornsak, "Studies on pectins as potential hydrogel matrices for controlled-release drug delivery," *Drug Development and Industrial Pharmacy*, vol. 25, no. 12, pp. 1271–1276, 1999.

[11] B. R. Thakur, R. K. Singh, A. K. Handa, and M. A. Rao, "Chemistry and uses of pectin—a review," *Critical Reviews in Food Science and Nutrition*, vol. 37, no. 1, pp. 47–73, 1997.

[12] C. E. Beneke, A. M. Viljoen, and J. H. Hamman, "Polymeric plant-derived excipients in drug delivery," *Molecules*, vol. 14, no. 7, pp. 2602–2620, 2009.

[13] T. W. Wong, G. Colombo, and F. Sonvico, "Pectin matrix as oral drug delivery vehicle for colon cancer treatment," *AAPS PharmSciTech*, vol. 12, no. 1, pp. 201–214, 2011.

[14] K. Ofori-Kwakye and J. T. Fell, "Biphasic drug release from film-coated tablets," *International Journal of Pharmaceutics*, vol. 250, no. 2, pp. 431–440, 2003.

[15] X. Wei, N. Sun, B. Wu, C. Yin, and W. Wu, "Sigmoidal release of indomethacin from pectin matrix tablets: effect of in situ crosslinking by calcium cations," *International Journal of Pharmaceutics*, vol. 318, no. 1-2, pp. 132–138, 2006.

[16] K. Ofori-Kwakye, J. T. Fell, H. L. Sharma, and A.-M. Smith, "Gamma scintigraphic evaluation of film-coated tablets intended for colonic or biphasic release," *International Journal of Pharmaceutics*, vol. 270, no. 1-2, pp. 307–313, 2004.

[17] C. Mollea, F. Chiampo, and R. Conti, "Extraction and characterization of pectins from cocoa husks: a preliminary study," *Food Chemistry*, vol. 107, no. 3, pp. 1353–1356, 2008.

[18] D. Adomako, "Cocoa pod husk pectin," *Phytochemistry*, vol. 11, no. 3, pp. 1145–1148, 1972.

[19] L. C. Vriesmann, R. F. Teófilo, and C. L. D. O. Petkowicz, "Optimization of nitric acid-mediated extraction of pectin from cacao pod husks (*Theobroma cacao* L.) using response surface methodology," *Carbohydrate Polymers*, vol. 84, no. 4, pp. 1230–1236, 2011.

[20] M. Arlorio, J. D. Coisson, P. Restani, and A. Martelli, "Characterization of pectins and some secondary compounds from *Theobroma cacao* hulls," *Journal of Food Science*, vol. 66, no. 5, pp. 653–656, 2001.

[21] G. K. Jani, D. P. Shah, V. D. Prajapatia, and V. C. Jain, "Gums and mucilages: versatile excipients for pharmaceutical formulations," *Asian Journal of Pharmaceutical Sciences*, vol. 4, no. 5, pp. 309–323, 2009.

[22] B. M. Yapo and K. L. Koffi, "Extraction and characterization of gelling and emulsifying pectin fractions from cacao pod husk," *Nature*, vol. 1, no. 4, pp. 46–51, 2013.

[23] R. Malviya, P. Srivastava, M. Bansal, and P. K. Sharma, "Mango peel pectin as a superdisintegrating agent," *Journal of Scientific and Industrial Research*, vol. 69, no. 9, pp. 688–690, 2010.

[24] United States Pharmacopoeia and National Formulary, *United States Pharmacopoeia XXIII*, U.S.P Convention, Rockville, Md, USA, 2007.

[25] N. Raaman, *Phytochemical Techniques*, New India Publishing Agency, New Delhi, India, 2006.

[26] British Pharmacopoeia, *British Pharmacopoeia Commission*, Her Majesty's Stationery Office, London, UK, 2007.

[27] World Health Organization (WHO), "Determination of swelling index," in *Quality Control Methods for Plant Materials*, p. 51, World Health Organization (WHO), Geneva, Switzerland, 1998, http://apps.who.int/iris/bitstream/10665/41986/1/9241545100.pdf.

[28] National Research Council, *Food Chemicals Codex*, National Academy of Sciences, Washington, DC, USA, 3rd edition, 1981.

[29] L. C. Vriesmann, R. D. de Mello Castanho Amboni, and C. L. de Oliveira Petkowicz, "Cacao pod husks (*Theobroma cacao* L.): composition and hot-water-soluble pectins," *Industrial Crops and Products*, vol. 34, no. 1, pp. 1173–1181, 2011.

[30] C. D. May, "Industrial pectins: Sources, production and applications," *Carbohydrate Polymers*, vol. 12, no. 1, pp. 79–99, 1990.

[31] P. C. Sharma, A. Gupta, and P. Kaushal, "Optimization of method for extraction of pectin from apple pomace," *Indian Journal of Natural Products and Resources*, vol. 5, no. 2, pp. 184–189, 2014.

[32] W. R. Blakemore, E. T. Dewar, and R. A. Hodge, "Polysaccharides of the cocoa pod husk," *Journal of the Science of Food and Agriculture*, vol. 17, no. 12, pp. 558–560, 1966.

[33] M. Arlorio, J. D. Coïsson, F. Travaglia et al., "Antioxidant and biological activity of phenolic pigments from *Theobroma cacao* hulls extracted with supercritical CO_2," *Food Research International*, vol. 38, no. 8-9, pp. 1009–1014, 2005.

[34] F. Sánchez-Rabaneda, O. Jáuregui, I. Casals, C. Andrés-Lacueva, M. Izquierdo-Pulido, and R. M. Lamuela-Raventós, "Liquid chromatographic/electrospray ionization tandem mass spectrometric study of the phenolic composition of cocoa (*Theobroma cacao*)," *Journal of Mass Spectrometry*, vol. 38, no. 1, pp. 35–42, 2003.

[35] J. Wollgast and E. Anklam, "Review on polyphenols in *Theobroma cacao*: changes in composition during the manufacture of chocolate and methodology for identification and quantification," *Food Research International*, vol. 33, no. 6, pp. 423–447, 2000.

[36] E. Lecumberri, R. Mateos, M. Izquierdo-Pulido, P. Rupérez, L. Goya, and L. Bravo, "Dietary fibre composition, antioxidant capacity and physico-chemical properties of a fibre-rich product from cocoa (*Theobroma cacao* L.)," *Food Chemistry*, vol. 104, no. 3, pp. 948–954, 2007.

[37] Y. Wan, J. A. Vinson, T. D. Etherton, J. Proch, S. A. Lazarus, and P. M. Kris-Etherton, "Effects of cocoa powder and dark chocolate on LDL oxidative susceptibility and prostaglandin concentrations in humans," *American Journal of Clinical Nutrition*, vol. 74, no. 5, pp. 596–602, 2001.

[38] E. Akpabio, C. Jackson, P. Ubulom, M. Adedokun, R. Umoh, and C. Ugwu, "Formulation and in vitro release properties of va plant gum obtained from *Sesamum indicum* (Fam. pedaliaceae," *International Journal of Pharmaceutical and Biomedical Research*, vol. 2, no. 3, pp. 166–171, 2011.

[39] P. Sriamornsak, "Chemistry of pectin and its pharmaceutical uses: a review," *Silpakorn University International Journal*, vol. 3, no. 1-2, pp. 206–228, 2003.

[40] M. E. Aulton, *Aulton's Pharmaceutics: The Design and Manufacture of Medicines*, Churchill Livingstone, London, UK, 2007.

[41] E. Sallam, H. Ibrahim, M. Takieddin, M. A. Shamat, and T. Baghal, "Dissolution characteristics of interactive powder mixtures. Part two: effect of surface characteristics of excipients," *Drug Development and Industrial Pharmacy*, vol. 14, no. 9, pp. 1277–1302, 1988.

[42] L. Pachuau, H. Lalhlenmawia, and B. Mazumder, "Characteristics and composition of *Albizia procera* (Roxb.) Benth gum," *Industrial Crops and Products*, vol. 40, no. 1, pp. 90–95, 2012.

[43] S. W. Cui, *Food Carbohydrates: Chemistry, Physical Properties, And Applications*, CRC Press, Boca Raton, Fla, USA, 2005.

[44] A. Sinitsya, J. Copiková, and H. Pavliková, "^{13}C CP/MAS NMR spectroscopy in the analysis of pectins," *Journal of Carbohydrate Chemistry*, vol. 17, no. 2, pp. 279–292, 1998.

[45] W. A. Bubb, "NMR spectroscopy in the study of carbohydrates: characterizing the structural complexity," *Concepts in Magnetic Resonance—Part A: Bridging Education and Research*, vol. 19, no. 1, pp. 1–19, 2003.

[46] B. O. Petersen, S. Meier, J. Ø. Duus, and M. H. Clausen, "Structural characterization of homogalacturonan by NMR spectroscopy-assignment of reference compounds," *Carbohydrate Research*, vol. 343, no. 16, pp. 2830–2833, 2008.

[47] B. Westereng, T. E. Michaelsen, A. B. Samuelsen, and S. H. Knutsen, "Effects of extraction conditions on the chemical structure and biological activity of white cabbage pectin," *Carbohydrate Polymers*, vol. 72, no. 1, pp. 32–42, 2008.

[48] G. S. Hutomo, D. W. Marseno, S. Anggrahini, and Supriyanto, "Synthesis and characterization of sodium carboxymethylcellulose from pod husk of cacao (*Theobroma cacao* L.)," *African Journal of Food Science*, vol. 6, no. 6, pp. 180–185, 2012.

[49] A. Belščak, D. Komes, D. Horžić, K. K. Ganić, and D. Karlović, "Comparative study of commercially available cocoa products in terms of their bioactive composition," *Food Research International*, vol. 42, no. 5-6, pp. 707–716, 2009.

[50] S. Martins, S. I. Mussatto, G. Martínez-Avila, J. Montañez-Saenz, C. N. Aguilar, and J. A. Teixeira, "Bioactive phenolic compounds: production and extraction by solid-state fermentation—a review," *Biotechnology Advances*, vol. 29, no. 3, pp. 365–373, 2011.

[51] K. E. Kalra, "Nutraceutical-definition and introduction," *AAPS PharmSci*, vol. 5, no. 3, pp. 27–28, 2003.

[52] R. E. Wildman, R. Wildman, and T. C. Wallace, *Handbook of Nutraceuticals and Functional Foods*, CRC Press, New York, NY, USA, 2006.

[53] N. K. Fuchs, *Modified Citrus Pectin (MCP): A Super Nutraceutical*, Basic Health Publications, Laguna Beach, Calif, USA, 2004.

[54] K. Kolodziejczyk, J. Markowski, M. Kosmala, B. Król, and W. Plocharski, "Apple pomace as a potential source of nutraceutical products," *Polish Journal of Food and Nutrition Sciences*, vol. 57, no. 4, pp. 291–295, 2007.

[55] M. Harris, *Pharmaceutical Microbiology*, Bailliere, Tindall & Cox, London, UK, 1964.

[56] R. X. Santos, D. A. Oliveira, G. A. Sodré, G. Gosmann, M. Brendel, and C. Pungartnik, "Antimicrobial activity of fermented theobroma cacao pod husk extract," *Genetics and Molecular Research*, vol. 13, no. 3, pp. 7725–7735, 2014.

[57] K. Osawa, T. Matsumoto, T. Maruyama, Y. Naito, K. Okuda, and I. Takazoe, "Inhibitory effects of aqueous extract of cacao bean husk on collagenase of *Bacteroides gingivalis*," *The Bulletin of Tokyo Dental College*, vol. 31, no. 2, pp. 125–128, 1990.

[58] P. J. P. Espitia, W.-X. Du, R. De Jesús Avena-Bustillos, N. D. F. F. Soares, and T. H. McHugh, "Edible films from pectin: physical-mechanical and antimicrobial properties—a review," *Food Hydrocolloids*, vol. 35, pp. 287–296, 2014.

10

In Vitro and In Vivo Correlation of Colon-Targeted Compression-Coated Tablets

Siddhartha Maity,[1] **Amit Kundu,**[2] **Sanmoy Karmakar,**[2] **and Biswanath Sa**[1]

[1]*Division of Pharmaceutics, Department of Pharmaceutical Technology, Jadavpur University, Kolkata 700032, India*
[2]*Division of Pharmacology, Department of Pharmaceutical Technology, Jadavpur University, Kolkata 700032, India*

Correspondence should be addressed to Biswanath Sa; biswanathsa2003@yahoo.com

Academic Editor: Jae Hyung Park

This study was performed to assess and correlate in vitro drug release with in vivo absorption of prednisolone (PDL) from a colon-targeted tablet prepared by compression coating of core tablet. In vivo drug absorption study was conducted using a high performance liquid chromatographic (HPLC) method, which was developed and validated for the estimation of PDL in rabbit plasma. The calibration curve showed linearity in the concentration range of 0.05 to 50 μg/mL with the correlation coefficient (r) of 0.999. The method was specific and sensitive with the limit of detection (LOD) and lower limit of quantification (LLOQ) of 31.89 ± 1.10 ng/mL and 96.63 ± 3.32 ng/mL, respectively. The extraction recovery (ER) of PDL from three different levels of quality control (QC) samples ranged from 98.18% to 103.54%. In vitro drug release study revealed that less than 10% drug was released in 6.34 h and almost complete (98.64%) drug release was achieved in the following 6 h. In vivo drug absorption study demonstrated lower values of C_{max}, AUC_{total}, and protracted T_{max} from compression-coated tablet. The results confirmed the maximum release of drug in the colon while minimizing release in the upper gastrointestinal tract (GIT). An excellent in vitro and in vivo correlation (IVIVC) was also achieved after considering the lag time.

1. Introduction

In recent years, colon-targeted oral drug delivery systems have been investigated extensively to achieve better therapeutic response of anticancer, anti-inflammatory, steroidal, and anthelmintic drugs, which are used in various colon-related diseases [1]. The most important advantage of colon-targeted drug delivery system is to provide a high concentration of therapeutic agent at the site of action while minimizing premature drug release in the upper gastrointestinal tract (GIT), namely, stomach and small intestine, and thus reducing the emergence of adverse effects to nontarget areas [2]. Different technologies based on site-specific triggering have been developed to drive the drug molecules to the colon bypassing the upper GIT and to provide a sigmoidal drug release pattern involving a longer lag time (T_{lag}) followed by burst release in the colon. The approaches include coating with pH-sensitive polymers, time dependent release systems, and compression coating with polysaccharides [3].

Several pH-sensitive microspheres dosage forms for colon targeting of drugs have been reported. pH-sensitive poly(3-hydroxybutyrate) based microspheres blended with cellulose acetate phthalate (CAP) [4] and polyethylene glycol cross-linked chitosan microspheres coated with CAP [5] have been reported to bypass the release of 5-fluorouracil (5-FU), an anticancer drug, in the gastric acidic environment and to provide slow release in intestinal condition. Polyhydroxybutyrate blended with CAP microsphere has also been found to provide prolongation of cytotoxic effect of 5-FU [6].

However, pH-sensitive and time dependent release systems exhibit unpredictable site specificity, respectively, because of large inter- and intrasubject variation and almost similar pH values of small intestinal and colonic fluids [7] and wide variation in gastric retention time [8]. Among the various technologies, compression-coated systems based on natural polysaccharides appear to be promising because they are degraded by the enzymes produced by the anaerobic microflora of colon [7, 9].

Natural polysaccharides have been used extensively in designing colon-targeted tablet dosage forms because they are biocompatible and biodegradable [10], highly stable, safe, nontoxic, and hydrophilic and fall under the category "generally regarded as safe" (GRAS) [11, 12]. Additionally, chemical modifications impart many important functionalities over the native polysaccharides for diverse application [13]. Frequently, a blend of polysaccharides provides more desirable drug release profile than a single polymer [14, 15]. Several polysaccharides such as guar gum, pectin, sodium alginate, and locust bean gum which remain undigested in the upper GIT but degrade by the enzymes secreted by colonic microflora have found applications in the formulation of compression-coated tablets [12, 16].

It has, however, been reported that the composition of human gut ecosystem may vary depending on the age, geographic provenance, dietary habit, disease, and intake of antibiotics and probiotics [17]. Moreover, degradation of certain polysaccharides like xanthan gum by colonic bacteria is questionable due to rigid structural framework [18–20]. Hence, it is rational to design a colon-targeted tablet by compression coating with polysaccharides that erodes slowly enough to retard premature drug release in the upper GIT and then provides burst release of the drug from the core tablet in the colon in the absence of colonic bacterial enzymes.

Xanthan gum, an exopolysaccharide obtained from *Xanthomonas campestris*, chemically consists of β,1-4-D-glucose backbone and a trisaccharide side chain consisting of two mannose residues separated by a glucuronic acid, attached with alternate glucose residues. The terminal D-mannose residue may contain a pyruvate group and the mannose closest to the backbone contains an acetyl function [21]. Sustained release of drugs from native xanthan gum tablets is well documented [21, 22]. We previously reported that matrix tablets composed of Ca^{+2} ion cross-linked carboxymethyl xanthan gum retarded the initial release of prednisolone for a considerable period of time, although complete drug release even in 10 h was not achievable [23]. Subsequently, we developed a compression-coated tablet in which core tablet of prednisolone containing microcrystalline cellulose (MCC, 55 mg), crospovidone (CP, 9 mg), trisodium citrate (TSC, 10 mg), and prednisolone (PDL, 15 mg) was coated with 225 mg of a blend of carboxymethyl xanthan gum (CMXG) and sodium alginate (SAL) in a ratio of 1.5 : 3.5, and the resulting tablet provided T_{lag}, the time required to release 10% or less drug, of 6.06 h followed by a pulse release within 4.36 h, and, thus, the optimized tablet appeared suitable for colon specific delivery of PDL without the intervention of colonic bacterial enzymes in dissolution fluid [24].

Therefore, the objective of this study was to assess and correlate preclinical pharmacokinetic profiles of PDL with in vitro release from the compression-coated tablet. In order to facilitate oral administration of the tablet in rabbit, a minitablet having the same composition of the previously optimized tablet was prepared and was subjected to in vitro drug release study under dynamic pH shift condition and in vivo drug absorption study on rabbit's model. An HPLC method was developed and validated to estimate the concentration of PDL obtained from rabbit's plasma.

Prednisolone (PDL), a synthetic glucocorticoid, is most widely used in the treatment of human ailment [25], such as rheumatoid arthritis, inflammatory bowel diseases, psoriasis, and asthma [26–28]. It is used for controlling the symptoms/inducing remission in both ulcerative colitis (UC) and Crohn's disease (CD) [29]. In spite of desired pharmacological responses, it also induces a larger number of multifarious adverse effects when absorbed from the upper GIT [30, 31] and hence appears to be a suitable drug for targeting into the colon [32].

2. Materials and Methods

2.1. Materials. Prednisolone (PDL) and dexamethasone as internal standard (IS) were obtained from Mepro Pharmaceuticals, Mumbai, India. Carboxymethyl xanthan gum (CMXG) having a degree of substitution 0.8 was synthesized in our laboratory. Sodium alginate (SAL), $CaCl_2$, $2H_2O$ ($CaCl_2$), microcrystalline cellulose, PH 102 (MCC), polyplasdone XL (crospovidone, CP), trisodium citrate (TSC), magnesium stearate (MS), and trisodium orthophosphate dodecahydrate (TSP) were purchased commercially. Methanol (HPLC-grade) was obtained from Rankem Pvt. Ltd. Dimethyl sulfoxide (DMSO), ethyl acetate (EA), ammonium acetate (AA), formic acid (FA), polyethylene glycol (PEG-400), and EDTA were purchased from Merck Specialties Pvt. Ltd., Mumbai, India. HPLC-grade Milli-Q water was used throughout the study. All other reagents and solvents of analytical grade were used as received.

2.2. Animals. The in vivo absorption study was conducted on 18 adult healthy male New Zealand rabbits weighing 1.5–2.0 Kg. The study was carried out as per the standard guidelines of "Committee for the Purpose of Control and Supervision of Experiments on Animals (CPCSEA)," Ministry of Social Justice and Empowerment, Government of India, and was approved by the Institutional Ethics Committee, Department of Pharmaceutical Technology, Jadavpur University, Kolkata (Approved Protocol number AEC/PHARM/1407/2014). Rabbits were acclimatized with 12 h light and dark cycles for 15 days and were given free access to standard food and water *ad libitum*. Rabbits were divided into three groups each consisting of six animals ($n = 6$) and were kept in fasted state 24 h prior to the experiment. Group I animals were given 0.1 mL of intravenous bolus of PDL (10 mg/mL PDL in 50% v/v of PEG-400 in sterile water for injection). Group II and Group III animals received, respectively, an immediate release core tablet and a compression-coated tablet both containing 5 mg of PDL.

2.3. Preparation of Core and Compression-Coated Tablets. The core and compression-coated tablets were prepared using 1/3rd of the ingredients used in the formulation of the optimized tablet having a larger size [24]. Initially, immediate release core tablets having a crushing strength of about 4 Kg, the composition and physical characteristics of which are shown in Table 1, were prepared by directly compressing

TABLE 1: Composition and physical characteristics of core tablet.

Ingredients	Weight (mg)
PDL	5
MCC	18.33
CP	3
TSC	3.33
MS	0.34
Total	30
Physical characteristics	
Thickness (mm)	2.95 ± 0.06
Friability (%)	0.89%
Drug content (mg)	5.05 ± 0.25
Weight variation (%)	-4.08 to 4.84

TABLE 2: Composition and physical characteristics of compression-coated tablet.

Composition of coating material	Weight (mg)
CMXG	18.75
SAL	43.75
CaCl$_2$	12.50
Total	75
Physical characteristics of coated tablet	
Thickness (mm)	3.62 ± 0.04
Friability (%)	0.78
Weight variation (%)	-3.26 to 2.00

a blend of drug and excipients with 3 mm punch in a 10-station rotary minipress tablet machine (RIMEK, Karnavati Engineering Ltd., Gujarat, India).

Granules, the composition of which is shown in Table 2, were prepared by wet massing a blend of CMXG and SAL with required amount of CaCl$_2$ solution. The resulting damp mass was passed through #22 BS screen (width of aperture 0.710 mm) and dried at 60°C to a residual moisture content of 2–4%. The compression-coated tablets having a crushing strength of about 6 Kg were prepared in the following way: core tablet was placed centrally in 40% of the granules kept in a 5.5 mm die and remaining 60% granules were placed over the core tablet and compressed into tablet using a flat face 5.5 mm punch in a 10-station rotary minipress tablet machine (RIMEK, Karnavati Engineering Ltd., Gujarat, India). Fifty core tablets and compression-coated tablets were prepared in duplicate.

2.3.1. Evaluation of Physical Characteristics of Tablets. The weight variation and friability of both the core and compression-coated tablets were evaluated following the methods as described in Indian Pharmacopoeia [33]. Drug contents of the core tablets were determined as per the method described elsewhere [23].

2.3.2. In Vitro Drug Release Study. In vitro drug release study was performed as per the method described previously [23]. Six compression-coated tablets were placed in 700 mL 0.1 (M) HCl solution (37 ± 0.5°C) of pH 1.2 contained in 6 vessels of

USP-II dissolution rate test apparatus (TDP-06P, Electro Lab, Mumbai, India) and rotated with paddles at 100 rpm. The pH of the solution was increased after 2 h to 7.4 by adding 200 mL 0.2 (M) trisodium orthophosphate dodecahydrate. After an additional 3 h period, the pH of the solution was changed to 6.8 by adding 5 mL 2 (M) HCl. Aliquots were removed at predetermined times and replenished immediately after each withdrawal with the same volume of fresh media maintained at 37°C. The aliquots following suitable dilution were analyzed at 248 nm using Microplate Spectrophotometer (Multiskan Go, Thermo Scientific, USA). The amount of PDL released from the tablets was calculated using calibration curves drawn in the respective dissolution medium.

2.4. Bioanalytical Method Development

2.4.1. Instrumentation and Chromatographic Conditions. The HPLC system (Shimadzu, Kyoto, Japan) consisted of a LC-20AD solvent delivery unit, a SPD-M20A photodiode array detector, and Rheodyne injector with a 100 μL loop. Detection and quantification were performed using LC solution. Chromatographic separation was performed isocratically at a flow rate of 1.0 mL/min using a Phenomenex C18 column (particle size 5 μm; 250 mm × 4.6 mm i.d.; Phenomenex, Torrance, USA) at 25°C. The mobile phase consisted of methanol and buffer (5 mM ammonium acetate and 0.1% formic acid in Milli-Q water, pH 3.0) in a volume ratio of 58 : 42. 40 μL of sample was injected into the loop of injector and the eluted peaks were measured at 245 nm using UV detector.

2.4.2. Preparation of Stock and Working Solutions. Stock solutions of PDL and IS were prepared at a concentration of 2 mg/mL in DMSO and were stored at 2–8°C until being used. The working stocks of PDL were prepared from 2 mg/mL stock of PDL in DMSO by diluting the stock solution with 50% v/v DMSO solution in Milli-Q water afresh before use. The working stock (25.00 μg/mL) of IS in ethyl acetate was also prepared from the stock solution of IS in DMSO (2 mg/mL).

2.4.3. Preparation of Calibration Standards and Quality Control (QC) of Samples. In order to construct calibration curve, eleven calibration points in the analytical ranges from 0.05 to 50.00 μg/mL of PDL with a fixed concentration of IS at 83.33 μg/mL were selected. 10 μL aliquot of PDL working solution (spiking solution) was spiked with 90 μL of blank plasma and 500 μL of IS (25 μg/mL) in ethyl acetate (EA). The samples of spiked plasma were vortexed for 5 min for complete extraction of PDL and IS in EA fraction, centrifuged (RMI2C, Remi Cooling Centrifuge, Mumbai, India) at 7000 rpm for 10 min and allowed to stand for 30 min. The supernatant EA fraction was collected carefully and evaporated to dryness under a stream of nitrogen. The residues were reconstituted with 150 μL of freshly prepared mobile phase. Finally, the samples were filtered through 0.2 μm syringe filter, and 40 μL was injected into the HPLC system. Three levels of QC samples at lower, middle, and higher concentration (LQC, MQC, and HQC), for example,

0.150 μg/mL (LQC), 20.00 μg/mL (MQC), and 40.00 μg/mL (HQC), were also prepared in a similar way.

2.5. Bioanalytical Method Validation.

2.5. Bioanalytical Method Validation. The method was validated for specificity, linearity, accuracy and precision, extraction recovery, and stability according to the guidelines and protocols of the United States Food and Drug Administration [34].

2.5.1. Specificity. The determination of specificity was performed by comparing the chromatograms of sample containing analyte (PDL) and IS against the blank plasma spiked with IS.

2.5.2. Linearity. The linearity of calibration curve was assessed by eleven different concentrations of analyte (PDL) ranges from 0.05 to 50.00 μg/mL with a constant concentration of IS (83.33 μg/mL) in spiked plasma samples. Peak area ratios for each concentration level of analytes to IS were measured in six replicates ($n = 6$) and the calibration curve was constructed from the least square linear regression analysis. The linearity was represented as correlation coefficient (r).

2.5.3. Accuracy and Precision. To determine the accuracy and precision, three QC samples (LQC, MQC, and HQC) were analysed for three consecutive days. Precision and accuracy were expressed in terms of coefficient of variation (% CV) and relative error (% RE), respectively. In case of precision, the values of CV ≤ 15% for MQC and HQC and CV ≤ 20% for LQC are acceptable. Similarly, in case of accuracy, the values of RE ≤ 15% for MQC and HQC and RE ≤ 20% for LQC are acceptable [34].

2.5.4. Sensitivity. The limit of detection (LOD) and lower limit of quantification (LLOQ) were determined according to the following equation:

$$\text{LOD or LLOQ} = \delta\left(\frac{S_D}{S}\right), \tag{1}$$

where δ is a constant (3.3 for LOD and 10 for LLOQ), S_D is the standard deviation of the analytical signal, and S is the slope of the concentration versus response graph.

2.5.5. Extraction Recovery. The extraction recovery (ER) of analyte (PDL) at three different levels of QC samples ($n = 6$) was evaluated by comparing the peak area responses from the plasma samples spiked with analyte before extraction with those from blank plasma samples extracted and spiked with the same concentration of analyte after extraction. Similarly, the extraction recovery for IS was also performed for a particular concentration of 83.33 μg/mL.

2.5.6. Stability. Blank plasma, spiked with three different levels of QC samples, namely, LQC (0.150 μg/mL), MQC (20.00 μg/mL), and HQC (40.00 μg/mL), was stored at different conditions: at room temperature for 24 h for short term, −20°C for one month and 3 months for long term,

and 3 cycles for freeze-thaw stability studies. Area under the curves (AUCs) of the three levels of QC samples were measured.

2.6. In Vivo Absorption Study. Blood samples (0.5 mL) after intravenous (IV) bolus and oral administration of the respective formulations were collected carefully from the rabbit's marginal ear vein at 5, 15, 30, 60, 90, 120, 180, and 240 min intervals for Group I, at 5, 15, 30, 60, 120, 180, 240, 300, and 360 min intervals for Group II, and at 5, 15, 30, 60, 120, 240, 360, 420, 480, 540, 600, 630, 660, and 720 min intervals for Group III animals. The samples were collected in 1.5 mL microcentrifuge tube (Eppendorf, USA) containing 10% (w/v) of EDTA solution, immediately centrifuged at 3000 rpm for 5 min at 15°C in a Cold Centrifuge (Heraeus Megafuge 1.0R, Thermo Scientific, USA), and the supernatant plasma layers were separated and stored at −4°C until being used. The pharmacokinetic parameters including maximum plasma concentration (C_{max}), the time required to reach C_{max} (T_{max}), and mean residence time (MRT) were calculated using a software package (Kinetica 5.1).

2.7. In Vitro and In Vivo Correlation (IVIVC). In vitro and in vivo correlation (IVIVC) is a predictive mathematical model, which describes the correlation between an in vitro (amount of drug released) and in vivo (amount of drug absorbed) results of a dosage form. Level A correlation is generally described as linear and represents a point-to-point relationship between in vitro drug release and the in vivo absorption of drugs. Level A IVIVC model using deconvolution method [35] has been adopted in this study design. In order to establish the IVIVC, percentage of drug absorbed in the systemic circulation after oral administration of various formulations was calculated based on the following model independent deconvoluted equation [36]:

$$C(t) = \int_0^t C_{\delta iv}(t - u) \cdot \Gamma_{\text{abs-vivo}}(u) \cdot du, \tag{2}$$

where $C(t)$ is the plasma concentration after oral administration of different tablets at time t, $C_{\delta iv}$ represents the plasma concentration after intravenous bolus injection, $\Gamma_{\text{abs-vivo}}$ represents in vivo absorption rate, and u is the variable of integration.

3. Results and Discussion

3.1. Preparation, Evaluation, and Drug Release from Compression-Coated Tablet. In order to facilitate animal feeding, minicore (3 mm) and compression-coated (5.5 mm) tablets were prepared by 1/3rd reduction in the composition of the larger tablets optimized previously [24]. The immediate release core tablets and compression-coated tablets intended for colon specific delivery of PDL complied with the Pharmacopoeial requirement [34] with respect to weight variation, drug content, and friability (Tables 1 and 2).

In vitro drug release studies were conducted in a condition mimicking the pH and transit time in GIT. Drug release from the core tablets was rapid and complete within 45 min

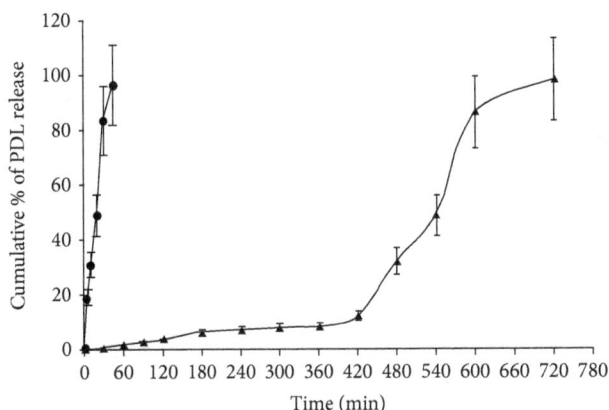

FIGURE 1: In vitro drug release profiles of immediate release core tablet (●) and compression-coated tablet (▲).

TABLE 3: Summary of the calibration standards at different levels of concentration.

Nominal concentration (μg/mL)	Observed concentration (μg/mL) (mean ± SD, $n = 6$)	% CV	% RE
50.00	50.296 ± 0.0077	0.02	0.59
25.00	25.124 ± 0.0037	0.01	0.50
12.50	12.559 ± 0.0031	0.02	0.48
6.25	6.271 ± 0.0021	0.03	0.34
3.125	3.145 ± 0.0007	0.02	0.64
1.56	1.568 ± 0.0011	0.07	0.54
0.80	0.785 ± 0.0002	0.02	−1.82
0.40	0.395 ± 0.0008	0.20	−1.26
0.20	0.198 ± 0.0000	0.01	−0.81
0.10	0.100 ± 0.0001	0.13	0.02
0.05	0.050 ± 0.0004	0.74	−0.77

(Figure 1) indicating that total amount of drug was released in gastric pH. On the other hand, only 3.9% and 8.69% drug were released from the compression-coated tablets, respectively, in 2 h and 6 h. In order to ascertain that drug release from the minitablet did not differ considerably from the previously optimized tablet having larger size, similarity (f_2) and dissimilarity (f_1) factors were determined and compared [37]. It was found that f_2 value was 57.03 ± 1.02, whereas f_1 value was 8.92 ± 0.41. This indicates that the release profile of tablet in reduced form did not change appreciably.

T_{lag}, defined as the time required to release 10% or less drug, was found to be 6.34 h. During the next 6 h period almost complete (98.64%) drug release was achieved (Figure 1). T_{rap}, the time required for rapid release following the lag time, was calculated by subtracting T_{lag} from the time required for complete release and was found to be about 6 h. This indicates an effective shielding of PDL release for an initial 6 h period during which the tablet may be located in the upper GIT and a rapid and complete release within the subsequent 6 h period when the tablet remains in the colon. Based on the results of in vitro drug release study it may be presumed that compression-coated tablets coated with a blend of Ca^{+2} ion cross-linked CMXG and SAL (1.5 : 3.5) might be suitable for colon targeting of PDL without the need of colonic bacterial enzymes.

3.2. Bioanalytical Method Development and Validation.
The HPLC method developed was sufficiently sensitive and suitable for estimation of PDL in rabbit's plasma. The specificity of an analytical method is the ability to differentiate and quantify the analyte (PDL) in the presence of any kind of interfering substances in the sample. The HPLC chromatograms of blank plasma spiked with IS and spiked with IS and PDL have been shown in Figure 2.

The retention time (R_t) of IS and PDL varied from 15.86 ± 0.15 min to 15.98 ± 0.05 min and 10.91 ± 0.06 min to 11.00 ± 0.026 min, respectively. It was also noted that the chromatogram of PDL was not interfered by the endogenous substances of plasma as most of the interferences were found within 4 min. The calibration curve exhibited excellent

linearity in the concentration range of 0.05 to 50 μg/mL with correlation coefficient of 0.999. The calibration equation shows the average slope of 0.00693 (±0.00001, range: 0.00692 to 0.00694) and intercept of −0.000014 ± 0.000005. Table 3 showed that all back calculated values of eleven calibration points were excellent in terms of accuracy (% RE) and precision (% CV).

The intraday and interday run precision (% CV) and accuracy (% RE) of PDL for three levels of QC sample (LQC, MQC, and HQC) ranged from 1.82 to 6.44% and −0.38 to 5.63%, respectively, and were within the acceptable limits (Table 4).

The limit of detection (LOD) and lower limit of quantification (LLOQ) were found to be, respectively, 31.89 ± 1.10 ng/mL and 96.63 ± 3.32 ng/mL indicating adequate sensitivity of the method for pharmacokinetic study. Moreover, the mean recoveries of PDL at LQC (0.150 μg/mL), MQC (20.00 μg/mL), and HQC (40.00 μg/mL) samples were, respectively, 100.50 ± 1.34%, 98.22 ± 2.36%, and 103.77 ± 8.26%. The mean recovery of IS was 102.79 ± 3.79% of the concentration used in the assay procedure. Finally, the % CV and % RE under short term and long term stability studies varied from 1.67 to 7.30% and −0.56 to 4.14%, respectively, and were within the acceptable limits (Table 5).

3.3. In Vivo Drug Absorption Study.
Intravenous bolus injection of PDL was given in Group I animals to obtain data for in vitro and in vivo correlation (IVIVC). Immediate release core tablets and compression-coated tablets each containing 5 mg of PDL were given orally to Group II and Group III animals, respectively. The plasma concentration time profiles obtained following administration of the drug in different dosage forms are shown in Figure 3, and in vivo absorption parameters are depicted in Table 6.

The first sign of appearance of PDL in plasma in a concentration of 515.65 ± 4.48 ng/mL was recorded within 5 min following the administration of core tablets. The peak plasma concentration (C_{max}) and the time (T_{max}) required

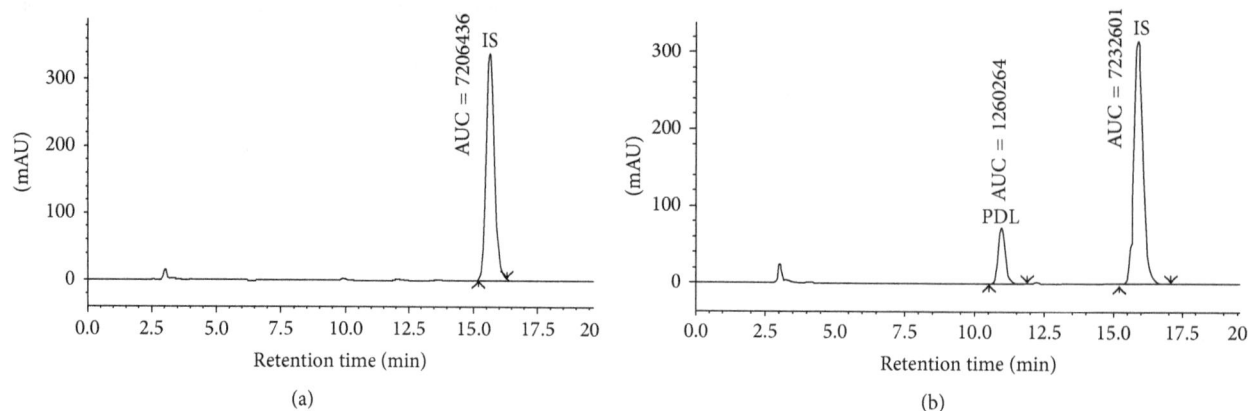

Figure 2: HPLC chromatogram of (a) plasma spiked with IS (83.33 μg/mL) and (b) plasma spiked with PDL (25.00 μg/mL) and IS (83.33 μg/mL).

Table 4: Summary of the intraday (n = 3) and interday (n = 9) precision (% CV) and accuracy (% RE) of the three levels of quality control (QC) samples.

Nominal concentration (μg/mL)	Mean observed concentration (μg/mL)	% CV	% RE
1st day (n = 3)			
0.150	0.151 ± 0.0028	1.85	−0.38
20.00	19.45 ± 0.48	2.48	2.73
40.00	38.10 ± 2.41	6.31	4.76
2nd day (n = 3)			
0.150	0.151 ± 0.0028	1.83	−0.47
20.00	19.53 ± 0.75	3.83	2.33
40.00	40.46 ± 1.46	3.60	−1.15
3rd day (n = 3)			
0.150	0.151 ± 0.0038	2.54	−0.68
20.00	18.87 ± 1.11	5.88	5.63
40.00	38.78 ± 2.50	6.44	3.05
Interday (n = 9)			
0.150	0.151 ± 0.0027	1.82	−0.51
20.00	19.29 ± 0.78	4.03	3.56
40.00	39.11 ± 2.15	5.51	2.22

Table 5: Summary of the short term and long term stability study data in three different levels of QC samples.

Nominal concentration (μg/mL)	Mean observed concentration (μg/mL)	% CV	% RE
3 freeze/thaw cycles (n = 6)			
0.150	0.144 ± 0.01	7.30	4.14
20.00	20.11 ± 0.81	4.02	−0.56
40.00	37.93 ± 2.03	5.36	5.17
Room temperature at 24 h (n = 6)			
0.150	0.148 ± 0.0073	4.91	1.11
20.00	19.56 ± 1.33	6.80	2.19
40.00	40.80 ± 2.47	6.06	−1.99
1 month at −20°C (n = 6)			
0.150	0.153 ± 0.0026	1.67	−2.05
20.00	19.23 ± 1.33	6.91	3.83
40.00	39.32 ± 1.73	4.41	1.69
3 months at −20°C (n = 6)			
0.150	0.145 ± 0.0046	3.13	3.12
20.00	19.74 ± 0.93	4.71	1.31
40.00	38.59 ± 1.45	3.75	3.53

to reach C_{max} were, respectively, 1172.28 ± 22.98 ng/mL and 60 min. The drug concentration in plasma declined to 114.92 ± 6.28 ng/mL at the end of 5 h. On oral administration of the compression-coated tablets, quantifiable amount of PDL (100.42 ± 2.81 ng/mL) in plasma was found at 6 h. The plasma drug concentration increased slowly and C_{max} of 245.40 ± 10.42 ng/mL was reached at 10 h (T_{max}) following which concentration declined and reached a level of 109.35 ± 4.29 ng/mL after 12 h. The results indicated that while PDL was rapidly absorbed from the stomach from the core tablets, compression-coated tablets released very small amount of drug in upper GIT within 6 h. This correlates well with the in

vitro drug release where the drug tended to increase rapidly only after 6 h and almost complete drug release occurred within 12 h. Comparison of AUC_{total} values revealed that availability of the drug in systemic circulation from the compression-coated tablets was less than that from the core tablet. This was due to difference in anatomical region of drug release [38]. Compression-coated tablets released the drug in the colon as evident from considerable delay in the appearance of the drug in the plasma. Lower AUC_{total} value is an indication of reduced drug absorption from the limited absorptive surface of colon [39]. MRT of compression-coated

TABLE 6: In vivo absorption parameters of PDL from various dosage form.

Parameters	Intravenous (IV)	Core tablet	Compression-coated tablet
C_{max} (ng/mL)	1624.29 ± 15.22	1172.28 ± 22.98	245.40 ± 10.42
T_{max} (min)	5	60	600
AUC_{total} (min·ng/mL)	104537 ± 1292.80	146075 ± 4133.50	83926.37 ± 1469.03
MRT (min)	130.05 ± 2.25	138.33 ± 5.74	572.33 ± 7.90

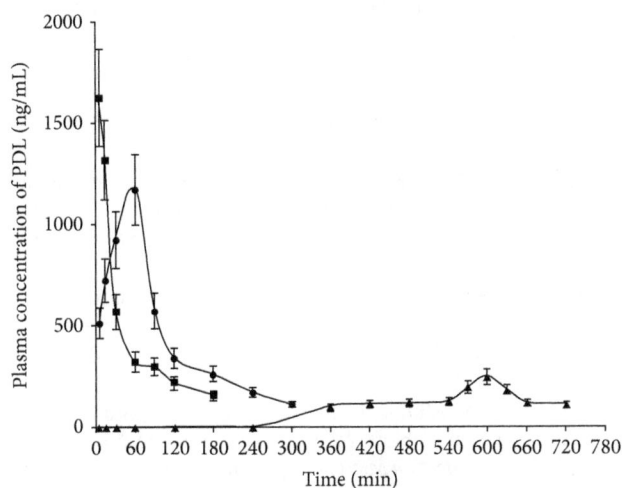

FIGURE 3: Plasma concentration versus time profiles of PDL obtained after oral administration of intravenous (IV) bolus administration (■), immediate release core tablet (●), and colon-targeted compression-coated tablet (▲).

tablets increased about 4 times in comparison to the core tablets suggesting that compression-coated tablet remained in the GIT for a prolonged period and did not expose the enclosed core tablet until it reached the colon.

3.4. In Vitro and In Vivo Correlation (IVIVC). To assess the correlation between in vitro drug release and in vivo drug absorption data, IVIVC study was carried out using immediate release core tablet and colon-targeted compression-coated tablet. When the cumulative percentage of drug released in vitro from immediate release core tablet was plotted against the percentage of drug absorbed in vivo, a good linear correlation (0.997) was observed (Figure 4).

In case of compression-coated tablet, when the cumulative percentage of drug released was plotted against percentage of drug absorbed in vivo, a poor correlation (0.842) was observed. However, a good correlation (0.992) was observed when the cumulative percentage of drug released in vitro versus percentage of drug absorbed in vivo was plotted after considering the lag time of 360 min. Moreover, the IVIVC of colon-targeted compression-coated tablet appeared to be a hockey-stick curve that corresponds to nonlinear characteristics of drug release, and drug absorbed from the compression-coated tablet indicates that the mixed function of drug dissolution and permeation through colonic mucosa is the rate limiting step for drug absorption [40].

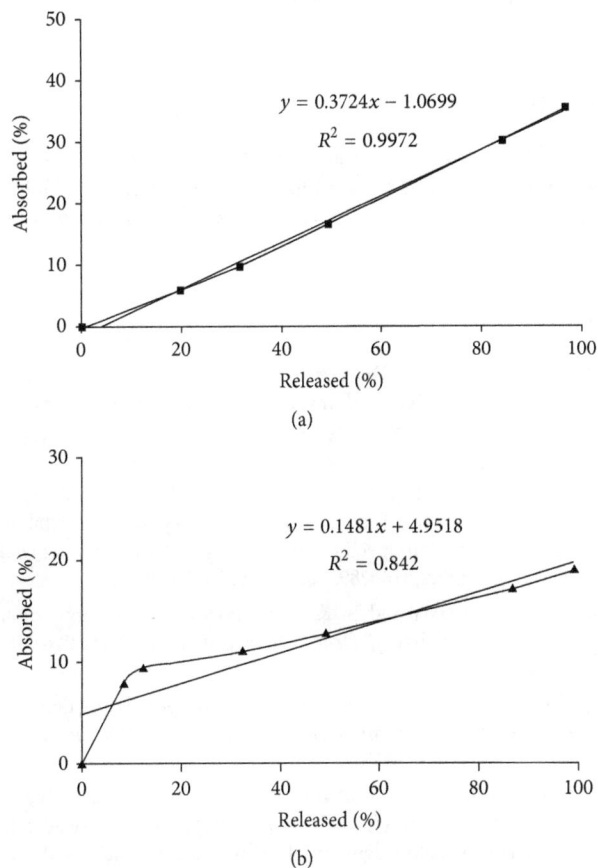

FIGURE 4: In vitro and in vivo correlation (IVIVC) of (a) immediate release core tablet and (b) colon-targeted compression-coated tablet.

4. Conclusion

The results of this study indicated that in vitro release of PDL from the mini-compression-coated tablets was less than 10% in 6 h during which the tablets are supposed to be located in upper GIT and complete release was achieved in the following 6 h in the absence of colonic fluid. In vivo preclinical pharmacokinetic parameters determined by the validated HPLC method reflected the same pattern wherein the plasma concentration was considerably less in 6 h period and reached a maximum value in 10 h. The lower values of C_{max}, AUC_{total}, and protracted T_{max} in comparison to immediate release tablet indicated that PDL was released in the colonic region of rabbit with minimal drug release in the upper GIT from the compression-coated tablet. A good level A in vitro and in vivo correlation (IVIVC) was also achieved after the lag time of drug release in vitro and absorption in vivo. It may be concluded that a blend of natural and modified polysaccharides such as SAL and CMXG both cross-linked with Ca^{+2} ion to an optimum extent could be a suitable coating material for the development of colon-targeted tablets of PDL.

Conflict of Interests

The authors declare that there is no conflict of interests regarding the publication of this paper.

Acknowledgment

One of the authors (S. Maity) wishes to express thanks to the Council of Scientific and Industrial Research, New Delhi, India, for the financial support as CSIR-SRF (Grant no. 9/96 (0727)2K12/EMR-1).

References

[1] M. L. Zema, M. D. Del Curto, A. Foppoli, and A. Gazzaniga, "Oral colon delivery of insulin with the aid of functional adjuvants," *Advanced Drug Delivery Reviews*, vol. 64, no. 6, pp. 540–556, 2012.

[2] V. R. Sinha, B. R. Mittal, and R. Kumria, "In vivo evaluation of time and site of disintegration of polysaccharide tablet prepared for colon-specific drug delivery," *International Journal of Pharmaceutics*, vol. 289, no. 1-2, pp. 79–85, 2005.

[3] M. K. Chourasia and S. K. Jain, "Polysaccharides for colon targeted drug delivery," *Drug Delivery*, vol. 11, no. 2, pp. 129–148, 2004.

[4] V. R. Sinha and R. Kumria, "Microbially triggered drug delivery to the colon," *European Journal of Pharmaceutical Sciences*, vol. 18, no. 1, pp. 3–18, 2003.

[5] K. Chaturvedi, A. R. Kulkarni, and T. M. Aminabhavi, "Blend microspheres of poly(3-hydroxybutyrate) and cellulose acetate phthalate for colon delivery of 5-fluorouracil," *Industrial and Engineering Chemistry Research*, vol. 50, no. 18, pp. 10414–10423, 2011.

[6] K. Ganguly, T. M. Aminabhavi, and A. R. Kulkarni, "Colon targeting of 5-fluorouracil using polyethylene glycol cross-linked chitosan microspheres enteric coated with cellulose acetate phthalate," *Industrial and Engineering Chemistry Research*, vol. 50, no. 21, pp. 11797–11807, 2011.

[7] K. Chaturvedi, S. K. Tripathi, A. R. Kulkarni, and T. M. Aminabhavi, "Cytotoxicity and antitumour activity of 5-fluorouracil-loaded polyhydroxybutyrate and cellulose acetate phthalate blend microspheres," *Journal of Microencapsulation*, vol. 30, no. 4, pp. 356–368, 2013.

[8] L. Yang, J. S. Chu, and J. A. Fix, "Colon-specific drug delivery: new approaches and in vitro/in vivo evaluation," *International Journal of Pharmaceutics*, vol. 235, no. 1-2, pp. 1–15, 2002.

[9] B. Bharaniraja, K. Jayaram Kumar, C. M. Prasad, and A. K. Sen, "Modified katira gum for colon targeted drug delivery," *Journal of Applied Polymer Science*, vol. 119, no. 5, pp. 2644–2651, 2011.

[10] A. G. Sullad, L. S. Manjeshwar, and T. M. Aminabhavi, "Microspheres of carboxymethyl guar gum for in vitro release of abacavir sulfate: preparation and characterization," *Journal of Applied Polymer Science*, vol. 122, no. 1, pp. 452–460, 2011.

[11] L. Pachuau and B. Mazumder, "Evaluation of *Albizia procera* gum as compression coating material for colonic delivery of budesonide," *International Journal of Biological Macromolecules*, vol. 61, pp. 333–339, 2013.

[12] V. R. Sinha and R. Kumria, "Polysaccharide matrices for microbially triggered drug delivery to the colon," *Drug Development and Industrial Pharmacy*, vol. 30, no. 2, pp. 143–150, 2004.

[13] P. G. Yeole, U. C. Galgatte, I. B. Babla, and P. D. Nakhat, "Design and evaluation of Xanthan gum-based sustained release matrix tablets of diclofenac sodium," *Indian Journal of Pharmaceutical Sciences*, vol. 68, no. 2, pp. 185–189, 2006.

[14] S. C. Jagdale, S. A. Patil, and B. S. Kuchekar, "Design, development and evaluation of floating tablets of tapentadol hydrochloride using chitosan," *Asian Journal of Pharmaceutical and Clinical Research*, vol. 5, no. 4, pp. 163–168, 2012.

[15] M. M. Meshali and K. E. Gabr, "Effect of interpolymer complex formation of chitosan with pectin or acacia on the release behaviour of chlorpromazine HCl," *International Journal of Pharmaceutics*, vol. 89, no. 3, pp. 177–181, 1993.

[16] S. L. Kosaraju, "Colon targeted delivery systems: review of polysaccharides for encapsulation and delivery," *Critical Reviews in Food Science and Nutrition*, vol. 45, no. 4, pp. 251–258, 2005.

[17] J.-C. Lagier, M. Million, P. Hugon, F. Armougom, and D. Raoult, "Human gut microbiota: repertoire and variations," *Frontiers in Cellular and Infection Microbiology*, vol. 2, no. 136, pp. 1–19, 2012.

[18] J. Daly, J. Tomlin, and N. W. Read, "The effect of feeding xanthan gum on colonic function in man: correlation with in vitro determinants of bacterial breakdown," *British Journal of Nutrition*, vol. 69, no. 3, pp. 897–902, 1993.

[19] A. M. Oprea, M. T. Nistor, L. Profire, M. I. Popa, C. E. Lupusoru, and C. Vasile, "Evaluation of the controlled release ability of theophylline from xanthan/chondroitin sulfate hydrogels," *Journal of Biomaterials and Nanobiotechnology*, vol. 4, no. 2, pp. 123–131, 2013.

[20] T. Ramasamy, U. D. S. Kandhasami, H. Ruttala, and S. Shanmugam, "Formulation and evaluation of xanthan gum based aceclofenac tablets for colon targeted drug delivery," *Brazilian Journal of Pharmaceutical Sciences*, vol. 47, no. 2, pp. 299–311, 2011.

[21] F. García-Ochoa, V. E. Santos, J. A. Casas, and E. Gómez, "Xanthan gum: production, recovery, and properties," *Biotechnology Advances*, vol. 18, no. 7, pp. 549–579, 2000.

[22] R. Kar, S. Mohapatra, S. Bhanja, D. Das, and B. Barik, "Formulation and in vitro characterization of xanthan gum-based sustained release matrix tables of isosorbide-5-mononitrate," *Iranian Journal of Pharmaceutical Research*, vol. 9, no. 1, pp. 13–19, 2010.

[23] S. Maity and B. Sa, "Development and evaluation of Ca^{+2} ion cross-linked carboxymethyl xanthan gum tablet prepared by wet granulation technique," *AAPS PharmSciTech*, vol. 15, no. 4, pp. 920–927, 2014.

[24] S. Maity and B. Sa, "Compression-coated tablet for colon targeting: impact of coating and core materials on drug release," *AAPS PharmSciTech*, pp. 1–12, 2015.

[25] A. C. Liberman, J. Druker, M. J. Perone, and E. Arzt, "Glucocorticoids in the regulation of transcription factors that control cytokine synthesis," *Cytokine and Growth Factor Reviews*, vol. 18, no. 1-2, pp. 45–56, 2007.

[26] J. Q. Del Rosso Do, "Combination topical therapy for the treatment of psoriasis," *Journal of Drugs in Dermatology*, vol. 5, no. 3, pp. 232–234, 2006.

[27] S. G. Hillier, "Diamonds are forever: the cortisone legacy," *Journal of Endocrinology*, vol. 195, no. 1, pp. 1–6, 2007.

[28] M. Schwartz and R. Cohen, "Optimizing conventional therapy for inflammatory bowel disease," *Current Gastroenterology Reports*, vol. 10, no. 6, pp. 585–590, 2008.

[29] K. D. Tripathi, "Hormones and related drugs," in *Essential of Medical Pharmacology*, section 5, Jaypee Brothers Medical Publishers, New Delhi, India, 5th edition, 2003.

[30] A. K. De, P. Bhattacharya, S. Datta, and A. Mukherjee, "Evaluation of in vivo efficacy and toxicity of prednisolone-loaded hydrogel-based drug delivery device," *International Journal of Pharmaceutical Investigation*, vol. 3, no. 4, pp. 225–233, 2013.

[31] M. Kusunoki, G. Möeslein, Y. Shoji et al., "Steroid complications in patients with ulcerative colitis," *Diseases of the Colon & Rectum*, vol. 35, no. 10, pp. 1003–1009, 1992.

[32] F. Dasankoppa, S. Patwa, H. Sholapur, and G. Arunkumar, "Formulation and characterization of colon specific drug delivery system of prednisolone," *Saudi Journal for Health Sciences*, vol. 1, no. 3, pp. 143–150, 2012.

[33] The Indian Pharmacopoeia Commission, *Indian Pharmacopoeia*, 2010.

[34] United States Food and Drug Administration, *Bioanalytical Method Validation*, 2001.

[35] J. M. Cardot, E. Beyssac, and M. Alric, "In vitro-in vivo correlation: importance of dissolution in IVIVC," *Dissolution Technologies*, vol. 14, no. 1, pp. 15–19, 2007.

[36] United States Food and Drug Administration, *Extended Release Oral Dosage Forms: Development, Evaluation, and Application of In Vitro/In Vivo Correlations*, 1997.

[37] N. Yuksel, A. E. Kanik, and T. Baykara, "Comparison of in vitro dissolution profiles by ANOVA-based, model-dependent and -independent methods," *International Journal of Pharmaceutics*, vol. 209, no. 1-2, pp. 57–67, 2000.

[38] T. Ishibashi, H. Hatano, M. Kobayashi, M. Mizobe, and H. Yoshino, "In vivo drug release behavior in dogs from a new colon-targeted delivery system," *Journal of Controlled Release*, vol. 57, no. 1, pp. 45–53, 1999.

[39] Y. S. R. Krishnaiah, P. V. Raju, B. D. Kumar, V. Satyanarayana, R. S. Karthikeyan, and P. Bhaskar, "Pharmacokinetic evaluation of guar gum-based colon-targeted drug delivery systems of mebendazole in healthy volunteers," *Journal of Controlled Release*, vol. 88, no. 1, pp. 95–103, 2003.

[40] J. E. Polli, J. R. Crison, and G. L. Amidon, "Novel approach to the analysis of in vitro-in vivo relationships," *Journal of Pharmaceutical Sciences*, vol. 85, no. 7, pp. 753–760, 1996.

11

Freeze Dried Quetiapine-Nicotinamide Binary Solid Dispersions: A New Strategy for Improving Physicochemical Properties and Ex Vivo Diffusion

Ahmed Mahmoud Abdelhaleem Ali[1,2] **and Mayyas Mohammad Ahmad Al-Remawi**[1,3]

[1]*Department of Pharmaceutics and Pharmaceutical Technology, College of Pharmacy, Taif University, Taif, Saudi Arabia*
[2]*Department of Pharmaceutics and Industrial Pharmacy, Faculty of Pharmacy, Beni-Suef University, Beni-Suef, Egypt*
[3]*Department of Pharmaceutics and Pharmaceutical Technology, Faculty of Pharmacy and Medical Sciences, Petra University, Amman, Jordan*

Correspondence should be addressed to Ahmed Mahmoud Abdelhaleem Ali; ahmed.mahmoud3@yahoo.com

Academic Editor: Sanyog Jain

Improving the physicochemical properties and oral bioavailability of quetiapine fumarate (QF) enabling enhanced antipsychotic attributes are the main aims of this research. The freeze dried solid dispersion strategy was adopted using nicotinamide (NIC) as highly soluble coformer. The prepared dispersions were characterized using scanning electron microscopy (SEM) differential scanning calorimetry (DSC), Fourier transform infrared spectroscopy (FTIR), and X-ray diffraction (XRD). Static disc intrinsic dissolution rate and ex vivo diffusion through intestinal tissues were conducted and compared to pure quetiapine fumarate. The results demonstrated a highly soluble coamorphous system formed between quetiapine fumarate and nicotinamide at 1:3 molar ratio through H-bonding interactions. The results showed >14-fold increase in solubility of QF from the prepared dispersions. Increased intrinsic dissolution rate (from 0.28 to 0.603 mg cm^{-2} min^{-1}) and faster flux rate through duodenum (from 0.027 to 0.041 mg cm^{-2} h^{-1}) and jejunum (0.027 to 0.036 mg cm^{-2} h^{-1}) were obtained. The prepared coamorphous dispersion proved to be effective in improving the drug solubility and dissolution rate and ex vivo diffusion. Therefore, binary coamorphous dispersions could be a promising solution to modify the physicochemical properties, raise oral bioavailability, and change the biopharmaceutics classification (BCS) of some active pharmaceutical ingredients.

1. Introduction

Quetiapine fumarate (QF) is a dibenzothiazepine antipsychotic drug used in treatment of schizophrenia and mania associated with type I bipolar disorders [1]. The drug has a relatively short half-life (6 hr) and undergoes extensive first-pass metabolism. The high frequency of administration of quetiapine (2–4 times daily) often results in numerous side effects including panic attacks, dyspnea, and swelling of lips and face [2]. Quetiapine is marketed under the brand name Seroquel™ in different strengths (25–300 mg) and shown to be effective up to a dose of 750 mg/day [3]. Quetiapine pharmacokinetics may change when concomitantly administered with some drugs such as ketoconazole,

phenytoin, or rifampicin which affect the activity of CYP3A4 enzymes [4]. Quetiapine has high affinity to serotonin 5-HT$_2$ than dopamine receptors which makes it suitable for successful control of psychotic symptoms associated with Parkinson's disease without worsening of body movements [5]. Quetiapine is soluble in acidic pH (2–4); however, due to its low water solubility over the physiological pH and high permeability, it was classified as BCS class II drug [6]. Therefore, solid state modification approaches which will increase its water solubility are expected also to improve its bioavailability and enable bypassing hepatic metabolism if administered in suitable dosage form such as orodispersible or sublingual tablets or films. The increased solubility by new formulation will enable development of new and predictable quality oral and/or parenteral sustained release dosage forms of the drug.

Stabilized amorphous solid dispersions of poorly soluble active ingredients are considered new emerging technology for improvement of water solubility and bioavailability for biopharmaceutics classification system (BCS) class II drugs. Amorphous polymeric glass solutions were used for long time as the favorable system for improving the solubility, dissolution rate, and stabilization of amorphous drugs [7, 8]. However, these types of systems are hygroscopic and more liable to reduction of glass transition temperature (T_g) and recrystallization upon storage [9–11]. Also, large amounts of polymers are often needed to produce effective systems. In addition a predetermined miscibility of the drug with the selected polymer is required [12]. All these challenging problems make it hard to manufacture amorphous dispersions [13–15]. As more promising alternative to polymers, low molecular weight excipients that could interact with the drug and lower the melting point and increase the T_g such as sugars, amino acids, and hydrotropic organic acids are currently used for drug amorphization [9, 16, 17].

Although the above-mentioned alternatives produced highly dissolving amorphous systems, yet some systems showed partial crystallinity observed from remaining unreacted drugs or excipients [18, 19]. Binary amorphous systems that are composed of two pharmacologically related low molecular weight drugs were recently introduced as effective coamorphous dispersions (COADs) that overcome the drawbacks of drug-polymer glass solutions [20, 21]. Many physically stable coamorphous dispersions with high solubility and dissolution rate were reported in the literature such as those formed between nateglinide and metformin, simvastatin and glipizide prepared by ball milling [22, 23], and naproxen and indomethacin by quench cooling [24]. Other methods such as solvent evaporation or spray drying could also be used for COAD formation [25]. However, due to the limited numbers of drug combinations that could interact at the molecular level with hydrogen or ionic bonding and produce coamorphous mixtures, other substitutes to one of the drugs can be made [26].

Amino acids and neutral molecules such as saccharin or nicotinamide, which are often used for cocrystal formation, can also be applied for COAD preparation using fast methods of solvent evaporation [15]. In this research amorphization of QF was undertaken through combination of with nicotinamide in different molar ratios using hot and cold approaches for rapid solvent evaporation in an attempt to enhance oral bioavailability and change the BCS classification of QF. The produced coamorphous dispersions were evaluated by solid state characterization, equilibrium solubility, intrinsic dissolution rate (IDR), and gut permeation compared to the pure drug.

2. Materials and Methods

2.1. Materials. Quetiapine fumarate (QF) was obtained as free sample from the Jordanian Pharmaceutical Manufacturing, Amman, Jordan. Nicotinamide (NIC) was purchased from Sigma Aldrich, UK. Acetonitrile and methanol (HPLC

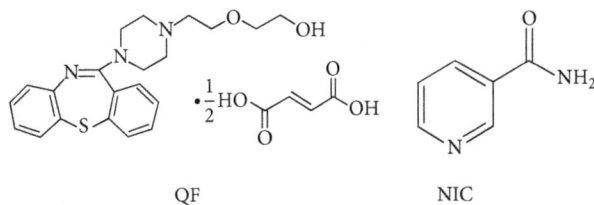

FIGURE 1: Chemical structure of quetiapine fumarate (QF) and nicotinamide (NIC).

grades) were purchased from Fluka, UK. Absolute ethanol, sodium dihydrogen phosphate, sodium hydroxide, and phosphoric acid were obtained from Natco Pharma, Hyderabad, India.

2.2. Preparation of Quetiapine Fumarate-Nicotinamide Coamorphous Dispersions. The coamorphous dispersions were prepared by a previously published coprecipitation method using fast solvent evaporation with some modifications [27]. Mixtures of QF and NIC based on their molar mass (441.5 and 122.12 g/mole) and electron donner/acceptor functional groups (Figure 1) were prepared as shown in Table 1. Two solvent systems, ethanol and 50% v/v mixture of ethanol and water (20 mL), were used for dissolving the drug and the conformer using 250 mL round bottom flask. QF dissolves well in ethanol but nicotinamide takes relatively longer time (30 min) on the sonicator before complete dissolution. As the formulations were dried using freeze drying, QF was dissolved in 20 mL ethanol and separately nicotinamide was added to an equal volume of water and the two solutions were admixed just before drying. Freeze drying (cold evaporation) was applied using Christ freeze dryer model Alpha 2–4 LD plus (Osterode, Germany). The fast and controlled cold evaporation increases the chances of contact and molecular H-bonding interaction between quetiapine and nicotinamide in concentrated solutions during freeze drying and could result in amorphous solid dispersions. The obtained powders were kept under completely dry conditions using silica gel desiccators until further investigation.

2.3. Scanning Electron Microscopy (SEM). The morphology of the prepared dispersions was examined using scanning electron microscopy (Analytical Scanning Microscope, JEOL-JSM-6510LA, JEOL, Japan). Few specks from each formulation were placed on the carbon stubs and then coated using a gold sputter (SPI-Module Sputter Coater, SPI Supplies Inc., USA) followed by microscopical scanning.

2.4. Differential Scanning Calorimetry (DSC). Samples of pure QF and NIC and the prepared COAD formulations (5 mg each) were individually filled into aluminum flat bottomed pans and heated using a simultaneous thermogravimetry-differential scanning calorimeter model STA 449 F3 Jupiter (Nietzsche, Germany) in an atmosphere of nitrogen. The heating temperature used for the crystalline components was set between 20 and 300°C with a heating rate 10°C min^{-1}. The percentage crystallinity Xc (%) of the prepared samples

TABLE 1: Molar ratio composition of QF-NIC coamorphous dispersions.

Formula number	Drug (mg)	Nicotinamide (mg)	**Mr	Solvent system	Evaporation method
F1	150	41.49	1:1	Ethanol	Cold evap.
F2	150	41.49	1:1	*Eth/W	Cold evap.
F3	150	82.98	1:2	Ethanol	Cold evap.
F4	150	82.98	1:2	*Eth/W	Cold evap.
F5	150	124.47	1:3	Ethanol	Cold evap.
F6	150	124.47	1:3	*Eth/W	Cold evap.

*: Eth/W: ethanol/water system 50 : 50 v/v; **Mr: molar ratio.

was calculated from the enthalpy of fusion of the sample (ΔH) compared to that of 100% crystalline QT (ΔH_0) according to the following equation [28]:

$$Xc\,(\%) = \left(\frac{\Delta H}{\Delta H_0}\right) \times 100. \tag{1}$$

2.5. Fourier Transform Infrared Analysis (FTIR). Small samples (2-3 mg) of QF and NIC and the prepared COADs were individually mixed with 500 mg dry potassium bromide. The powder mixtures were compressed into discs under a pressure of 68.5–103.4 MPa using a hydrostatic press. The infrared spectrum was determined at a scanning range of 1000–3500 cm^{-1} to detect major characteristic bands in QT and NIC using a Fourier transform infrared instrument (IR Prestige-21, Shimadzu, Japan).

2.6. X-Ray Diffraction (XRD). Samples of QF powder and NIC as well as the COAD formulations were subjected to X-ray diffraction analysis. A Shimadzu XRD-6000 X-ray powder diffractometer (Shimadzu, Japan) coupled with a standard Cu sealed X-ray tube with voltage, current (40 kV and 40 mA), was used to characterize the amorphous or crystalline state of formulations [29]. Data collection was performed at 2θ of 5–60° in steps of 0.04 and scanning speed of 0.4 degrees per step. Any change in the crystalline pattern of the prepared coamorphous dispersions compared to those of the parent crystalline components was recorded and evaluated. The index of crystallinity was calculated according to the ratio of the relative intensity of the sample (Is) compared to that of the pure crystalline component (Ic) with highest peak [30, 31] according to the following equation:

$$\%\ \text{Crystallinity index} = \left(\frac{Is}{Ic}\right) \times 100. \tag{2}$$

2.7. Drug Content and Equilibrium Solubility. Samples of the prepared amorphous dispersions equivalent to 5 mg QF were dissolved in methanol and adjusted to volume using a standard 50 mL volumetric flask. Then, 2 mL was taken and diluted to 10 mL with mobile phase. Drug content was then determined using a photodiode array automated HPLC analysis system model DGU-20A3/LC-20AT/SIL-20A/CTO-20A/SPD-M20A (Shimadzu, Japan). For equilibrium solubility, an amount of the prepared COAD formulations

equivalent to 10 mg QF was weighed, placed into 2 mL Eppendorf tubes, and dispersed into 250 μL of distilled water. The dispersions were then placed on an orbital shaker model SSM (Stuart, UK) operated at a rate of 300 cycles per min. The process was continued for 72 hr followed by sonication for 30 minutes; then, 10 μL of the filtered supernatant was taken and diluted to 10 mL with methanol. The diluted sample solutions (n = 3) were measured by HPLC analysis. The mobile phase was composed of a mixture of acetonitrile and 0.02 M phosphate buffer (50 : 50 v/v) at pH 5.5 adjusted by 0.02 M orthophosphoric acid and 0.02 M NaOH. The flow rate was adjusted to 0.8 mL/min and the detector wave length was set at 247 nm [32].

2.8. In Vitro Intrinsic Dissolution Rate Studies. Fixed-disc method was applied to determine the intrinsic dissolution rate [33]. In this test, an amount of pure QF (15–20 mg) and an equivalent amount from the selected COAD formulations (F6) were compressed into small tablets inside aluminum discs (0.4 cm in diameter) using a manual mini hand press model MHP-1 (Shimadzu, Japan). The backs of the discs (n = 3) were covered with a layer of molted hard paraffin which were permitted to solidify before immersion into the dissolution medium. The study was performed using full automated dissolution system model UDT-804 paddle dissolution apparatus (Logan, USA) with vessels containing 500 mL of phosphate buffer pH 6.8 and rotation speeds of 50, 75, and 100 rpm in three runs. The temperature of the media was kept at 37 ± 0.5°C and at predetermined time intervals (15, 30, 60, 90, and 120 min); samples were automatically withdrawn and taken for HPLC analysis. The intrinsic dissolution per unit area of the disc (G_ω) was determined as a function of dissolution time and the intrinsic dissolution rate at infinite rotation speed (K_1), that is, at zero diffusion layer (mg·cm^{-2}·sec^{-1}), was obtained from the following equation resulting from plotting the reciprocal of G_ω against the reciprocal of the angular velocity ω [34]:

$$\frac{1}{G_\omega} = \frac{1}{K_1} + K_2\frac{1}{\omega}, \tag{3}$$

where G_ω is the intrinsic dissolution rate at ω (mg·cm^{-2}·sec^{-1}), K_1 is the intrinsic dissolution rate at infinite rotation speed (mg·cm^{-2}·Sec^{-1}), K_2 is a constant, and ω is the angular velocity of the disc (radians·sec^{-1}).

TABLE 2: Thermal analysis and % crystallinity data of QF coamorphous dispersions compared to pure QF and NIC.

| Formula | DSC | | | | TGA | **Degree of crystallinity (%) | |
| | Peak 1 | | Peak 2 | | | | |
	Melting maximum (°C)	Heat of fusion (μV/mg)	Melting maximum (°C)	Heat of fusion (μV/mg)	Onset of degradation (°C)	DSC	XRD
F1	120.10	37.77	152.00	60.14	186.00	67.34	51.00
F2	117.0	31.42	150.60	65.89	184.00	66.93	53.40
F3	120.00	38.70	142.30	21.67	192.60	39.63	73.30
F4	119.50	73.20	*NA	*NA	182.70	48.05	51.50
F5	122.00	128.40	*NA	*NA	199.50	81.69	38.60
F6	117.0	31.0	*NA	*NA	172.00	19.72	24.00
QF	175.40	134.60	*NA	*NA	267.30	—	—
NIC	131.80	184.40	*NA	*NA	200.00	—	—

*NA: not available; **degree of crystallinity (%) calculated from DSC and XRD data.

2.9. Ex Vivo Diffusion Studies.

The test was performed to compare the rate of diffusion of pure QF to that of the prepared coamorphous dispersions using parts of a fresh cattle gut. The excised tissues of duodenum and jejunum were placed on 3.5 cm in diameter plastic diffusion cells (SES GmbH, Germany) filled to top with 8 mL phosphate buffer (pH 6.8) containing 20 mg pure drug or equivalent amount of the dispersion. The units were placed at the bottom of the dissolution flasks containing 250 mL of the buffer solution. The paddles were rotated at a speed of 100 rpm and the temperature was adjusted to $37 \pm 0.5°C$. After 0.5, 1, 2, 3, 4, 5, and 6 hr intervals samples were automatically withdrawn and taken for HPLC analysis using the same method mentioned under the drug content and equilibrium solubility section. The flux rate J_0 (mg·cm^{-2} hr^{-1}) was obtained from the slope of the plotted line relating cumulative amount of QF permeated (mg/cm^2) to time (hr) as shown in Figure 8 [35].

3. Results

3.1. Solid State Characterization

3.1.1. DSC Studies.

The DSC thermograms of QF and NIC and the solid dispersions are shown in Figure 2. Characteristic melting peaks at specific temperatures for QF and NC were observed at 175.40 and 131.80°, respectively. The prepared dispersions showed lower melting temperatures compared to parent components as displayed in Table 2 containing the thermal data of QF/NIC coamorphous dispersions. From Table 2, it could be noticed that two peaks with different melting points were recorded with various heats of fusion (ΔH_f) from the DSC thermograms of COAD formulations F1, F2, and F3 whilst single peaks were observed for F4, F5, and F6. In addition, the sharp decrease in weight was monitored using TGA to indicate the decomposition temperature. The coamorphous dispersion F6 showed the lowest melting temperature (117°C), lowest heat of fusion ($\Delta H_f = 31$ μV/mg), and decomposition temperature (172°C). The % crystallinity was also calculated from the DSC data and the results showed that the dispersion F6 (1 : 3 Mr) demonstrated the lowest crystallinity (19%) as shown in Table 2.

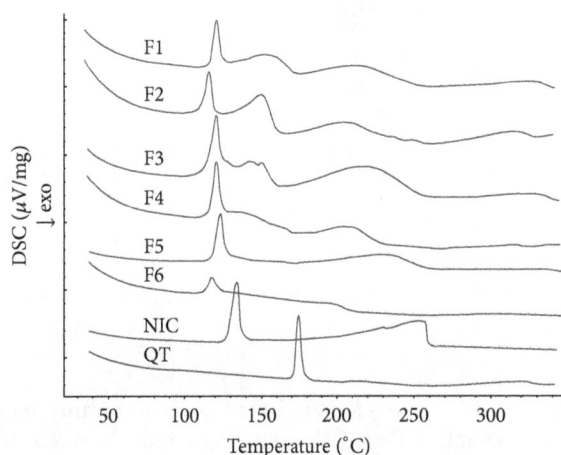

FIGURE 2: DSC thermograms of quetiapine fumarate (QT), nicotinamide (NIC), and solid dispersions (F1–F6).

3.1.2. FTIR Studies.

FTIR results collected for COAD samples as well as pure QF and NIC were shown in Figure 3. The FTIR spectra of NIC indicated the appearance of the characteristic amino group –NH2 symmetric stretching vibrations at 3379 cm^{-1} (Figure 3(a)). The C=O stretching also appeared at 1628 and the –CN stretching vibrations also appeared at 1427 cm^{-1} which correspond well with the recorded values in the literature [36]. Other characteristic peaks were noticed such as the amide band at 1703 and C–O stretching at 1032 cm^{-1}. The FTIR spectra of QF (Figure 3(a)) showed characteristic peaks at 3313, 3072, 3045, 3012, 2941, 2866, 2870, 2738, 2627, 2347, 1942, 1608, 1568, 1460, 1342, and 1305 cm^{-1}. These peaks also are highly similar to those of QF Form I polymorph reported in the literature [37]. The peak at 3313 corresponded to –OH stretching vibrations, between 3072 and 3130 cm^{-1} corresponding to –CH aromatic stretching, whilst –CH aliphatic stretching vibrations were observed at bands in the region between 2900 and 2940 cm^{-1}. The aromatic amino (secondary and tertiary) showed absorption bands between 1300 and 1340 cm^{-1}. The fumarate salt

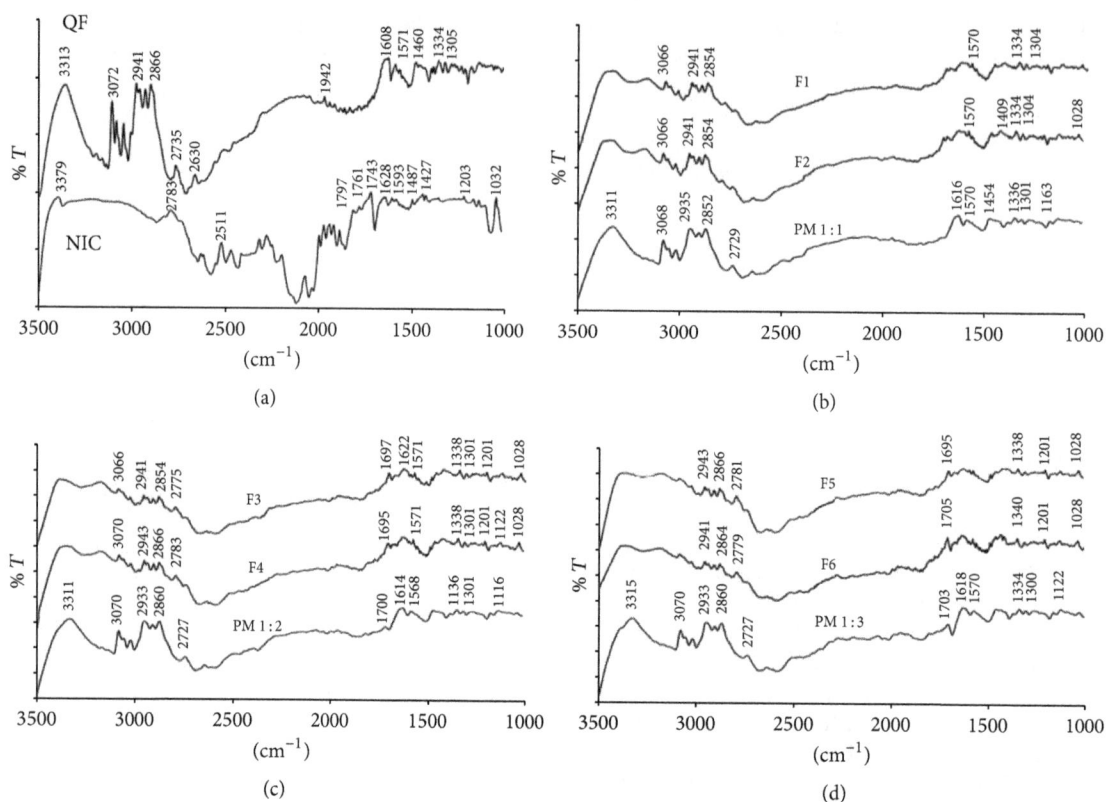

FIGURE 3: IR spectra of quetiapine fumarate (QF), nicotinamide (NIC), physical mixtures (PM1–3), and the prepared dispersions (F1–F6).

moiety showed characteristic broad –OH stretching band which overlapped the –CH stretching region between 300 and 3300 cm^{-1}. The prepared dispersions showed IR bands shorter than those of parent components and also demonstrated shifting of some peaks and formation of shoulders in others as observed in Figures 3(b)–3(d).

3.1.3. XRD Studies. The results of XRD data collected for QF and NIC and the coamorphous samples are shown in Figures 4 and 5. The highly crystalline QF showed sharp diffraction lines at 2θ 7.3, 9.1, 11.5, 13.2, 14.9, 15.3, 16.2, 17.6, 19.9, 21, 21.7, 22.3, 23.2, 24.8, 25.1, 25.5, 27.1, 28.4, 29.2, 30.6, 33.1, 40.3, and 42.7 degrees. The XRD pattern of NIC showed characteristic diffraction lines at 2θ values of 21.67°, 22.63°, 24.81°, 26.43°, 29.91°, 31.57°, 33.55°, 35.88°, 37.52°, and 40.28° (Figure 4). The degree of crystallinity was obtained by calculating the ratio of highest intensity of the solid dispersion sample to that of the pure crystalline component (Table 2). The XRD patterns of the dispersions shown in Figure 5 demonstrated lower intensity (counts 25000–15000) compared to the physical mixtures (counts >45000). It was observed that sample F6 showed the lowest degree of crystallinity (24.0%) compared to other dispersions (Table 2).

3.2. Morphology of the Prepared Dispersions Compared to Parent Components. Scanning electron micrographs of QF and NIC (Figure 6) demonstrated crystalline shape of both compounds. The SEM images of the physical mixture showed

small rod like crystals of QF dispersed on large prismatic crystals of NIC (Figure 6(a)). The binary coamorphous dispersion F6 (prepared at 1 : 3 molar ratio) showed lack of defined crystals and appearance of a homogenous dispersion lacking defined crystals (Figure 6(b)).

3.3. Drug Content and Equilibrium Solubility. The results of measured equilibrium solubility of the prepared dispersions obtained after HPLC analysis are shown in Table 3. The analysis data showed separate and sharp peaks for both components after injection of the dispersion formulation (Figure 7) indicating chemical stability of separated QF from the dispersion. Formula F6 composed of QF and NIC in 1 : 3 molar ratio and prepared by cold evaporation method demonstrated the highest relative percentage increase in QF water solubility (1363%) with more than 16-fold increase in concentration compared to the pure crystalline QF (Table 3). Formula F5 which had similar composition and evaporation method to F6 also showed comparable percentage increase in solubility (1303%). The drug content per 5 mg of the dispersion was calculated for each formula and the results were found to be comparable to the theoretical content with insignificant differences between the two ($P > 0.05$).

3.4. Intrinsic Dissolution Rate and Ex Vivo Diffusion Studies. The calculated IDR for pure QF and F6 under the abovementioned experimental conditions was found to be 0.284

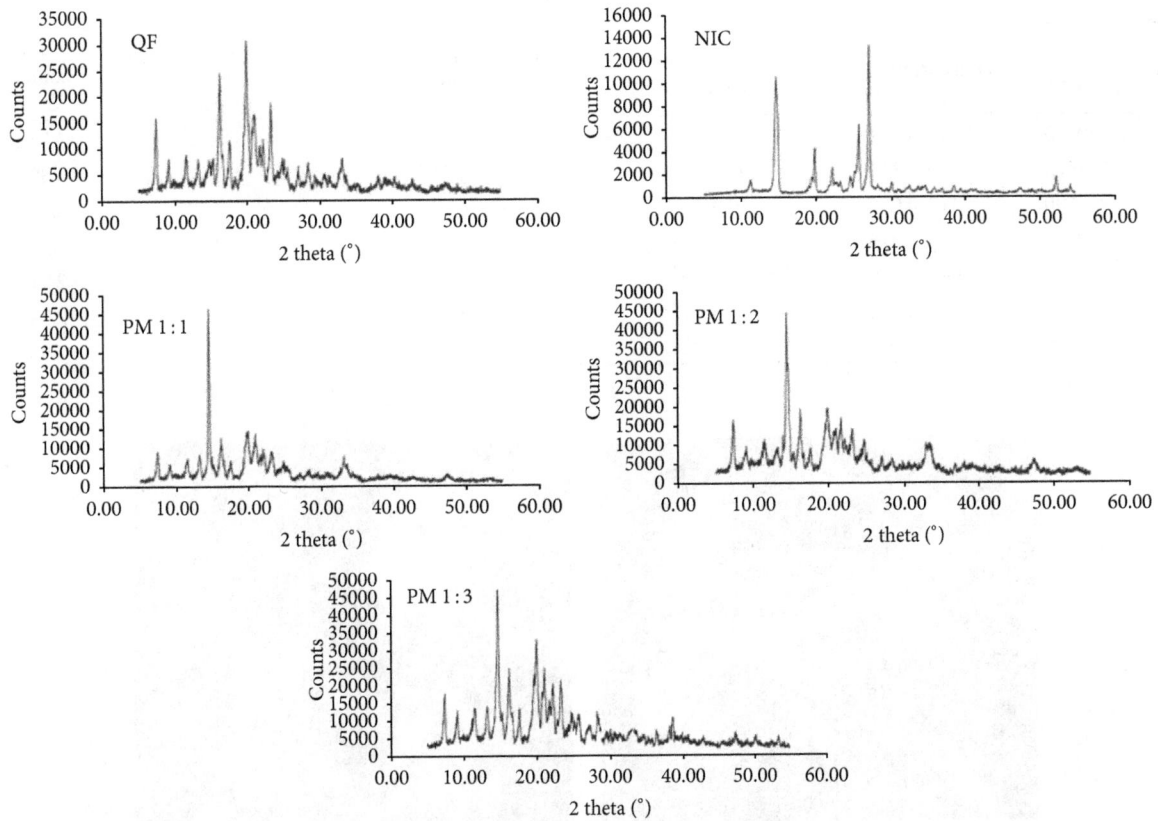

FIGURE 4: X-ray diffractograms of quetiapine fumarate (QF), nicotinamide (NIC), and physical mixtures (PM1–3).

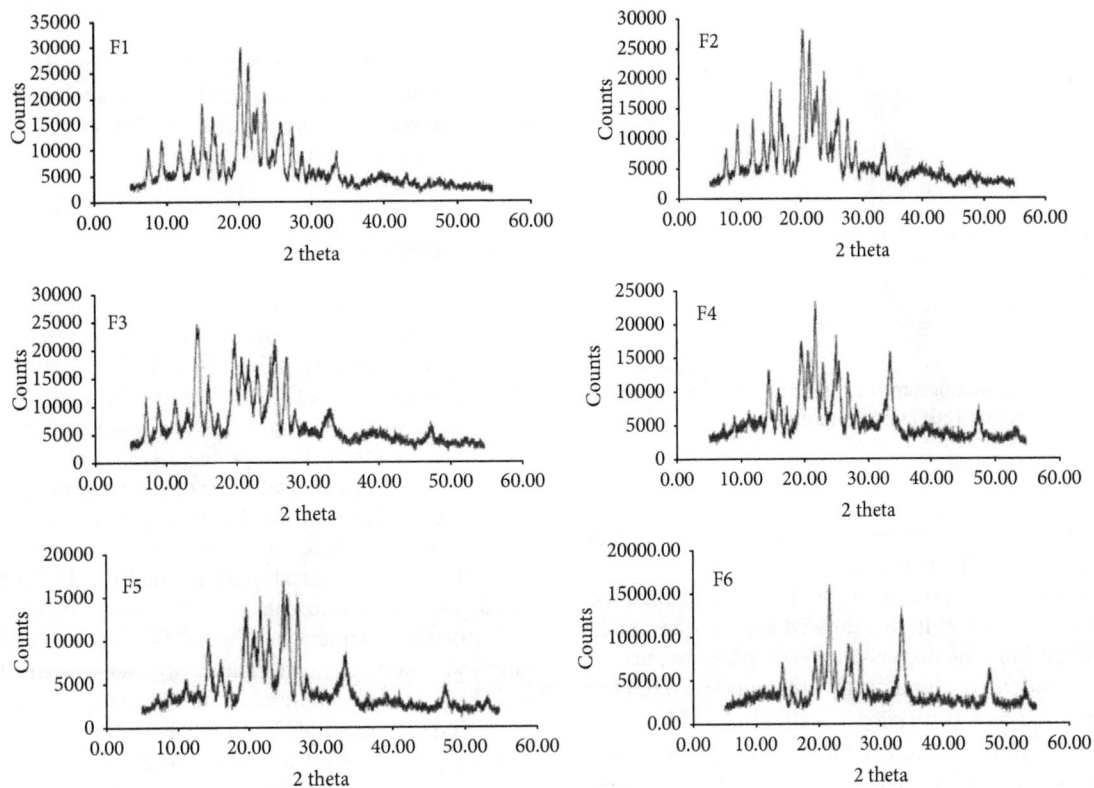

FIGURE 5: X-ray diffractograms of QF-NIC binary coamorphous dispersions (F1–F6).

TABLE 3: Results of equilibrium solubility of QF coamorphous dispersions compared to pure QF.

Formula	HPLC peak area	Average concentration (mcg/mL ± SD)	Number of folds' increase in solubility	% Increase in solubility (% ± SD)	Theoretical drug content/5 mg dispersion	Actual drug content/5 mg dispersion
F1	569475	10.22 ± 0.102	5.97	497 ± 2.15	3.92	3.94 ± 0.001
F2	578628	10.38 ± 0.337	6.07	507 ± 7.07	3.92	3.89 ± 0.002
F3	963690	17.25 ± 0.080	10.09	909 ± 1.67	3.22	3.18 ± 0.002
F4	792933	14.20 ± 0.076	8.31	731 ± 1.60	3.22	3.21 ± 0.001
F5	1341763	23.99 ± 0.000	14.03	1303 ± 0.00	2.73	2.71 ± 0.003
F6	1398833	**25.01 ± 0.032**	**14.63**	**1363 ± 0.66**	2.73	2.74 ± 0.002
*QF	92868	1.71 ± 0.035	1.00	0.00	5.00	4.98 ± 0.001

*Quetiapine fumarate.

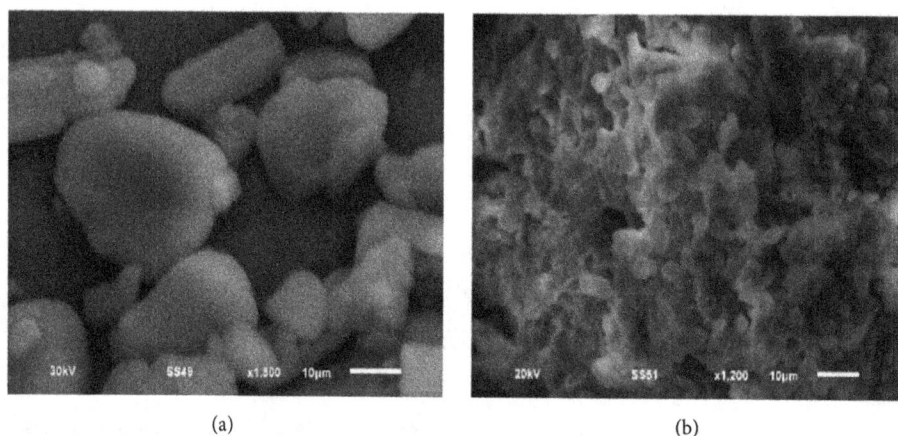

(a)   (b)

FIGURE 6: Scanning electron micrographs (SEM) of QF-NIC physical mixture (a) and binary coamorphous dispersion F6 (b).

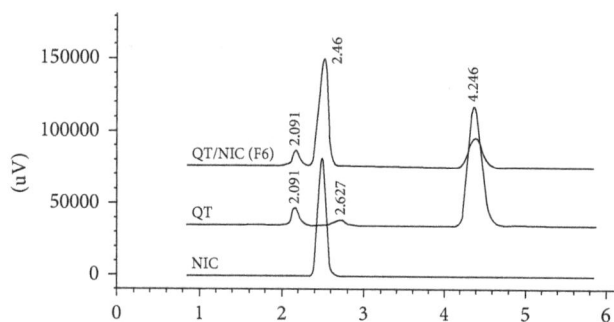

FIGURE 7: HPLC chromatograms of QF and NIC and the binary coamorphous dispersion (F6) after dissolution.

and 0.603 mg·cm^{-2}·min^{-1}, respectively, indicating more than twofold increase in IDR (Figure 8).

The in vitro diffusion studies through cattle intestinal sections (duodenum and jejunum) showed superior and faster diffusion of QF from the dispersion F6 compared to pure QF (Figures 9(a) and 9(b)). Significantly different ($P < 0.05$) flux rates (J_0) for the new dispersion (0.041 mg cm^{-1} h^{-1}) compared to pure QF (0.027 mg cm^{-1} h^{-1}) through duodenum and (0.036 mg cm^{-1} h^{-1} to 0.028 mg cm^{-1} h^{-1}) for jejunum were observed, respectively (Table 4). The data also showed statistically significant difference in the lag times prior to commencement of diffusion in both cases in favor of the F6 which showed substantially lower lag times than pure QF and the reported values in the literature [38].

4. Discussion

The crystalline nature of QF and NIC was confirmed by sharp melting endotherms which were found to coincide with those previously published 174°C [39] and 128–131°C [40], respectively. The COAD F6 demonstrated a single short endotherm with minimum melting temperature indicating miscibility of the two components [41]. The lowest heat of fusion (31 μV/mg) of this formula among other prepared COADs may also indicate that such preparation could have the maximum degree of amorphousness. The IR spectra showed that the physical mixtures had much shorter peaks which represent summation of the peaks of QF and NC with possible interactions (Figure 3). The binary dispersion samples, however, showed much broader and shorter peaks and disappearance of some characteristic peaks of QF. The characteristic peaks at 3313 of QT and 3379 cm^{-1} of NIC which represent –OH and –NH stretching vibrations were found to form a bridge in all binary solid dispersions (Figures 3(b)–3(d)) indicating H-bonding interactions [42].

TABLE 4: Results of in vitro gut permeation of QF through duodenum and jejunum compared to the coamorphous dispersion F6.

Formula	Duodenum			Jejunum		
	Flux rate (mg/cm^2/h)	Lag time (min)	Regression R^2	Flux rate (mg/cm^2/h)	Lag time (min)	Regression R^2
Pure QF	0.027	38.22	0.97	0.028	32.51	0.98
QF-NIC (F6)	0.041	12.15	0.99	0.036	17.72	0.99

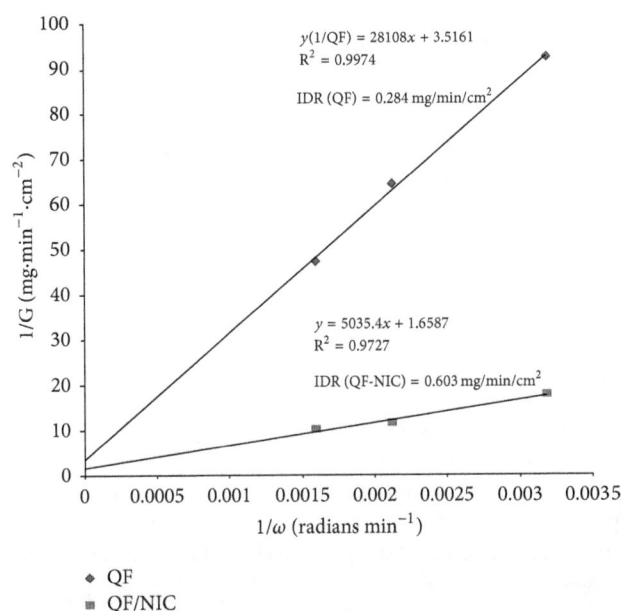

FIGURE 8: Plot of the reciprocal of the dissolution rate $1/G$ (mg cm^{-2} min^{-1}) versus reciprocal of angular velocity ($1/\omega$) (radians·min^{-1}) for determination of IDR from QF and coamorphous dispersion F6 (QF-NIC).

Complete disappearance of the characteristic amide peaks of NIC between 1628 and 1797 cm^{-1} and C=O asymmetric stretching of QT salt at 1608 cm^{-1} have been observed in almost all dispersions also suggesting H-bonding formation [43, 44]. The coamorphous sample F6 (Figure 3(d)) showed shifting of the characteristic peaks of QT from 2735 to 2775 which may support the suggestion of formation of a true coamorphous dispersion. However, in order to get another proof of amorphousness, the degree of crystallinity was calculated from both DSC and X-ray diffraction data. From the XRD diffraction pattern of QF (Figure 4), it was shown that the diffraction lines were highly identical to those observed for QF Form I polymorph cited in the literature [45]. For nicotinamide also, numerous diffraction lines were similar to those found in previous research works [46]. For the prepared dispersions (Figure 5) the intensity of the diffraction lines was highly shortened especially with the dispersions formulated at 1 : 2 and 1 : 3 molar ratios (F5 and F6). The lowest degrees of crystallinity (31%) observed for F6 from XRD data and 19% as obtained from DSC data support the point of view of formation of substantially amorphous or semicrystalline dispersion [47]. Also the obtained data from SEM (Figure 6) indicated differences in the shape of the final

coamorphous dispersion being a homogenous aggregate with undefined edges compared to the clearly identified crystalline parent components. This dispersion also showed the highest equilibrium solubility with more than 14-fold increase in solubility compared to pure crystalline QF.

Therefore, by combining the results of DSC, FTIR, equilibrium solubility, and XRD data, it becomes clear that the coamorphous dispersion F6 had a single and short DSC endotherm, lowest melting temperature, lowest heat of fusion, shorter and broader IR bands, and lowest degree of crystallinity. Hence, this QF/NIC (1 : 3 Mr) coamorphous dispersion could be considered the best obtained amorphous sample with limited crystallinity and consequently it was selected for in vitro intrinsic dissolution and ex vivo diffusion studies.

For equilibrium solubility, F6 obtained the largest value followed by F5 which also support the above hypothesis of COAD formation. The difference between F6 and F5 is in the solvent used during preparation of the dispersion, being ethanol and ethanol/water for F5 and F6, respectively. This small difference in solubility (both showed >14-fold increase in solubility) may indicate that the ethanol/water solvent system has higher support to formation of H-bonding during freeze drying leading to formation of a highly soluble dispersion. The differences in the degrees of crystallinity of F5 (38.6%) compared to F6 (31%) also confirm that the molar ratio 1 : 3 was the best between other ratios (Tables 1 and 2).

The importance of the calculation of the intrinsic dissolution rate (IDR) of drugs evolves from the roles of both drug solubility and IDR in the FDA updated determination of biopharmaceutics classification system of drugs [48, 49]. Although the results of IDR obtained for QF and COAD F6 were found to be a bit lower than the universally suggested values of IDR (1.00 mg·cm^{-2}·min^{-1} or 0.017 mg·cm^{-2}·Sec^{-1}) for drugs classified as highly soluble [38, 50], yet the COAD system showed promising results by approaching that value (Figure 8 and Table 4). It is well known that the measurement of IDR of drugs may vary by variation of the dissolution conditions such as the media composition, pH, and volume; however under the same testing conditions differences between F6 and the reference pure QF were highly evident. In a similar study but under somewhat different conditions, quetiapine benzoate IDR was tested in comparison with quetiapine hemifumarate (using 900 mL degassed water and US Pharmacopoeia 2 apparatus with device for intrinsic testing, at 100 rpm). In this test, quetiapine benzoate demonstrated more than 6-fold increase in IDR compared to quetiapine hemifumarate [51]. In another study for determination of IDR, numerous active pharmaceutical ingredients in the salt

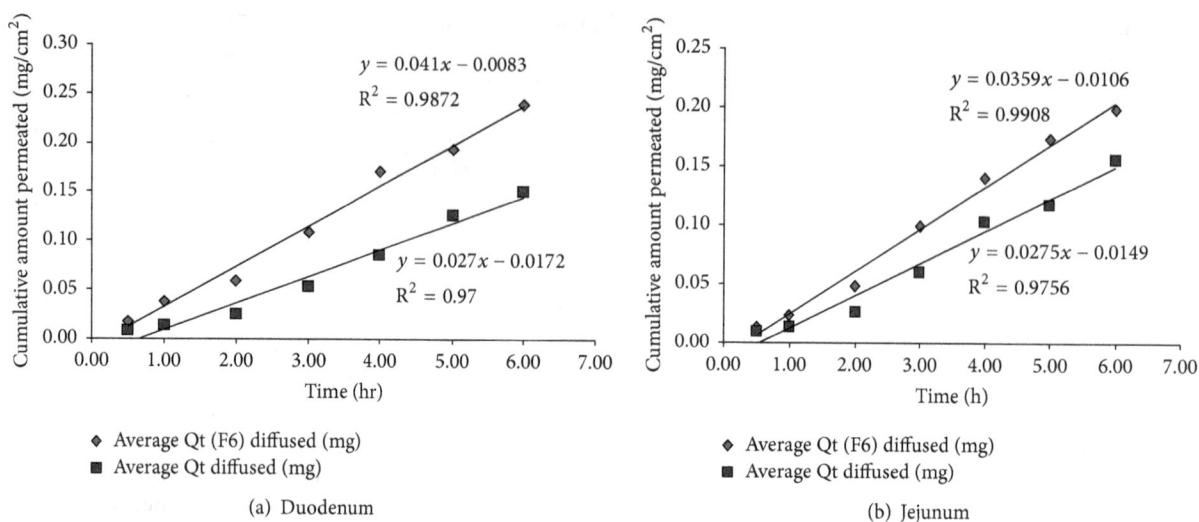

FIGURE 9: Ex vivo gut permeation profile of quetiapine fumarate (QF) compared to the binary coamorphous dispersion (F6).

form demonstrated IDR values which were not substantially higher than that observed for the prepared COAD [52]. In this study, nicotinamide has been selected as a coformer due to its high solubility, neutral structure, low melting temperature, and capability of interacting at molecular level with H-bonding formation. Such properties were used to obtain stable coamorphous dispersions. The benefits of increased solubility and dissolution rate were tested for impact on the drug diffusion through gut tissues. The results of ex vivo diffusion through duodenum and jejunum showed faster rate of diffusion from F6 (>51%) and >28% compared to QF, respectively (Figure 9 and Table 4). Also, a lower lag time was observed indicating that the new combination is expected to have successful role in improving the oral bioavailability following in vivo administration.

5. Conclusions

The above results of preparation and characterization of QF/NIC coamorphous dispersions indicated feasibility of the preparation method and applicability of the dispersion at a molar ratio of 1 : 3 in improving the physicochemical properties of QF. The increased solubility by 14-fold and intrinsic dissolution rate of the drug by 22-fold can be considered an important achievement that will inevitably result in enhanced oral bioavailability. This new formulation could also be used as in-mouth instantly dissolving dosage form which could enable bypassing of first-pass metabolism. The improved ex vivo diffusion (high flux and low lag time) observed with the COAD also provides another proof of success for this new formulation in raising the expected bioavailability and possibly changing of the FDA BCS classification of QF.

Competing Interests

The authors of this manuscript report no declaration of interests.

Acknowledgments

The authors of this research acknowledge Taif University research deanship, KSA, for the institutional support provided under the program of research project funding. A special acknowledgment is also directed to Dr. Mohamed Ghazi for his sincere help during HPLC analysis of the samples.

References

[1] A. J. Cutler, J. M. Goldstein, and J. A. Tumas, "Dosing and switching strategies for quetiapine fumarate," *Clinical Therapeutics*, vol. 24, no. 2, pp. 209–222, 2002.

[2] K. Krishnaraj, M. J. N. Chandrasekar, M. J. Nanjan, S. Muralidharan, and D. Manikandan, "Development of sustained release antipsychotic tablets using novel polysaccharide isolated from Delonix regia seeds and its pharmacokinetic studies," *Saudi Pharmaceutical Journal*, vol. 20, no. 3, pp. 239–248, 2012.

[3] C. L. DeVane and C. B. Nemeroff, "Clinical pharmacokinetics of quetiapine: an atypical antipsychotic," *Clinical Pharmacokinetics*, vol. 40, no. 7, pp. 509–522, 2001.

[4] S. W. Grimm, N. M. Richtand, H. R. Winter, K. R. Stams, and S. B. Reele, "Effects of cytochrome P450 3A modulators ketoconazole and carbamazepine on quetiapine pharmacokinetics," *British Journal of Clinical Pharmacology*, vol. 61, no. 1, pp. 58–69, 2006.

[5] M. A. Parsa and B. Bastani, "Quetiapine (Seroquel) in the treatment of psychosis in patients with Parkinson's disease," *Journal of Neuropsychiatry and Clinical Neurosciences*, vol. 10, no. 2, pp. 216–219, 1998.

[6] G. Garbacz, A. Kandzi, M. Koziolek, J. Mazgalski, and W. Weitschies, "Release characteristics of quetiapine fumarate extended release tablets under biorelevant stress test conditions," *AAPS PharmSciTech*, vol. 15, no. 1, pp. 230–236, 2014.

[7] S. Prodduturi, K. L. Urman, J. U. Otaigbe, and M. A. Repka, "Stabilization of hot-melt extrusion formulations containing solid solutions using polymer blends," *AAPS PharmSciTech*, vol. 8, no. 2, pp. E152–E161, 2007.

[8] P. Gupta and A. K. Bansal, "Devitrification of amorphous celecoxib," *AAPS PharmSciTech*, vol. 6, no. 2, pp. E223–E230, 2005.

[9] Q. Lu and G. Zografi, "Phase behavior of binary and ternary amorphous mixtures containing indomethacin, citric acid, and PVP," *Pharmaceutical Research*, vol. 15, no. 8, pp. 1202–1206, 1998.

[10] A. Forster, J. Hempenstall, and T. Rades, "Characterization of glass solutions of poorly water-soluble drugs produced by melt extrusion with hydrophilic amorphous polymers," *Journal of Pharmacy and Pharmacology*, vol. 53, no. 3, pp. 303–315, 2001.

[11] A. C. F. Rumondor and L. S. Taylor, "Effect of polymer hygroscopicity on the phase behavior of amorphous solid dispersions in the presence of moisture," *Molecular Pharmaceutics*, vol. 7, no. 2, pp. 477–490, 2010.

[12] O. A. Sammour, M. A. Hammad, N. A. Megrab, and A. S. Zidan, "Formulation and optimization of mouth dissolve tablets containing rofecoxib solid dispersion," *AAPS PharmSciTech*, vol. 7, no. 2, pp. E167–E175, 2006.

[13] P. Srinarong, H. de Waard, H. W. Frijlink, and W. L. J. Hinrichs, "Improved dissolution behavior of lipophilic drugs by solid dispersions: the production process as starting point for formulation considerations," *Expert Opinion on Drug Delivery*, vol. 8, no. 9, pp. 1121–1140, 2011.

[14] E. Karavas, G. Ktistis, A. Xenakis, and E. Georgarakis, "Miscibility behavior and formation mechanism of stabilized felodipine-polyvinylpyrrolidone amorphous solid dispersions," *Drug Development and Industrial Pharmacy*, vol. 31, no. 6, pp. 473–489, 2005.

[15] K. Löbmann, K. T. Jensen, R. Laitinen, T. Rades, C. J. Strachan, and H. Grohganz, "Stabilized amorphous solid dispersions with small molecule excipients," in *Amorphous Solid Dispersions*, pp. 613–636, Springer, Berlin, Germany, 2014.

[16] T. Masuda, Y. Yoshihashi, E. Yonemochi, K. Fujii, H. Uekusa, and K. Terada, "Cocrystallization and amorphization induced by drug-excipient interaction improves the physical properties of acyclovir," *International Journal of Pharmaceutics*, vol. 422, no. 1-2, pp. 160–169, 2012.

[17] F. Qian, J. Wang, R. Hartley et al., "Solution behavior of PVP-VA and HPMC-AS-Based amorphous solid dispersions and their bioavailability implications," *Pharmaceutical Research*, vol. 29, no. 10, pp. 2766–2776, 2012.

[18] S. C. Arora, P. K. Sharma, R. Irchhaiya, A. Khatkar, N. Singh, and J. Gagoria, "Development, characterization and solubility study of solid dispersions of cefuroxime axetil by the solvent evaporation method," *Journal of Advanced Pharmaceutical Technology and Research*, vol. 1, no. 3, pp. 326–329, 2010.

[19] A. K. Aggarwal and S. Jain, "Physicochemical characterization and dissolution study of solid dispersions of ketoconazole with nicotinamide," *Chemical and Pharmaceutical Bulletin*, vol. 59, no. 5, pp. 629–638, 2011.

[20] N. Chieng, J. Aaltonen, D. Saville, and T. Rades, "Physical characterization and stability of amorphous indomethacin and ranitidine hydrochloride binary systems prepared by mechanical activation," *European Journal of Pharmaceutics and Biopharmaceutics*, vol. 71, no. 1, pp. 47–54, 2009.

[21] M. Allesø, N. Chieng, S. Rehder, J. Rantanen, T. Rades, and J. Aaltonen, "Enhanced dissolution rate and synchronized release of drugs in binary systems through formulation: amorphous naproxen-cimetidine mixtures prepared by mechanical activation," *Journal of Controlled Release*, vol. 136, no. 1, pp. 45–53, 2009.

[22] K. Löbmann, C. Strachan, H. Grohganz, T. Rades, O. Korhonen, and R. Laitinen, "Co-amorphous simvastatin and glipizide combinations show improved physical stability without evidence of intermolecular interactions," *European Journal of Pharmaceutics and Biopharmaceutics*, vol. 81, no. 1, pp. 159–169, 2012.

[23] S. Wairkar and R. Gaud, "Co-Amorphous Combination of Nateglinide-Metformin Hydrochloride for Dissolution Enhancement," *AAPS PharmSciTech*, 2015.

[24] K. Löbmann, R. Laitinen, H. Grohganz, K. C. Gordon, C. Strachan, and T. Rades, "Coamorphous drug systems: enhanced physical stability and dissolution rate of indomethacin and naproxen," *Molecular Pharmaceutics*, vol. 8, no. 5, pp. 1919–1928, 2011.

[25] A. Paudel, Z. A. Worku, J. Meeus, S. Guns, and G. Van Den Mooter, "Manufacturing of solid dispersions of poorly water soluble drugs by spray drying: formulation and process considerations," *International Journal of Pharmaceutics*, vol. 453, no. 1, pp. 253–284, 2013.

[26] R. Laitinen, K. Löbmann, C. J. Strachan, H. Grohganz, and T. Rades, "Emerging trends in the stabilization of amorphous drugs," *International Journal of Pharmaceutics*, vol. 453, no. 1, pp. 65–79, 2013.

[27] A. M. A. Ali, A. A. Ali, and I. A. Maghrabi, "Clozapine-carboxylic acid plasticized co-amorphous dispersions: preparation, characterization and solution stability evaluation," *Acta Pharmaceutica*, vol. 65, no. 2, pp. 133–146, 2015.

[28] B. Shah, V. K. Kakumanu, and A. K. Bansal, "Analytical techniques for quantification of amorphous/crystalline phases in pharmaceutical solids," *Journal of Pharmaceutical Sciences*, vol. 95, no. 8, pp. 1641–1665, 2006.

[29] A. Newman, D. Engers, S. Bates, I. Ivanisevic, R. C. Kelly, and G. Zografi, "Characterization of amorphous API:polymer mixtures using X-ray powder diffraction," *Journal of Pharmaceutical Sciences*, vol. 97, no. 11, pp. 4840–4856, 2008.

[30] O. Rewthong, S. Soponronnarit, C. Taechapairoj, P. Tungtrakul, and S. Prachayawarakorn, "Effects of cooking, drying and pretreatment methods on texture and starch digestibility of instant rice," *Journal of Food Engineering*, vol. 103, no. 3, pp. 258–264, 2011.

[31] J. Reyes-Gasga, E. L. Martínez-Piñeiro, G. Rodríguez-Álvarez, G. E. Tiznado-Orozco, R. García-García, and E. F. Brès, "XRD and FTIR crystallinity indices in sound human tooth enamel and synthetic hydroxyapatite," *Materials Science and Engineering: C*, vol. 33, no. 8, pp. 4568–4574, 2013.

[32] F. Belal, A. Elbrashy, M. Eid, and J. J. Nasr, "Stability-indicating HPLC method for the determination of quetiapine: application to tablets and human plasma," *Journal of Liquid Chromatography and Related Technologies*, vol. 31, no. 9, pp. 1283–1298, 2008.

[33] L. X. Yu, A. S. Carlin, G. L. Amidon, and A. S. Hussain, "Feasibility studies of utilizing disk intrinsic dissolution rate to classify drugs," *International Journal of Pharmaceutics*, vol. 270, no. 1-2, pp. 221–227, 2004.

[34] M. Nicklasson and A. B. Magnusson, "Program for evaluating drug dissolution kinetics in preformulation," *Pharmaceutical Research*, vol. 2, no. 6, pp. 262–266, 1985.

[35] P. Dixit, D. K. Jain, and J. Dumbwani, "Standardization of an ex vivo method for determination of intestinal permeability of drugs using everted rat intestine apparatus," *Journal of Pharmacological and Toxicological Methods*, vol. 65, no. 1, pp. 13–17, 2012.

[36] S. Bayarı, A. Ataç, and Ş. Yurdakul, "Coordination behaviour of nicotinamide: an infrared spectroscopic study," *Journal of Molecular Structure*, vol. 655, no. 1, pp. 163–170, 2003.

[37] R. Lifshitz-Liron, E. Kovalevski-Ishai, B.-Z. Dolitzky, S. Wizel, and R. Lidor-Hadas, Crystalline forms of quetiapine hemifumarate, Google Patents, 2003.

[38] P. Zakeri-Milani, M. Barzegar-Jalali, M. Azimi, and H. Valizadeh, "Biopharmaceutical classification of drugs using intrinsic dissolution rate (IDR) and rat intestinal permeability," *European Journal of Pharmaceutics and Biopharmaceutics*, vol. 73, no. 1, pp. 102–106, 2009.

[39] P. Deshpande, A. Holkar, O. Gudaparthi, and J. Kumar, Such as 11-[4-[2-(2-hydroxyethoxy) ethyl]-1-pinerazinyl] dibenzo [b, f][1, 4] thiazepine (quetiapine) via reduction, cyclization, and deprotection, Google Patents, 2004.

[40] R. V. Heinzelmann, Purification of nicotinamide, Google Patents, 1951.

[41] D. J. Greenhalgh, A. C. Williams, P. Timmins, and P. York, "Solubility parameters as predictors of miscibility in solid dispersions," *Journal of Pharmaceutical Sciences*, vol. 88, no. 11, pp. 1182–1190, 1999.

[42] J. Coates, "Interpretation of infrared spectra, a practical approach," in *Encyclopedia of Analytical Chemistry*, R. A. Meyers, Ed., pp. 10815–10837, John Wiley & Sons, Chichester, UK, 2000.

[43] L. Liu and X. Wang, "Improved dissolution of oleanolic acid with ternary solid dispersions," *AAPS PharmSciTech*, vol. 8, no. 4, pp. 267–271, 2007.

[44] A. A. Ambike, K. R. Mahadik, and A. Paradkar, "Spray-dried amorphous solid dispersions of simvastatin, a low Tg drug: in vitro and in vivo evaluations," *Pharmaceutical Research*, vol. 22, no. 6, pp. 990–998, 2005.

[45] R. Parthasaradhi, R. Rathnakar, R. R. Raji, R. Muralidhara, and R. K. S. Chander, "Polymorphs of quetiapine fumarate," Google Patents, 2007.

[46] Z. Rahman, C. Agarabi, A. S. Zidan, S. R. Khan, and M. A. Khan, "Physico-mechanical and stability evaluation of carbamazepine cocrystal with nicotinamide," *AAPS PharmSciTech*, vol. 12, no. 2, pp. 693–704, 2011.

[47] W. Rowe, P. Hurter, C. Young et al., Pharmaceutical composition and administration thereof, Google Patents, 2009.

[48] M. G. Issa and H. G. Ferraz, "Intrinsic dissolution as a tool for evaluating drug solubility in accordance with the biopharmaceutics classification system," *Dissolution Technologies*, vol. 18, no. 3, pp. 6–11, 2011.

[49] G. L. Amidon, H. Lennernas, V. P. Shah, and J. R. Crison, "A theoretical basis for a biopharmaceutic drug classification: the correlation of in vitro drug product dissolution and in vivo bioavailability," *Pharmaceutical Research*, vol. 12, no. 3, pp. 413–420, 1995.

[50] L. X. Yu, G. L. Amidon, J. E. Polli et al., "Biopharmaceutics classification system: the scientific basis for biowaiver extensions," *Pharmaceutical Research*, vol. 19, no. 7, pp. 921–925, 2002.

[51] A. Danilovski, H. Ceric, Z. Siljkovic, A. Kwokal, and I. Grebenar, Salts of quetiapine, Google Patents, 2006.

[52] Z. Rahman, A. S. Zidan, R. Samy, V. A. Sayeed, and M. A. Khan, "Improvement of physicochemical properties of an antiepileptic drug by salt engineering," *AAPS PharmSciTech*, vol. 13, no. 3, pp. 793–801, 2012.

12

Combined Effect of Synthetic and Natural Polymers in Preparation of Cetirizine Hydrochloride Oral Disintegrating Tablets: Optimization by Central Composite Design

Chandra Sekhar Patro and Prafulla Kumar Sahu

Raghu College of Pharmacy, Dakamarri, Visakhapatnam, Andhra Pradesh 531 162, India

Correspondence should be addressed to Chandra Sekhar Patro; c.patro@rediffmail.com

Academic Editor: Sanyog Jain

Our aim was to employ experimental design to formulate and optimize cetirizine hydrochloride oral disintegrating tablets (ODTs) by direct compression technique, using the mutual effect of synthetic croscarmellose sodium (CCS) and natural *Hibiscus rosa-sinensis* mucilage (HRM) as disintegrants in the formulation. Central composite design (CCD) was applied to optimize the influence of three levels each of CCS (X_1) and HRM (X_2) concentrations (independent variables) for investigated responses: disintegration time (DT) (Y_1), % friability (F) (Y_2), and % cumulative drug release (DR) (Y_3) (dependent variables). This face-centered second-order model's reliability was verified by the probability and adequate precision values from the analysis of variance, while the significant factor effects influencing the studied responses were identified using multiple linear regression analysis. Perturbation and response surface plots were interpreted to evaluate the responses' sensitivity towards the variables. During optimization, the concentrations of the processed factors were evaluated, and the resulting values were in good agreement with predicted estimates endorsing the validity. Spectral study by Fourier Transform Infrared Spectroscopy (FTIR) and thermograms from Differential Scanning Calorimetry (DSC) demonstrated the drug-excipients compatibility of the optimized formulation. The optimized formulation has concentrations of 9.05 mg and 16.04 mg of CCS and HRM each, respectively, and the model predicted DT of 13.271 sec, F of 0.498, and DR of 99.768%.

1. Introduction

The conventional formulations like tablets and capsules play a major role in the oral drug-delivery system with many pros and cons. With respect to patient compliance, ease of swallow is one of the important factors that determine the acceptance of these formulations, especially in pediatric and geriatric patients. It was assessed that 40–50% of the population face the problem of dysphagia or difficulty in swallowing with frequent complaints of taste, surface, and size of the tablets which lead to noncompliance and poor treatment [1–3]. Technological advents in ODTs have drawn global attention during the last decades that can overcome these problems. Unlike conventional dosage forms, ODTs rapidly disintegrate in the mouth in presence of saliva and

are then swallowed comfortably into the stomach [4–7]. The drug release from ODTs has a prospect to be absorbed in oromucosal tissue followed by esophagus and pharynx resulting in potential rapid action, enhanced therapeutic efficacy devoid of gastric irritation, and partial first-pass effect [8].

For an ideal ODT, the disintegration time varies from several seconds to about a minute. Numerous unique properties of ODTs like fast disintegration, taste-masking ingredients, sensitiveness to moisture, tablet strength, and porosity make them distinct from conventional tablets. However, the best formula of ingredients' composition to achieve the desired properties has been a great challenge for the researchers since time immemorial. Recently, Response Surface Methodology (RSM) has become a widely accepted optimization

TABLE 1: Physicochemical parameters of mucilage powder (number of experiments = 3).

Parameters	Conditions	
Angle of repose		26.37°
Bulk density		0.56 g/cm^3
Tapped density		0.76 g/cm^3
Average particle size		152 μm
Compressibility ratio		26.31
Loss on drying		5%
Percentage yield		29%
Swelling ratio	In water	48
Solubility		Slowly soluble in water producing huge viscous solution
Total ash		20.35%
Acid insoluble ash		4.9%
Microbial load	Bacteria (CFUs/g)	6
	Fungi (CFUs/g)	3

technique to overwhelm the complexity in formulation and development of pharmaceutical preparations [9]. The aim of RSM is to design the way in which a response is affected by the independent variables or their interactions. The fitted model is used to reach the destination at the best operating conditions, which conclude in either maximum or minimum response. It is also useful to analyze the functional relation between completely dependent and wholly autonomous variables [10]. RSM has many types of experimental designs, which demonstrates polynomial equations and determines the optimal levels to formulate the dosage forms [11–13].

CTZ, an active hydroxyzine (H1-receptor antagonist) metabolite, is a drug of choice for the treatment of all types of allergies, rhinitis, hay fever, atopic dermatitis, asthma, allergic cough, and urticaria. Being a second-generation nonsedative antihistamine, it exhibits inhibition of several cytotoxic mediators, eosinophil chemotaxis, and release of histamines during allergies [14, 15]. In this paper, we have demonstrated the formulation and development of cetirizine hydrochloride (CTZ) ODTs using an optimized combination of CCS and HRM as disintegrants. Disintegration capacity of the natural mucilage (HRM) was studied when employed alone and in binary mixture with the synthetic superdisintegrant (CCS) and vice versa. During comparative evaluation, it was observed that the ODTs with optimal combination of CCS and HRM provide faster disintegration and better tablet strength.

2. Materials and Methods

2.1. Materials. CTZ was procured from Lotus Enterprises, Visakhapatnam (India). CCS, Pearlitol SD 200, magnesium stearate, sorbitol, aerosil, and flavour were purchased from Yarrow Chem Products, Mumbai, and aspartame was purchased from Loba Chemicals, Mumbai. Fresh leaves of *Hibiscus rosa-sinensis* were collected from the local source.

2.2. Methods

2.2.1. Extraction and Purification of Hibiscus rosa-sinensis Mucilage. The fresh and healthy leaves of *Hibiscus rosa-sinensis* were carefully cleaned. The dirt and dust particles were removed by washing with water, dried, and processed. Powdered leaves were set aside in water for a period of 5-6 hrs for soaking followed by boiling for 30 min. The mucilage was collected into water from the above mixture. Thereafter, the material was squeezed to remove the marc from the solution by an eight-folded muslin cloth bag. A sufficient quantity of acetone was added to the above filtrate to get the precipitate. The collected mucilage was dried at a temperature of 30°C in hot air oven. The dried mucilage was powdered, sieved through sieve (#80), and put aside in a desiccator at 30°C and 45% relative humidity until use. The common method of segregation of gums from food was used. About 1% of mucilage along with 5% of cold diluted trichloroacetic acid solution was homogenized, centrifuged, and neutralized by using sodium hydroxide and then dialyzed for 30 hrs against distilled water. The mucilage was reprecipitated using ethanol (three volumes) and washed successively with ethanol, acetone, and diethyl ether [16, 17]. The dried powder mucilage was characterized for physicochemical properties shown in Table 1.

2.2.2. Drug: Excipient Compatibility Study. Both FTIR and DSC analysis was carried out to evaluate the interfering between drug and excipients used for the CTZ ODTs formulation.

2.2.3. Formulation Development. CCS, a synthetic polymer, and natural mucilage of HRM were individually used as disintegrating promoting agents for preparing oral disintegrating tablets. Four different concentrations of the respected disintegrants were discreetly chosen for the formulation development. Each preliminary trial batch of the formulation

TABLE 2: Composition of preliminary trial batch with individual disintegrant and their evaluation parameters.

Ingredients (mg)	F_{A1}	F_{A2}	F_{A3}	F_{A4}	F_{A5}	F_{A6}	F_{A7}	F_{A8}
CTZ	10	10	10	10	10	10	10	10
CCS	5 (2.5%)	10 (5%)	15 (7.5%)	20 (10%)	—	—	—	—
HRM	—	—	—	—	10 (5%)	20 (10%)	30 (15%)	40 (20%)
Pearlitol SD 200	149	144	139	134	144	134	124	114
Sorbitol	20	20	20	20	20	20	20	20
Otherexcipients*	12	12	12	12	12	12	12	12
Aspartame	4	4	4	4	4	4	4	4
Evaluation Parameters								
DT (sec)	31 ± 2	18 ± 2.2	25 ± 1.3	28 ± 2.3	39 ± 0.33	28 ± 0.12	36 ± 0.23	49 ± 0.32
F (%)	0.93	0.91	1.11	1.34	0.49	0.31	0.79	0.87
Wetting time (sec)	27	16	24	22	36	25	33	47
DR at 25 min	98.24	98.99	98.72	97.47	93.32	98.32	89.45	87.33

Net tablet weight: 200 mg; batch size: 50 CTZ ODTs.
Note. The amount of all the ingredients was calculated on the basis of net weight of one tablet (200 mg). For the preliminary trial batch four varied concentrations of CCS and HRM (ΔCCS: 2.5%–10%; ΔHRM: 5%–20%) were trialed for desired tablet properties. D-sorbitol (10%) and aspartame (2%) as sweetening agent were used to mask the inherent bitter taste of cetirizine hydrochloride in all the trial formulations.
*Other excipients used were magnesium stearate, 2 mg (1%); aerosil, 2 mg (1%); talc, 2 mg (1%); and flavour, 6 mg (3%).

was composed of various proportions of drug and excipients as depicted in Table 2. ODTs of each batch of 50 tablets (each tablet weight is 200 mg ± 50 mg) were prepared by direct compression method using Cadmach single punch machine with 10 mm flat plane face punches. The drug and excipients sieved through #22 mesh and mixed accurately in a polyethylene bag for 30 minutes. To the resultant blend, lubricant was added and mixed well to get the uniform composite. The formulations were equipped to develop the tablets. Although additions of natural mucilage have shown satisfactory results, the formulations containing synthetic polymer exhibited better performance when evaluated [18, 19].

Further, a combination of both the above disintegrants in different ratios was screened to assess their mutual contribution on the formulation's performance. The proposed method aimed to establish a formulation containing an optimal ratio of both the disintegrants to exhibit their best synergistic effects on the investigated responses.

2.2.4. Formulation Design. To develop and optimize the formulation design of CTZ ODTs, a CCD with $\alpha = 1$ was used to recognize the significant factors' effects influencing the investigated responses in the proposed oral disintegrating tablet formulation. The concentrations of CCS (X_1) and HRM (X_2) as independent variables run at three levels were discretely screened for their major effect and interactions on the responses such as DT (Y_1), F (Y_2), and DR (Y_3) as dependent variables. The responses were optimized together by multiple response algorithms using Design-Expert® version-8.0.4 (Stat-Ease). To depict the interrelationship between

independent and dependent variables, the investigational data and model were fitted and evaluated by ANOVA.

As per the above-mentioned factors, a CCD was used, where the two independent factors converted to being dimensionless each at three levels (+1, 0, −1) to have control over the response pattern and their optimum variable combinations. The central point (0, 0) of the design was studied in quintuplicate to compute the reproducibility of the technique and also to countenance the valuation of error. Table 3 summarizes a version of 13 experimental runs, their independent variable's combination, and coded level version used during study.

During the design study, all the responses develop fitted polynomial models, along with their interactions and quadratic expressions utilizing multiple regression analysis methodologies. The fitting form of the second-order polynomial model is described as the following equation:

$$Y = \beta_0 + \beta_1 X_1 + \beta_2 X_2 + \beta_3 X_1 X_2 + \beta_4 X_1^2 + \beta_5 X_2^2 + \beta_6 X_1 X_2^2 + \beta_7 X_1^2 X_2 \tag{1}$$

Y is the predicted/measured response for the combination of each factor level, which correlates with β (regression coefficient): β_0, which is the intercept signifying the arithmetical mean of whole of quantifiable results of 13 runs; β_1 to β_7 are linear coefficients appraised from the contemplated values of the measured response; X_1 and X_2 are translated coded values for each independent variable. The expressions $X_1 X_2$ and X_i^2 signify the interaction between them and influence on response. The rationality of statistical polynomial models was predictable by ANOVA. Three-dimensional response surface plots (3D) were designed to

TABLE 3: Formulation trial carried out for oral disintegrating tablet formulation of CTZ ODTs with CCS/ HRM at different level as per experimental design.

Trial run	Coded factor levels	
	X_1	X_2
F 1	−1	−1
F 2	0	−1
F 3	1	−1
F 4	−1	0
F 5	0	0
F 6	1	0
F 7	−1	1
F 8	0	1
F 9	1	1
F 10	0	0
F 11	0	0
F 12	0	0
F 13	0	0
Translation coded values	−1	0	+1
X_1: CCS (%)	2.5	5	7.5
X_2: HRM (%)	5	10	15
Dependent variables			
Y_1	Disintegration time (sec)		
Y_2	Friability (%)		
Y_3	Cumulative drug released at 25 minutes (%)		

check the interaction of factors and their significant influence on responses [20–22].

2.2.5. Validation and Optimization of Proposed Model.

To validate the experimental design, eight checkpoint solutions were selected for investigation. The prepared formulations equivalent to each of the checkpoints were screened for the selected responses. The resultant observed responses were compared quantitatively with their corresponding foretold values. Subsequently, the linear regression plots were drawn between the obtained observed response properties and the consequent predicted values to observe the error.

3. Evaluation

3.1. Mechanical Properties of Tablets.

To determine the mechanical strength of a tablet, hardness and friability are measured as the two significant parameters. The crushing strength/hardness of the tablets was measured by using the hardness tester (Monsanto), whereas the friability F was evaluated using a Roche friabilator. For % friability, accurately weighed twenty tablets were allowed to rotate in the friabilator at 25 rpm for 5 minutes and change in tablet weight was analyzed.

3.2. Wetting Profile.

The wetting time of the formulations was calculated by standard procedure. Five circular pieces of filter papers of 10 cm diameter and 0.45 μm pore sizes (Hi-media) were placed in a Petri dish. 10 mL of eosin dye water solution was added to the dish; then a tablet was positioned on the filter paper and time taken for overall wetting of the tablet was noted down [23].

3.3. Disintegration Test of Tablets.

The USP disintegration apparatus is having six glass tubes 3″ long with top side open and detained beside 10″ screen at the opposite bottom side of the basket. After the tablet is sited in every tube, the basket frame is disillusioned in one-liter beaker of double distilled water at 37±2°C, in such a manner that the tablets stay behind the liquid surface on their uphill movement and downward not nearer than 2.5 cm from the bottom of the basket. The DT was recorded [24].

3.4. In vitro Dissolution Study.

The ODTs were evaluated for drug release studies by using phosphate buffer (pH-7.4) for one hour to contact the capability of the formulated tablets to furnish quick drug delivery. The eight-stage dissolution test apparatus (DISSO 2000, Lab India) was used to perform in vitro drug dissolution studies of ODTs by using 900 mL of the dissolution medium (pH-7.4 phosphate buffer) constantly well kept at 37±1°C. The tablets were placed in the cylindrical vessel, and the paddle type stirrer rotated at 50 rpm. Samples of 5 mL were withdrawn at each time interval (2, 5, 10, 15, 20, 30, 45, and 60 minutes) from the dissolution medium and replaced by 5 mL of fresh mediums each time to maintain sink condition. The drawn samples were filtered, and 1 mL was taken of each filtrate to dilute to 10 mL with same media. The absorbance of the samples was measured at λ_{max} 250 nm using UV spectrophotometer [25].

4. Results and Discussion

4.1. Drug-Excipients Interaction Study.

The interaction study between drug and excipients was carried out in order to get confirmation on the probable interaction for any interface using FTIR and DSC analysis. Figure 1 shows the infrared spectra of pure CTZ, CCS, and HRM and combination of these three ingredients. The unadulterated drug alone shows 3043, 3022, 2983 (aromatic C-H str), 1600, 1580 (aromatic (C⋯C)), 1741 (C=O), 1200–1100 (C-O-C), 1250–1310 (C-N), 2891–2741 (C-OH) (w, b), and 750–700 (C-Cl), respectively. The optimal ratio of CCS and HRM as the key excipients in the formulation showed almost all bands without affecting their peak position and trends, which indicates the absence of well-defined interaction between the drug and the two disintegrating agents.

The DSC thermograms of pure CTZ, CCS, and HRM and combination of these three are shown in Figure 2. The thermogram of pure CTZ exhibits a single endotherm corresponding to the melting point of the pure drug, which showed a sharp characteristic peak at 222.6°C (Tonset = 213.71°C, Tendset = 226.73°C, and heat of fusion is 600.06°C) due to melting point of the solid drug. The thermogram of

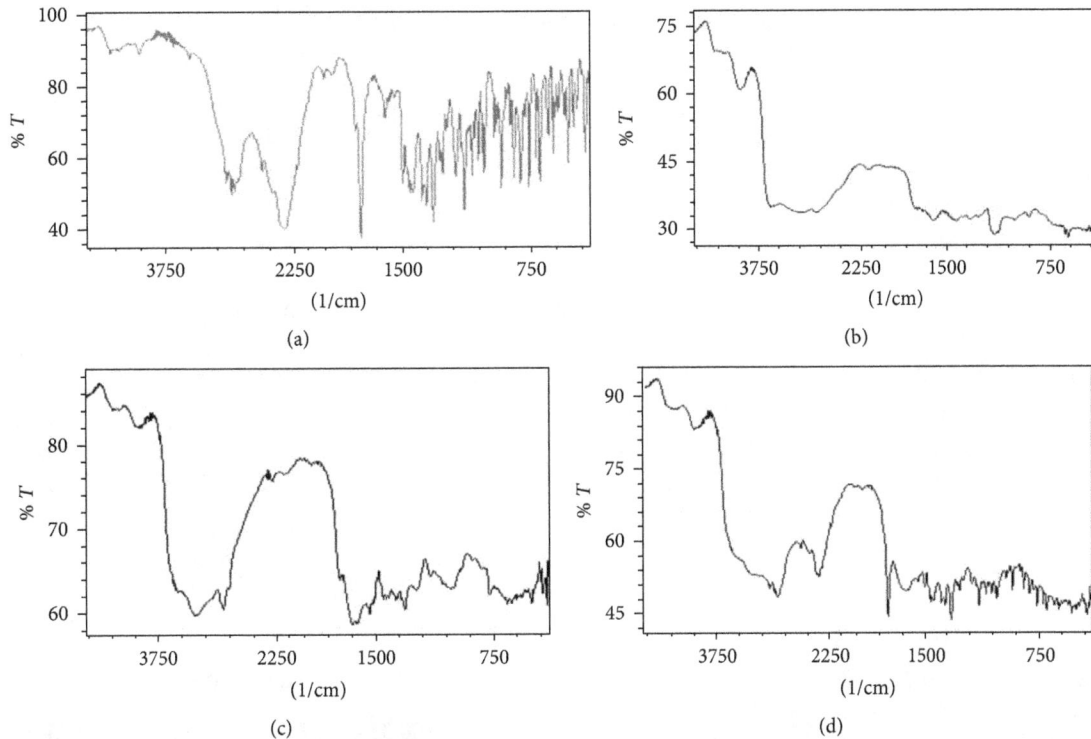

FIGURE 1: FTIR spectra for (a) cetirizine; (b) physical mixture of cetirizine with CCS; (c) physical mixture of cetirizine with HRM; and (d) optimized formulation, physical mixture of cetirizine with CCS and HRM.

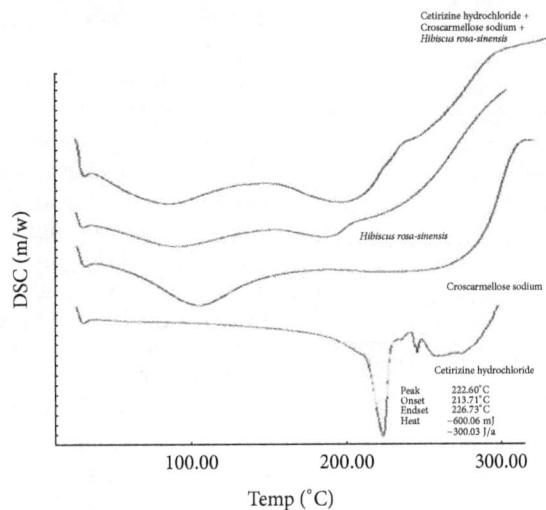

FIGURE 2: Overlaid DSC curve of cetirizine HCl, CCS, HRM, and their mixture.

mixture did not show any peak at 222.6°C, which confirms compatibility of drug and excipients. There is no melting endotherm of drug in the optimized formulation, which indicates that the drug was present in amorphous phase.

4.2. Experimental Design and Data Acquiring. The influence of both disintegrants used to formulate CTZ ODTs was

studied. Tablets were obtained employing direct compression method due to (i) ease of fabrication and (ii) economic (iii) faster disintegration or dissolution. HRM was used as disintegrating promoting agent due to its swelling property in water. After coming in contact with water the mucilage wicks the water into the matrix network and then swells, which reduces adhesiveness of other ingredients causing disintegration. CCS

TABLE 4: Response variables (Y_1–Y_3) obtained from trial formulations of CTZ ODTs.

Trial run	Croscarmellose sodium (mg) (X_1)	H. rosa-sinensis mucilage (mg) (X_2)	Disintegration time (sec) (Y_1)	Friability (%) (Y_2)	Cumulative drug released (%) (Y_3)
F1	5	10	22	0.61 ± 0.16	95.34 ± 1.9
F2	10	10	17	0.53 ± 0.13	96.12 ± 2.56
F3	15	10	16	0.32 ± 0.07	96.87 ± 1.96
F4	5	20	15	0.64 ± 0.10	96.50 ± 1.77
F5	10	20	12	0.47 ± 0.12	99.19 ± 2.24
F6	15	20	14	0.59 ± 0.09	98.50 ± 1.35
F7	5	30	16	0.35 ± 0.17	98.88 ± 1.71
F8	10	30	18	0.43 ± 0.03	97.76 ± 2.55
F9	15	30	20	0.29 ± 0.11	96.22 ± 1.33
F10	10	20	13	0.41 ± 0.30	97.39 ± 1.95
F11	10	20	12	0.39 ± 0.21	97.98 ± 1.28
F12	10	20	12	0.46 ± 0.05	98.01 ± 1.25
F13	10	20	12	0.49 ± 0.25	98.2 ± 1.11

used as disintegrating agent due to its cross network polymeric system water drawing capacity considerably increases. RSM with the aid of CCD was exploited methodically to estimate the impact of disintegrants as dependent variables and their interactions on the investigated responses. The experiment was aimed to identify the significant factor effects influencing the formulation performance and to establish their superlative levels for the desirability of responses shown in Table 4.

4.3. Statistical Analysis and Mathematical Modeling of Experimental Data. To estimate the quantitative effects of the combined ratio of factors and their levels on the selected responses, the experimental values of the flux were analyzed by Design-Expert software and mathematical models obtained for each response [26]. The statistical models were generated by the results obtained from investigation and regression of statistically significant factors [8]. The polynomial equations derived from multiple regression analysis for each flux are shown below.

Y_1 (Disintegration time)

$$= +12.38 - 0.50 * X_1 - 0.50 * X_2 + 2.50 * X_1$$
$$* X_2 + 1.67 * X_1^2 + 4.67 * X_2^2 - 1.00 * X_1^2 \quad (2)$$
$$* X_2 + 0.00 * X_1 * X_2^2$$

Y_2 (% Friabilty)

$$= +0.48 - 0.025 * X_1 - 0.050 * X_2 + 0.057 * X_1$$
$$* X_2 + 0.046 * X_1^2 - 0.089 * X_2^2 - 0.022 \quad (3)$$
$$* X_1^2 * X_2 - 0.062 * X_1 * X_2^2$$

Y_3 (Cumulative % drug released)

$$= +100.33 + 0.57 * X_1 + 0.32 * X_2 - 0.75 * X_1$$
$$* X_2 - 0.12 * X_1^2 - 1.75 * X_2^2 - 0.047 * X_1^2 \quad (4)$$
$$* X_2 - 0.40 * X_1 * X_2^2$$

The above equations reveal the assessable effect of the dependent variables, concentrations of CCS (X_1) and HRM (X_2) and their interaction on the responses such as DT (Y_1), F (Y_2), and DR (Y_3) as dependent variables. The polynomial equation includes the coefficients intercept, first order of individual factor's influence, interaction, and higher-order term [27]. In the equations, the positive signs indicate synergistic effect, and the negative sign signifies the antagonistic affect. The negative regression coefficient of both factors (X_1 and X_2) in (2) and (3) proposes a decrease in DT and F with an increase in concentration of the independent variables and in (4) an increase in DR with an increase in concentrations of factors. It is also concluded that variable X_2 had the most profound effect on % friability, whilst variable X_1 mostly affected % drug release. However, disintegration time experienced equal influence by both the variables (X_1 and X_2). In (2)–(4) coefficients of factors with higher-order term (X_1^2, X_1^2) represent quadratic correlation, while the coefficients having both factors (X_1, X_2) indicate an interaction effect on the selected responses. The positive regression coefficient of the quadratic term of X_1^2 in (2) and (3) signifies that the respective responses decrease slightly and later increase, whereas in (4) negative indicates the decrease in drug release. The quadratic term X_2^2 had significant effect on all the three responses (disintegration time, % friability, and % cumulative drug release). There is a positive influence on both DT and F by the interaction of both factors and negative impact on drug release [28, 29].

The analysis of variance (ANOVA) test on the quadratic response model was executed to signify the linear interaction

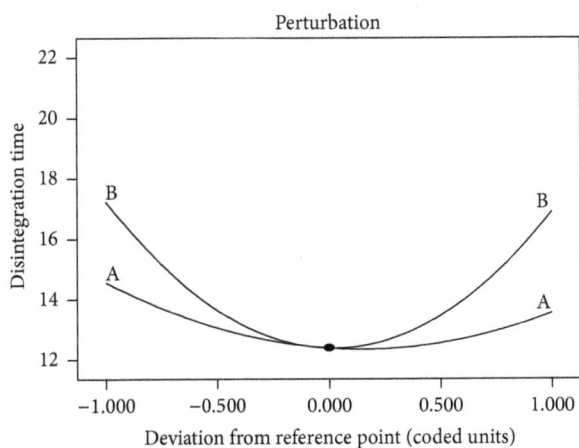

Design-Expert software
Factor coding: actual
Disintegration time

Actual factors
A: CCS = 10.00
B: HRM = 20.00

(a)

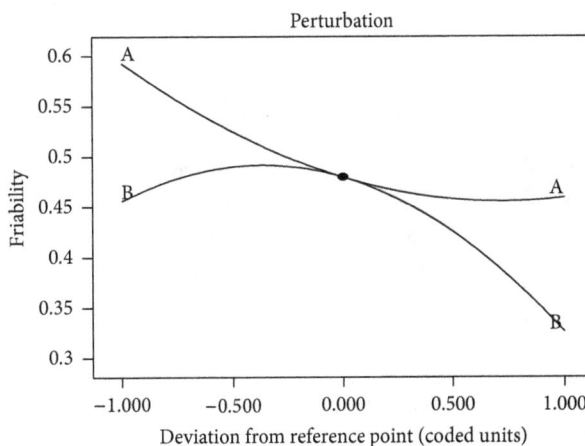

Design-Expert software
Factor coding: actual
Friability

Actual factors
A: CCS = 10.00
B: HRM = 20.00

(b)

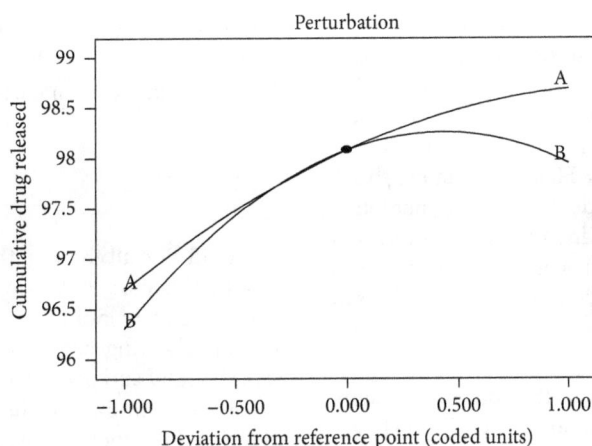

Design-Expert software
Factor coding: actual
Cumulative drug released

Actual factors
A: CCS = 10.00
B: HRM = 20.00

(c)

FIGURE 3: Perturbation plots showing the effects of the variables on the responses, (a) DT in sec and (b) F and DR in 25 minutes, where A is concentration of CCS (X_1) and B is concentration of HRM (X_2).

effect of the factors, the quadratic term on responses, and lack of fit [30]. The analysis of variance (ANOVA) was calculated by the Design-Expert software as shown in Table 5. At the significance level of 5%, the quadratic model was significant, as the p value is less than 0.05 [31].

4.4. Evaluation of Variable Effectiveness by Perturbation Plots. The resulting perturbation plots in Figure 3 help to competently study the effect of each independent factor at a certain point on a specific response, while the remaining

factor maintained constant at a particular mentioned point. A steep or curve slope specifies that the response is sensitive to the definite variable. Figures 3(a)–3(c) show that the concentration of HRM (X_2) had a maximum effect on DT, while concentration of CCS (X_1) significantly affected F and DR. Rising level of X_2 until the reference point results in decrease in DT (synergistic effect). Further increase of X_2 after the reference point results in an increase in DT (antagonistic effect), whilst the elevated concentration of X_1 had a synergistic effect on decrease in F and increases in DR.

TABLE 5: ANOVA for response surface quadratic model for responses.

Term	DT		F		DR	
	F value	p value	F value	p value	F value	p value
Model	46.08	0.0003*	1.25	0.0156*	7.52	0.0205*
X_1-CCS	1.27	0.3106	0.12	0.7457	2.46	0.1777
X_2-HRM	1.27	0.3106	0.47	0.5235	0.77	0.4191
$X_1 X_2$	63.60	0.0005*	1.24	0.3156	8.45	0.0335*
X_1^2	19.65	0.0068*	0.55	0.4901	0.15	0.7184
X_2^2	153.39	<0.0001*	2.05	0.2120	31.92	0.0024*
$X_1^2 X_2$	3.39	0.1249	0.063	0.8112	0.011	0.9192
$X_1 X_2^2$	0.000	1.0000	0.49	0.5154	0.82	0.4075

*$P < 0.05$ gives an indication of the significance of an effect $\alpha = 0.05$.

4.5. Formation of 3D Response Surface Plots. To envision the influence of independent factors on flux, three-dimensional (3D) plots in Figure 4 for (a) DT, (b) F, and (c) DR were formed based on the polynomial model. All of the observed response surfaces formed hillsides with large curvatures confirming that they were mostly influenced by the interaction effect of concentrations of HRM and CCS. From the response surface plots, it was concluded that the increase in concentration of both factors leads to significant decrease in DT, but at a certain point DT may increase due to the wicking problem. Figure 4(a) exhibits that DT varies in a largely curved nonlinear descending order upon increasing HRM and decreasing CCS concentrations. Figure 4(b) shows that F changes in a slightly curved linear descending manner when concentrations of HRM and CCS increased. However, it is illustrated that the DR (Figure 4(c)) alters in a largely curved nonlinear ascending model with increasing concentrations of HRM and CCS.

4.6. Optimization of the Model. From the above discussion, it fairly represents that the formulations of CTZ ODTs are very tough to forecast the overall output traits based on simple interpretation of significant factor deviation. Hence, the desirability function was employed to resolve the optimal default setting of the process parameters that will maximize the three responses. Optimization was performed to obtain the optimal values of X_1 and X_2 for achieving the desirability constraints in the range of disintegration time (12 to 14 seconds), % friability (0.29 to 0.5), and cumulative % drug release (99 to 101.32). The optimized amount of CCS and HRM was incorporated in Table 6.

4.7. Validation of RSM Results of CTZ ODTs Formulation. Eight checkpoint solutions were selected on the principles of optimal formulation specified by thorough grid search to validate the selected experimental design and nonlinear polynomial equations. These checkpoint solutions were prepared and evaluated for the dependent response properties. Table 7 lists the composition, experimental and predicted values of the three response variables, and their respective percentage errors. Moreover, the linear regression plots were constructed accurately between observed and predicted values to the individual response characteristics by MS-Excel, imposing

TABLE 6: Optimization of CTZ ODTs formulation by surface response method.

Name	Constraints		
	Goal	Lower limit	Upper limit
CCS	In range	−1	1
HRM	In range	−1	1
DT (sec)	In range	12	14
F (%)	In range	0.29	0.5
DR in 25 minutes	In range	99.0	101.32

the trend-line all the way through starting point to measure quantitatively as shown in Figures 5(a)–5(c). In the linear graph group of points are scattered above and below the 45° line showing better prediction and less error between experimental and predicted values. The formulation number $F * 4$ was optimized as the best formulation for CTZ ODTs in which the error was minimum for the dependent variables. The composition of optimized formulation $F * 4$ is given in Table 8. The powder flow properties and postcompression parameters are given in Tables 9 and 10, respectively.

5. Conclusion

In this experimental study, the synthetic and natural disintegrants were detected to have a reflective and collaborative influence upon the characteristics of ODTs of CTZ formulation. This system embraces the drug-delivery system that achieves fast and relatively quick release of the drug over agreeable period of time. The response variables of the formulation are optimized by RSM (CCD design), and the results observed indicated that this experimental design had been successfully applied to develop the combination of CCS and HRM to prepare ODTs with desirable rapid disintegration and drug release. Combination of synthetic and natural disintegrant using response surface methodology can be formulated in an ideal oral disintegrating tablet. Moreover, their mutual influences on studied parameters can be exploited and commercialized.

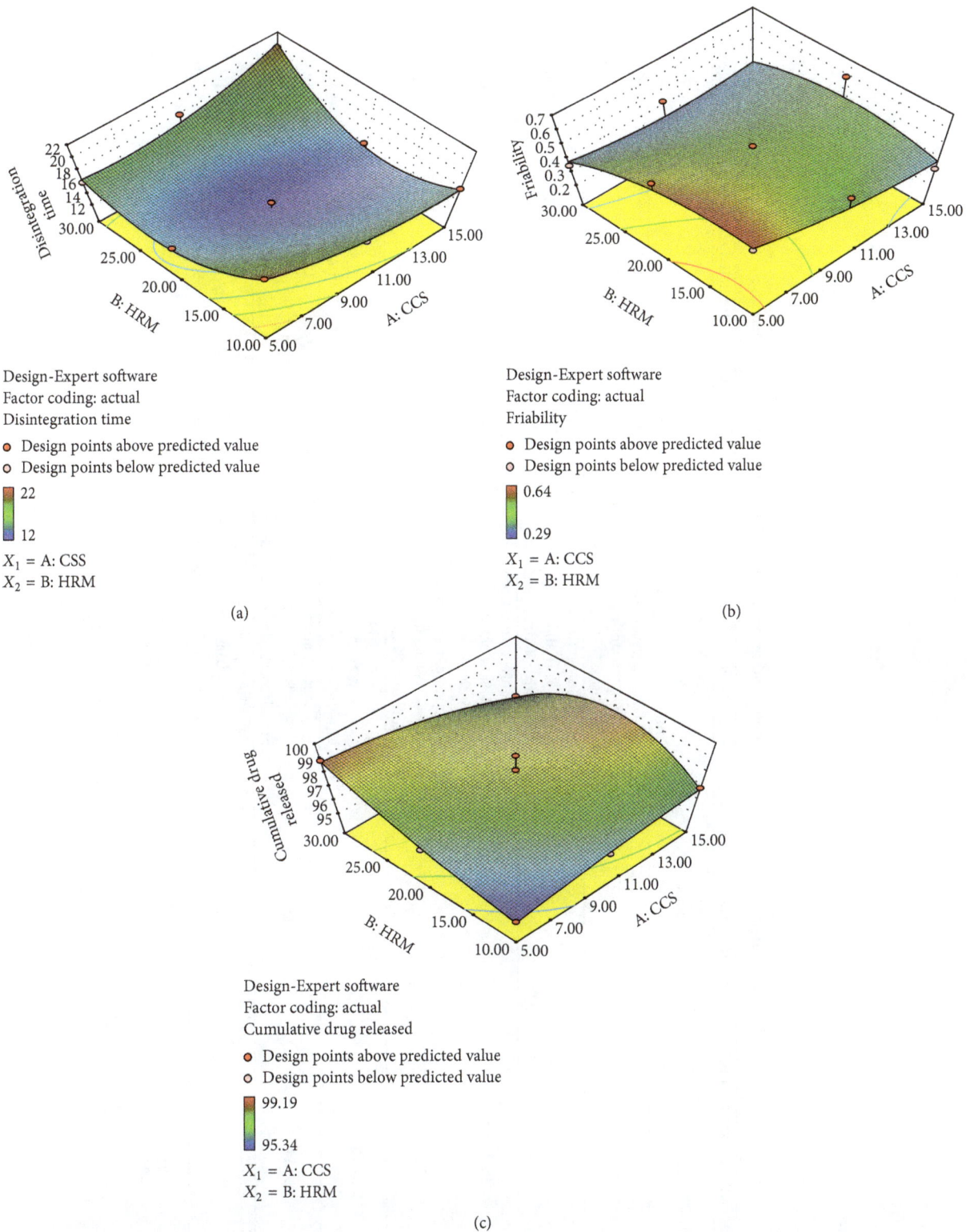

Design-Expert software
Factor coding: actual
Disintegration time

● Design points above predicted value
○ Design points below predicted value

■ 22

□ 12

X_1 = A: CSS
X_2 = B: HRM

(a)

Design-Expert software
Factor coding: actual
Friability

● Design points above predicted value
○ Design points below predicted value

■ 0.64

□ 0.29

X_1 = A: CCS
X_2 = B: HRM

(b)

Design-Expert software
Factor coding: actual
Cumulative drug released

● Design points above predicted value
○ Design points below predicted value

■ 99.19

□ 95.34

X_1 = A: CCS
X_2 = B: HRM

(c)

FIGURE 4: Response surface plot showing interaction of variable X_1 (concentration of CCS) and variable X_2 (concentration of HRM) influencing (a) disintegration time, (b) % friability, and (c) cumulative % drug release.

TABLE 7: Composition of the checkpoint formulations and the predicted and experimental values of response variables.

Number	Croscarmellose sodium (mg)	*H. rosa-sinensis* mucilage (mg)	Response variables	Observed response	Predicted response	Percentage error	Avg
F * 1	10.34	20.11	Disintegration time	12.392	12.361	0.031	2.231
			% friability	0.446	0.478	−0.032	
			Cumulative % drug released	100.031	100.367	−0.336	
F * 2	9.13	17.36	Disintegration time	12.932	12.834	0.763	1.008
			% friability	0.511	0.496	3.024	
			Cumulative % drug released	100.64	99.986	0.654	
F * 3	8.72	17.92	Disintegration time	12.993	12.861	1.026	1.67
			% friability	0.524	0.499	5.01	
			Cumulative % drug released	99.261	99.995	−0.734	
F * 4	9.05	16.04	Disintegration time	13.010	13.271	−1.96	**0.133**
			% friability	0.500	0.498	0.401	
			Cumulative % drug released	99.523	99.768	−0.245	
F * 5	10.61	14.23	Disintegration time	13.323	13.445	−0.907	1.48
			% friability	0.492	0.471	4.458	
			Cumulative % drug released	99.358	99.661	−0.304	
F * 6	10.40	16.71	Disintegration time	12.539	12.627	−0.696	2.282
			% friability	0.515	0.482	6.846	
			Cumulative % drug released	100.364	100.092	0.272	
F * 7	12.14	15.49	Disintegration time	12.528	12.796	−2.094	0.212
			% friability	0.498	0.467	6.638	
			Cumulative % drug released	100.548	100.161	0.386	
F * 8	11.50	13.00	Disintegration time	13.995	13.857	0.995	1.284
			% friability	0.461	0.447	3.131	
			Cumulative % drug released	99.125	99.505	−0.381	

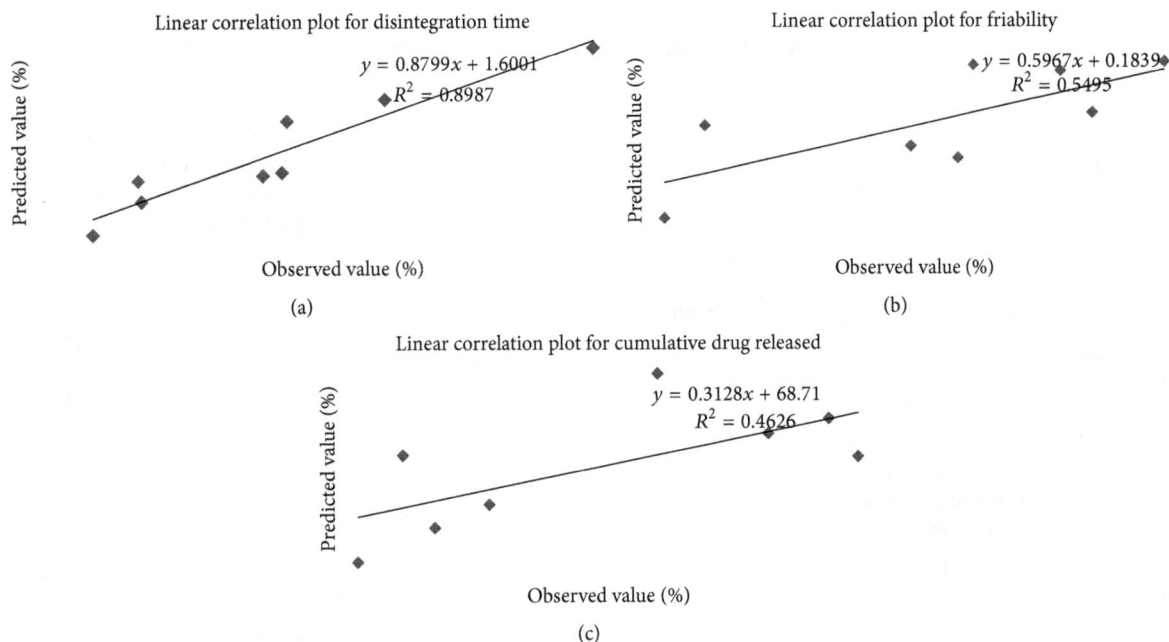

FIGURE 5: Linear correlation plots between observed and predicted values for (a) DT in sec, (b) percent of F, and (c) percent of cumulative drug release of cetirizine HCl oral disintegration tablet formulations.

TABLE 8: Final optimized formulation ($F * 4$) of CTZ ODTs formulation.

Composition	Amount
CTZ	10 mg
Pearlitol SD 100	128.91 mg
CCS	9.05 mg
HRM	16.04 mg
Sorbitol	20 mg
Other excipients	12 mg
Aspartame	4 mg

*Other excipients: magnesium stearate: 2 mg, aerosil: 2 mg, talc: 2 mg, flavour: 6 mg, total tablet weight: 200 mg, and batch size: 50 tablets.

TABLE 9: Powder flow properties of the optimized formulation ($F * 4$).

Properties	Optimized formulation ($F * 4$)
Angle of repose	26.46
Bulk density	0.487
Tapped density	0.581
Carr's Compressibility Index	16.71
Hausner's ratio	1.192

TABLE 10: Postcompression parameters of the optimized formulation ($F * 4$).

Parameters	Value
Wetting time (sec)**	10
Water absorption ratio (%)**	89.01 ± 0.05
Weight variation (%)#	0.71
Thickness (mm)*	3.1 ± 0.28
Hardness	3.1 ± 0.44
Content uniformity (%)#	99.99 ± 0.35
Residual remaining on the screen $\neq 22$#	No
Average weight**	199.81
Taste/mouth feel*	Palatable

*Each value was an average of six determinations. **Each value was an average of three determinations. #Results of one batch $n = 20$.

Acknowledgments

The authors are very grateful to Dr. Jagadeesh Panda, Principal of Raghu College of pharmacy, Visakhapatnam, for his encouragement and support.

Competing Interests

The authors declare no conflict of interests.

References

[1] J. Xu, L. L. Bovet, and K. Zhao, "Taste masking microspheres for orally disintegrating tablets," International Journal of Pharmaceutics, vol. 359, no. 1-2, pp. 63–69, 2008.

[2] H. Seager, "Drug-delivery products and the Zydis fast-dissolving dosage form," Journal of Pharmacy and Pharmacology, vol. 50, no. 4, pp. 375–382, 1998.

[3] L. Dobetti, "Fast melting tablets: developments and technologies," *Pharmaceutica. Technology Europe*, vol. 12, no. 9, pp. 32–42, 2000.

[4] S. Hamlen and K. MacGregor, "Patient compliance study: new data shows drug delivery has positive impact on patient compliance," *Drug Development & Delivery*, vol. 11, no. 7, pp. 30–33, 2011.

[5] M. Guhmann, M. Preis, F. Gerber, N. Pöllinger, J. Breitkreutz, and W. Weitschies, "Development of oral taste masked diclofenac formulations using a taste sensing system," *International Journal of Pharmaceutics*, vol. 438, no. 1-2, pp. 81–90, 2012.

[6] G. Abdelbary, P. Prinderre, C. Eouani, J. Joachim, J. P. Reynier, and P. Piccerelle, "The preparation of orally disintegrating tablets using a hydrophilic waxy binder," *International Journal of Pharmaceutics*, vol. 278, no. 2, pp. 423–433, 2004.

[7] S. Singh and D. Shah, "Development and characterization of mouth dissolving tablet of zolmitriptan," *Asian Pacific Journal of Tropical Disease*, vol. 2, no. 1, pp. S457–S464, 2012.

[8] S. G. Late, Y.-Y. Yu, and A. K. Banga, "Effects of disintegration-promoting agent, lubricants and moisture treatment on optimized fast disintegrating tablets," *International Journal of Pharmaceutics*, vol. 365, no. 1-2, pp. 4–11, 2009.

[9] A. Ghosh and P. Chakraborty, "Formulation and mathematical optimization of controlled release calcium alginate micro pellets of frusemide," *BioMed Research International*, vol. 2013, Article ID 819674, 14 pages, 2013.

[10] D. C. Montgomery, "Response surface methodology," in *Design and Analysis of Experiments*, John Wiley & Sons, New York, NY, USA, 2nd edition, 1996.

[11] B. Singh, S. K. Chakkal, and N. Ahuja, "Formulation and optimization of controlled release mucoadhesive tablets of atenolol using response surface methodology," *AAPS PharmSciTech*, vol. 7, no. 1, article no. 3, 2006.

[12] B. Singh, R. Kumar, and N. Ahuja, "Optimizing drug delivery systems using systematic "design of experiments." Part I: fundamental aspects," *Critical Reviews in Therapeutic Drug Carrier Systems*, vol. 22, no. 1, pp. 27–105, 2005.

[13] B. Singh, M. Dahiya, V. Saharan, and N. Ahuja, "Optimizing drug delivery systems using systematic 'design of experiments.' Part II: retrospect and prospects," *Critical Reviews in Therapeutic Drug Carrier Systems*, vol. 22, no. 3, pp. 215–294, 2005.

[14] S. C. Sweetman, *Martindale: The Complete Drug Reference*, 35th edition, 2007.

[15] R. Mishra and A. Amin, "Formulation and characterization of rapidly dissolving films of cetirizine hydrochloride using pullulan as a film forming agent," *Indian Journal of Pharmaceutical Education and Research*, vol. 45, no. 1, pp. 71–77, 2011.

[16] L. Prabakaran, V. S. N. Murthy, and M. Karpakavalli, "Extraction and characterization of Hybiscus Rosa-Sinensis leaves mucilage for Pharmaceutical applications," *RGUHS Journal of Pharmaceutical Sciences*, vol. 1, no. 3, pp. 232–238, 2011.

[17] H. A. Ahad, C. S. Kumar, P. Yesupadam, P. S. Rani, A. C. Sekhar, and G. V. Sivaramakrishna, "Fabrication and characterization of diclofenac sodium hibiscus rosa-sinensis leaves mucilage sustained release matrix tablets," *Der Pharmacia Lettre*, vol. 2, no. 1, pp. 452–456, 2010.

[18] S. Schiermeier and P. C. Schmidt, "Fast dispersible ibuprofen tablets," *European Journal of Pharmaceutical Sciences*, vol. 15, no. 3, pp. 295–305, 2002.

[19] S. C. Basak, B. M. J. Reddy, and K. P. L. Mani, "Formulation and release behaviour of sustained release ambroxol hydrochloride HPMC matrix tablet," *Indian Journal of Pharmaceutical Sciences*, vol. 68, no. 5, pp. 594–598, 2006.

[20] S. Chopra, G. V. Patil, and S. K. Motwani, "Release modulating hydrophilic matrix systems of losartan potassium: optimization of formulation using statistical experimental design," *European Journal of Pharmaceutics and Biopharmaceutics*, vol. 66, no. 1, pp. 73–82, 2007.

[21] P. R. Radhika, T. K. Pal, and T. Sivakumar, "Optimization of glipizide sustained release matrix tablet formulation by central composite design- response surface methodology," *Journal of Pharmacy Research*, vol. 2, no. 1, pp. 94–102, 2009.

[22] B. K. Sahoo, U. Chakraborty, J. Mukherjee, and T. K. Pal, "Optimization and validation of modulated release formulation of ranitidine HCl by response surface methodology," *Journal of Biomedical Sciences and Research*, vol. 2, no. 2, pp. 76–85, 2010.

[23] Y. X. Bi, H. Sunada, Y. Yonezawa, and K. Danjo, "Evaluation of rapidly disintegrating tablets prepared by a direct compression method," *Drug Development and Industrial Pharmacy*, vol. 25, no. 5, pp. 571–581, 1999.

[24] R. J. Jones, A. Rajabi-Siahboomi, M. Levina, Y. Perrie, and A. R. Mohammed, "The influence of formulation and manufacturing process parameters on the characteristics of lyophilized orally disintegrating tablets," *Pharmaceutics*, vol. 3, no. 3, pp. 440–457, 2011.

[25] D. D. Douroumis, A. Gryczke, and S. Schminke, "Development and evaluation of cetirizine HCl taste-masked oral disintegrating tablets," *AAPS PharmSciTech*, vol. 12, no. 1, pp. 141–151, 2011.

[26] J.-S. Chang, Y.-B. Huang, S.-S. Hou, R.-J. Wang, P.-C. Wu, and Y.-H. Tsai, "Formulation optimization of meloxicam sodium gel using response surface methodology," *International Journal of Pharmaceutics*, vol. 338, no. 1-2, pp. 48–54, 2007.

[27] M. Ahuja, M. Yadav, and S. Kumar, "Application of response surface methodology to formulation of ionotropically gelled gum cordia/gellan beads," *Carbohydrate Polymers*, vol. 80, no. 1, pp. 161–167, 2010.

[28] R. M. Pabari and Z. Ramtoola, "Application of face centred central composite design to optimise compression force and tablet diameter for the formulation of mechanically strong and fast disintegrating orodispersible tablets," *International Journal of Pharmaceutics*, vol. 430, no. 1-2, pp. 18–25, 2012.

[29] H. Sunada and Y. Bi, "Preparation, evaluation and optimization of rapidly disintegrating tablets," *Powder Technology*, vol. 122, no. 2-3, pp. 188–198, 2002.

[30] H. E. Gan, R. Karim, S. K. S. Muhammad, J. A. Bakar, D. M. Hashim, and R. A. Rahman, "Optimization of the basic formulation of a traditional baked cassava cake using response surface methodology," *LWT—Food Science and Technology*, vol. 40, no. 4, pp. 611–618, 2007.

[31] S. Furlanetto, M. Cirri, F. Maestrelli, G. Corti, and P. Mura, "Study of formulation variables influencing the drug release rate from matrix tablets by experimental design," *European Journal of Pharmaceutics and Biopharmaceutics*, vol. 62, no. 1, pp. 77–84, 2006.

13

Formulation and Evaluation of Antibacterial Creams and Gels Containing Metal Ions for Topical Application

Mei X. Chen, Kenneth S. Alexander, and Gabriella Baki

Department of Pharmacy Practice, College of Pharmacy and Pharmaceutical Sciences, University of Toledo, 3000 Arlington Ave., Toledo, OH 43614, USA

Correspondence should be addressed to Gabriella Baki; gabriella.baki@utoledo.edu

Academic Editor: Sumio Chono

Background. Skin infections occur commonly and often present therapeutic challenges to practitioners due to the growing concerns regarding multidrug-resistant bacterial, viral, and fungal strains. The antimicrobial properties of zinc sulfate and copper sulfate are well known and have been investigated for many years. However, the synergistic activity between these two metal ions as antimicrobial ingredients has not been evaluated in topical formulations. *Objective.* The aims of the present study were to (1) formulate topical creams and gels containing zinc and copper alone or in combination and (2) evaluate the *in vitro* antibacterial activity of these metal ions in the formulations. *Method.* Formulation of the gels and creams was followed by evaluating their organoleptic characteristics, physicochemical properties, and *in vitro* antibacterial activity against *Escherichia coli* and *Staphylococcus aureus. Results.* Zinc sulfate and copper sulfate had a strong synergistic antibacterial activity in the creams and gels. The minimum effective concentration was found to be 3 w/w% for both active ingredients against the two tested microorganisms. *Conclusions.* This study evaluated and confirmed the synergistic *in vitro* antibacterial effect of copper sulfate and zinc sulfate in a cream and two gels.

1. Introduction

Topical skin infections commonly occur and often present therapeutic challenges to practitioners, despite the numerous existing antimicrobial agents available today. The necessity for developing new antimicrobial means has increased significantly due to growing concerns regarding multidrug-resistant bacterial, viral, and fungal strains [1–4]. Consequently, attention has been devoted to safe, new, and/or alternative antimicrobial materials in the field of antimicrobial chemotherapy.

Common examples for topical skin infections include diaper rash, cold sores, and tinea (also called pityriasis) versicolor. Diaper rash is a form of irritant contact dermatitis. It is one of the most common dermatological conditions encountered in babies while using diapers [5] and is estimated to occur in 7–35% of babies between the ages of 9 and 12 months [6]. Its development is multifactorial, including skin wetness, friction, skin irritants, and pH change, which favors the growth of microorganisms including *Candida,*

Staphylococcus, and *Streptococcus* [7]. It has been shown that zinc and copper ions have antimicrobial activity against *Staphylococcus aureus* and *Candida albicans* [8]. Cold sores (also known as herpes labialis) are a common viral infection occurring on the lips, primarily caused by herpes simplex virus (HSV) type 1 [9]. Studies have shown that zinc and copper salts exhibit inactivation of HSV both *in vivo* and *in vitro* [10–13]. Zinc sulfate was found to have an antimicrobial effect in treating cold sores [14]. The molecular mechanism of its therapeutic effect was found to be the drastic inactivation of free virus in skin tissues, intercellular vesicles, and blisters [15]. Pityriasis versicolor is a superficial fungal infection of the skin, usually caused by *Malassezia* species. It is one of the most common skin diseases in tropical and subtropical areas and is characterized by fine scaly patches and macules [16]. Both zinc sulfate and copper sulfate have been found to be effective in treating this disease [17, 18].

In recent years, a number of metal ions have been studied as potential antimicrobial agents, including silver [19], copper [20], zinc [21], iron [22], magnesium [23], and titanium [24].

Zinc, alone or as an adjuvant, has been found to be advantageous in a number of dermatological infections and inflammatory diseases owing to its modulating actions on macrophage and neutrophil functions, natural killer cell/phagocytic activity, and various inflammatory cytokines. Zinc sulfate has been studied *in vivo* in a number of diseases, including warts [25], herpes genitalis [26], pityriasis versicolor [18], and acne vulgaris [27] in varying concentrations. Copper is well known for its antimicrobial properties. It has been used as an algicide, germicide, and fungicide for decades. Several antimicrobial mechanisms of copper were proposed in recent articles, including reactive hydroxyl radical formation leading to damaged cell integrity, denaturation of DNA by binding of copper to protein molecules, and inactivation of enzymes and obstruction of functional groups of proteins from displacement of essential ions [28–30]. Additionally, topically applied copper sulfate and hypericum perforatum were found to be efficacious *in vivo* in the treatment of herpes skin lesions [13].

The antimicrobial activity of zinc sulfate and copper sulfate has been investigated for many years. However, the synergistic activity between these two metal ions as antimicrobial ingredients has not been evaluated in topical formulations. The aim of the present study was to formulate topical creams and gels containing zinc sulfate or copper sulfate, and a combination of these, and to evaluate the *in vitro* antibacterial activity of these metal salts in the formulations against *Escherichia coli* and *Staphylococcus aureus*. The *in vitro* antibacterial activity of the formulated products was also compared to commercial products available for the treatment of diaper rash and cold sores.

Incorporating metal ions such as zinc and copper often creates a formulation challenge due to the high reactivity of these ions. Even trace amounts of metal ions are able to catalyze oxidation reactions in fatty compounds in products, leading to deterioration including odor formation, color change, and physical and/or chemical instability [31]. Metal ion reactions with the ingredients in the formulations can affect the quality, efficacy, consumer appeal, and shelf-life of formulations. Stability of product and of the antibacterial activity was studied for 12 weeks at two different temperatures in two different containers.

2. Materials and Methods

2.1. Materials. Copper sulfate pentahydrate was purchased from Fagron, Inc. (St. Paul, MN). Zinc sulfate heptahydrate, Carbomer 940, refined corn oil, almond oil sweet, lecithin soya granular, glycerin, and propylene glycol were purchased from Letco Medical (Decatur, AL). (*ι*)-Carrageenan was purchased from Sigma-Aldrich (St. Louis, MO). Hypromellose (Benecel, K4M PHARM, also known as hydroxypropylmethyl cellulose, HPMC), and Prolipid 141 (a mixture of glyceryl stearate, behenyl alcohol, palmitic acid, stearic acid, lecithin, lauryl alcohol, myristyl alcohol, and cetyl alcohol) were received as gifts from Ashland (Wilmington, DE). Kollidon® 90F (poly vinylpyrrolidone, PVP) was obtained from BASF (Ludwigshafen, Germany). Poloxamer 407 was

purchased from PCCA (Houston, TX). FlexiThix™ (2-pyrrolidinone-1-ethenyl homopolymer) was received as a free sample from ISP Technologies, Inc. (Wayne, NJ). Xanthan gum, guar gum, methylparaben, propylparaben, butylated hydroxytoluene (BHT), and citric acid monohydrate were obtained from Spectrum Chemical (Gardena, CA). Medium chain triglycerides (MCT) were obtained from Mead Johnson & Company (Evansville, Indiana). Soybean oil, Cithrol™ GMS 40 (glyceryl stearate), Arlacel™ 165 (a mixture of glyceryl stearate and PEG-100 stearate), Tween 60, and Span 80 were received as free samples from Croda, Inc. (Edison, NJ). PEG-16 Macadamia and PEG-10 Sunflower were obtained from FloraTech (Gilbert, Arizona). Cocoa butter was a gift from Koster Keunen, Inc. (Watertown, CT). Cetyl alcohol, stearic acid, stearyl alcohol, and isopropyl myristate were obtained from Sherman Research Labs (Toledo, OH). Coconut oil was purchased from Spectrum Organic Products, (Melville, NY). Tefose HC (a mixture of cetyl alcohol, glyceryl stearate, ceteth-20, and steareth-20) was a free sample from Gattefossé (Saint-Priest Cedex, France). PEG-8 beeswax was a gift from Koster Keunen, Inc. (Watertown, CT). Urea was purchased from Gallipot®, Inc. (St. Paul, MN). Triethanolamine was purchased from Making Cosmetics (Snoqualmie, WA). Mueller-Hinton agar and gentamicin 10 μg standard discs were purchased from Becton, Dickinson and Company (Sparks, MD). The marketed products included Equate® Diaper Rash Relief Cream (distributed by Walmart, Inc.), Nexcare™ Cold Sore Treatment Cream (distributed by 3M), and Campho-Phenique® Cold Sore Treatment Gel (distributed by Bayer Health Care LLC), which were all purchased at a local Walmart store (Toledo, OH). All ingredients used in the various formulations can be found in Tables 1 and 2.

2.2. Methods

2.2.1. Formulation of the Topical Cream. The oil phase was prepared by melting the waxes at 75°C and mixing the ingredients uniformly. The aqueous phase was prepared by dissolving the water-soluble ingredients in deionized water. The water phase was warmed to 75–80°C until all ingredients were dissolved. When the water and oil phase were at the same temperature, the aqueous phase was slowly added to the oil phase with moderate agitation and was kept stirred until the temperature dropped to 40°C. The emulsion was cooled to room temperature to form a semisolid cream base. Zinc sulfate and copper sulfate were dissolved in warmed deionized water, and the solutions were added to the cream base using an overhead stirrer (Talboys Engineering Corp, Emerson, NJ). The mixture was stirred for 15 min until the formulation became uniform. The drug-loaded cream was preserved with paraben concentrate. The exact concentration of each ingredient is shown in Table 1.

2.2.2. Formulation of the Topical Gels. When using (*ι*)-carrageenan, xanthan gum, and guar gum, the powder polymers were dispersed in 75°C warm deionized water with stirring. When all the polymers were dissolved, the mixture was removed from the hot plate. The desired amount of

TABLE 1: Composition of the topical cream formulations.

Ingredients	Amount of each ingredient (%); formulations are coded from 1 to 20																				
	C1	C2	C3	C4	C5	C6	C7	C8	C9	C10	C11	C12	C13	C14	C15	C16	C17	C18	C19	C20
Copper sulfate											3									
Zinc sulfate											3									
Corn oil	4	4	4	4	—	—	—	—	—	—	—	—	—	—	—	—	—	—	—	—
MCT	4	4	4	4	—	3	3	3	5	5	4	4	—	—	—	6	—	4	4	4
Sweet Almond oil	4	4	4	4	5	4	4	5	—	—	—	—	10	10	6	—	5	4	4	4
Coconut oil	—	—	—	—	—	—	—	—	5	5	4	4	—	—	—	4	5	4	4	4
Cocoa butter	—	—	—	—	—	—	—	—	—	—	—	—	—	—	—	3	—	—	—	—
Soy bean oil	—	—	—	—	5	6	6	6	5	5	4	4	—	—	6	4	4	—	—	—
PEG-16 Macadamia	—	—	—	—	—	—	—	—	—	—	—	—	—	—	—	4	—	—	—	—
PEG-10 Sunflower	—	—	—	—	—	—	—	—	—	—	—	—	2	2	—	—	—	—	—	—
Tefose HC	4	5	6	6	—	—	—	—	—	—	—	—	—	—	—	—	—	—	—	—
Prolipid 141	5	6	5	7	—	—	—	—	—	—	—	—	—	—	—	—	—	—	—	—
PEG-8 Beeswax	7	8	6	6	—	—	—	—	—	4	6	7	—	—	—	—	—	7	6	7
Cithrol GMS 40	5	6	6	6	—	—	—	—	—	—	—	—	—	—	—	—	—	—	—	3
Span 80	—	—	—	—	—	—	—	—	—	—	—	—	1.05	2.25	1.57	1.42	1.77	—	—	—
Tween 60	—	—	—	—	—	—	—	—	—	—	—	—	0.95	2.75	2.43	2.58	2.23	—	—	—
Stearyl Alcohol	—	—	—	—	—	—	—	—	—	—	—	—	—	—	—	4	5	—	5	2
Stearic acid	—	—	—	—	3	2	3	4	4	4	4	5	2	2	5	—	—	4	—	—
Cetyl alcohol	—	—	—	—	5	4	5	7	6	6	6	7	2	4	5	3	5	6	6	6
Arlacel 165	—	—	—	—	5	5	5	5	5	5	5	5	—	—	—	—	—	5	5	5
Urea	—	—	—	—	3	—	—	—	—	—	—	—	4	4	3	3	—	—	—	—
2% HPMC gel	—	—	—	—	—	—	—	—	—	—	—	—	—	—	—	—	—	5	—	—
Xanthan gum	—	—	—	—	—	0.5	0.25	0.25	0.25	0.25	0.25	0.25	—	—	0.5	0.5	—	—	—	—
Carrageenan	0.35	0.35	0.35	0.35	—	—	—	—	—	—	—	—	—	—	—	—	—	—	—	—
Glycerin											5									
Citric acid											1									
BHT											0.05									
DI water											qs ad to 100									

MCT: medium chain triglycerides; HPMC: hypromellose; BHT: butylated hydroxytoluene.

TABLE 2: Composition of the topical gel formulations.

Ingredients	Amount of each ingredient (%); formulations are coded from 1 to 18																		
	G1	G2	G3	G4	G5	G6	G7	G8	G9	G10	G11	G12	G13	G14	G15	G16	G17	G18
Zinc sulfate									3									
Copper sulfate									3									
ι-Carrageenan	2	1	—	—	—	—	—	—	—	—	—	—	—	—	—	—	—	—
5% HPMC gel	—	—	qs 100	qs 100	50	25	—	—	—	—	—	—	—	—	—	—	—	—
Xanthan gum	—	—	—	—	—	—	2	—	—	—	—	—	—	—	—	—	—	—
Guar gum	—	—	—	—	—	—	—	2	—	—	—	—	—	—	—	—	—	—
Poloxamer 407	—	—	—	—	—	—	—	—	32	24	16	—	—	—	—	—	—	—
Lecithin	—	—	—	—	—	—	—	—	10	10	10	—	—	—	—	—	—	—
Isopropyl myristate	—	—	—	—	—	—	—	—	10	10	10	—	—	—	—	—	—	—
Kollidon 90F	—	—	—	—	—	—	—	—	—	—	—	30	20	10	—	—	—	—
FlexiThix	—	—	—	—	—	—	—	—	—	—	—	—	—	—	6	4	2	—
Carbomer 940	—	—	—	—	—	—	—	—	—	—	—	—	—	—	—	—	—	1
Triethanolamine	—	—	—	—	—	—	—	—	—	—	—	—	—	—	—	—	—	1.35
BHT	—	—	—	—	—	—	—	—	0.05	0.05	0.05	—	—	—	—	—	—	—
DI water	qs ad to 100	—		25								qs ad to 100						

HPMC: hypromellose; BHT: butylated hydroxytoluene.

zinc sulfate and copper sulfate was dissolved in the clear gel with intensive stirring. The mixture was then cooled to room temperature and preserved with paraben concentrate.

In formulations where HPMC was the thickening agent, the polymer was dispersed in 75°C warm deionized water with stirring. The resulting solution was stored at room temperature overnight until a clear gel formed. Zinc sulfate crystals and then copper sulfate crystals, after complete dissolution, were dispersed into the gel with intensive agitation. Preservative was added to the formulation in the last step.

Poloxamer was dissolved in cold water and stored under refrigerated conditions at 4°C for a night. The oil phase was prepared by mixing lecithin and isopropyl myristate in a 1:1 ratio. The mixture was stored at room temperature overnight for the complete dissolution of lecithin. The active ingredients were then added directly to the aqueous phase. The gel was prepared by mixing 1 part of oil phase with 4 parts of aqueous phase (poloxamer gel) using a vortex mixer (VORTEX-T, Genie® 2, Bohemia, NY).

Kollidon 90F, FlexiThix, and Carbomer 940 were directly dispersed into deionized water at room temperature with intensive agitation. Active ingredients were incorporated into the gel uniformly. In order for Carbomer 940 to form a gel, triethanolamine was added to neutralize the pH to 6–6.5. Table 2 shows the amount of ingredients used for the gels.

2.2.3. Physical Evaluation of the Topical Formulations

(1) Organoleptic Characteristics. All blank formulations (i.e., formulations without any active ingredients or preservatives) and drug-loaded formulations were tested for physical appearance, color, texture, phase separation, and homogeneity. These characteristics were evaluated by visual observation. Homogeneity and texture were tested by pressing a small quantity of the formulated cream and gels between the thumb and index finger. The consistency of the formulations and presence of coarse particles were used to evaluate the texture and homogeneity of the formulations. Immediate skin feel (including stiffness, grittiness, and greasiness) was also evaluated.

(2) Spreadability. Spreadability of the formulations was determined by measuring the spreading diameter of 1 g of sample between two horizontal glass plates (10 cm × 20 cm) after one minute. The standard weight applied to the upper plate was 25 g. Each formulation was tested three times.

(3) pH Values. One gram of each formulation (including the blank, i.e., formulation without any active ingredients or preservatives, and drug-loaded formulation) was dispersed in 25 mL of deionized water, and the pH was determined using a pH meter (Mettler-Toledo Ingold Inc., Billerica, MA). Measurements were made in triplicate. The pH meter was calibrated with standard buffer solutions (pH 4, 7, and 10) before each use.

(4) Viscosity Measurement. A Brookfield viscometer DV-I (Brookfield Engineering Laboratories, Middleboro, MA) was used with a concentric cylinder spindle #29 to determine the viscosity of the different topical formulations. The tests were carried out at 21°C. The spindle was rotated at 0, 0.5, 1, 2, 2.5, 4, 5, 10, 20, 50, and 100 rpm values. All measurements were made in triplicate.

2.2.4. In Vitro Antibacterial Activity

(1) Preparation of Mueller-Hinton (MH) Agar Plates. Mueller-Hinton (MH) agar medium was prepared according to the manufacturer's instructions and autoclaved for 20 minutes at 20 psi. After autoclaving, the agar medium was cooled to 40–45°C in a water bath. Sixty mL of the cooled agar medium was poured onto the prepared 150 × 15 mm petri dish. The agar was allowed to cool to room temperature and stored in a refrigerator (2–8°C) until used.

(2) Preparation of Inoculum. Escherichia coli (ATCC 25922) and *Staphylococcus aureus* (ATCC 29213) were used to evaluate the antibacterial activity of the topical formulations containing zinc sulfate and copper sulfate. The microorganisms were subcultured the previous day to ensure that the tested microorganisms were in their log phase of growth and to ensure the validity of the results. One or two isolated colonies of the tested microorganisms were touched using a sterile cotton swab. The microorganisms were suspended in 2 mL of sterile saline medium and vortexed well until a uniform suspension was obtained. The turbidity of the suspension was measured at 625 nm using a UV-Vis spectrophotometer (Thermo Scientific, Waltham, MA). The turbidity of the suspension was adjusted to a 0.5 McFarland standard by adding more microorganism if the suspension was too light or diluting with sterile saline if the suspension was too heavy. The suspension was prepared before inoculating the microorganisms on the agar plate.

(3) Inoculation of the MH Plate. To inoculate the MH agar plates, a sterile cotton swab was dipped into the suspension and streaked over the surface of the agar plates. This procedure was repeated three times; each time, the plate was rotated approximately 60 degrees to ensure even distribution of the inoculum [32]. The plates were then allowed to dry at room temperature for 5 min before applying the drug.

(4) Preparation of Agar Well Diffusion Assay. The dried inoculated MH agar plates prepared above were used to perform the agar well diffusion assay. A sterile cork borer was used to make the wells by punching holes on the inoculated MH agar plates. Each well was 5 mm in diameter, and the cut-out of the agar was removed using a sterile needle. A desired amount of the formulations was weighed and placed into each well on an analytical balance. Gentamicin 10 μg standard discs were used as a control to ensure that the agar medium was appropriate to support the growth of the microorganism beyond the zone of inhibition. The gentamicin standard disc was placed and pressed gently onto the same inoculated agar plate by using sterile forceps. The inoculated agar plate was incubated at 37°C for 18 hours. The observed diameters of the zones of inhibition were measured by using a ruler to the nearest millimeter.

First, in order to observe how effective the active ingredients were alone versus combined, 20 μL of 3% copper sulfate, 3% zinc sulfate, 6% copper sulfate, 6% zinc sulfate, and 3 + 3% copper sulfate and zinc sulfate combined solutions were tested for antibacterial activity against *E. coli* and *S. aureus*. Next, the selected cream and gel formulations containing both active ingredients in a series of concentrations (including 0, 0.1, 0.25, 0.5, 1, 2, and 3% of each ingredient) were tested for antibacterial activity against *E. coli* and *S. aureus* to evaluate their effective concentration. Gentamicin 10 μg standard disc was used as the control. The sample size directly measured into the wells was 80.2 ± 0.3 μg in this study. Finally, the selected cream and gel formulations were directly compared to the marketed products, including Nexcare Cold Sore Treatment Cream, Campho-Phenique Cold Sore Treatment Gel, and Equate Diaper Rash Relief Cream, in terms of their antibacterial activity against *E. coli* and *S. aureus*. The sample size directly measured into the wells was 72.3 ± 1 μg in this study.

2.2.5. Stability Study. The antibacterial activity of all selected drug-loaded formulations was tested against *E. coli* using the above-described agar well diffusion assay for 12 weeks (measurements were made on day 1, week 3, week 6, week 9, and week 12). The antibacterial activity of the formulations was compared for samples stored at room temperature (25°C) and in the refrigerator (4°C) as well as those packaged into glass containers versus plastic containers. In addition to the antibacterial activity, pH values, color, physical appearance, and texture were also tested during the 12 weeks with the above-described methods.

2.2.6. Statistical Analysis. Statistical analysis of data was performed using one-way ANOVA (Tukey's *post hoc* test). A difference was considered statistically significant when $p < 0.05$.

3. Results

From the twenty different creams formulated, C1 was selected as the final formulation for further testing. Eighteen different gels were formulated in this study, from which G1 and G5 were selected as optimal formulations for further evaluation.

3.1. Physical Evaluation of Topical Cream and Gels

3.1.1. Organoleptic Characteristics. The organoleptic properties, including physical appearance, color, texture, phase separation, homogeneity, and immediate skin feel of the selected topical formulations, are displayed in Table 3. Results showed that the cream and both gels had a cosmetically appealing appearance and smooth texture, and they were all homogenous with no signs of phase separation. All formulations were blue due to copper sulfate.

3.1.2. Spreadability. Spreadability of semisolid formulations, that is, the ability of a cream or gel to evenly spread on the skin, plays an important role in the administration of a

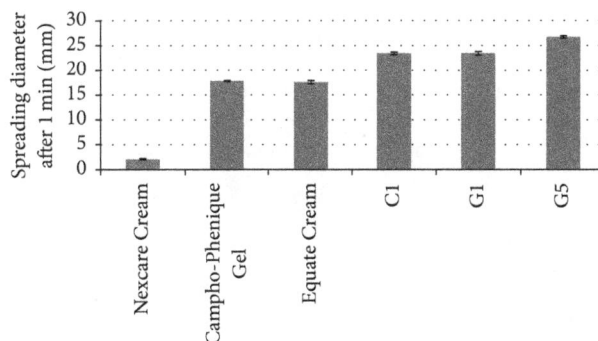

FIGURE 1: Spreadability values for the selected cream (C1) and gels (G1 and G5) compared to various marketed products ($n = 3$, results shown as mean ± SD).

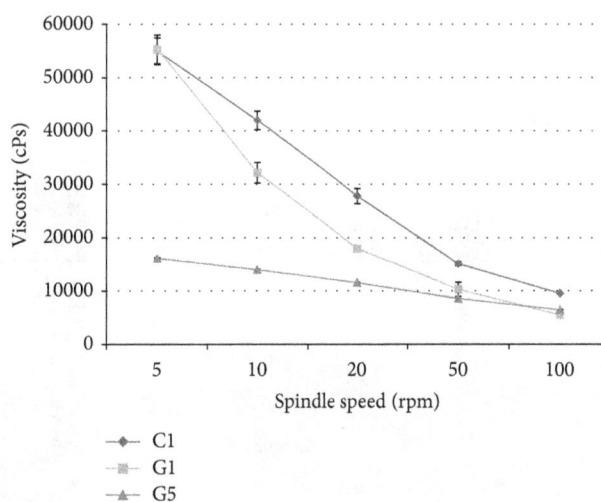

FIGURE 2: Viscosity curves for the selected cream (C1) and gels (G1 and G5) ($n = 3$, results shown as mean ± SD).

standard dose of a medicated formulation to the skin and the efficacy of a topical therapy. Figure 1 shows the spreading values, that is, diameters observed for the formulations, after one minute. The values refer to the extent to which the formulations readily spread on the application surface by applying a small amount of shear. Results indicated that our cream and gels had comparable spreadability to that of commercial products used as comparators in the study.

3.1.3. pH Values. The pH values for the blank and drug-loaded cream and gels are shown in Table 4. The pH of the formulations decreased when the active ingredients were added to the bases. The pH of the skin normally ranges from 4 to 6. The pH of the cream was more acidic than that of the skin, while the gels' pH values were similar to the skin's normal pH value. The pH values of the formulations did not change significantly over the period of 12 weeks.

3.1.4. Viscosity Measurement. Viscosity values for the drug-loaded cream and gels are shown in Figure 2. All products

TABLE 3: Physicochemical evaluation of selected topical formulations.

Formulation	Physical appearance	Color	Texture	Phase separation	Homogeneity	Immediate skin feel
C1	Opaque	Blue	Smooth	No	Homogeneous	Moisturizing, no grittiness, light, not greasy
G1	Transparent	Blue	Smooth	No	Homogeneous	Refreshing, cool, no grittiness or greasiness
G5	Transparent	Blue	Smooth	No	Homogeneous	Film formed after dry, cool, no grittiness or greasiness

TABLE 4: pH of blank and drug-loaded formulations at day 1 and at week 12.

Formulation	pH (mean ± SD)		
	Blank formulation	Drug-loaded formulations at day 1	Drug-loaded formulations at week 12
C1	3.07 ± 0.02	2.85 ± 0.03	2.90 ± 0.01
G1	6.47 ± 0.09	4.95 ± 0.06	4.96 ± 0.04
G5	6.39 ± 0.04	4.96 ± 0.04	5.05 ± 0.04

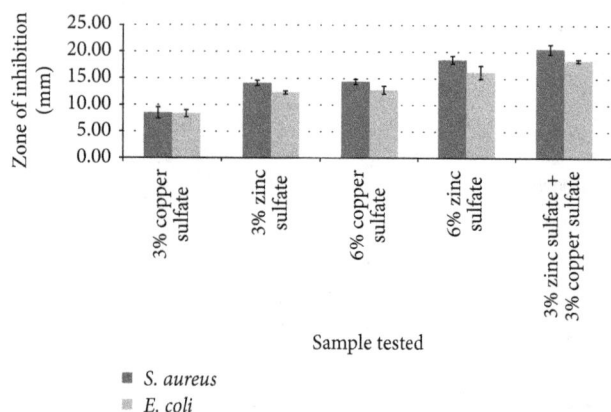

FIGURE 3: Antimicrobial activity of copper sulfate and zinc sulfate solutions in various concentrations against *Escherichia coli* and *Staphylococcus aureus* ($n = 3$, results shown as mean ± SD) ($p = 0.05$).

had a pseudoplastic behavior, as expected. C1 and G1 had a similar viscosity curve, while G5 had a lower initial viscosity.

3.1.5. In Vitro Antibacterial Activity. The *in vitro* antibacterial study was performed by measuring and comparing the diameter of zones of inhibition (in mm) for the various products. The zone of inhibition can be defined as the clear region around the well that contains an antimicrobial agent. It is known that the larger the zone of inhibition, the more potent the antimicrobial agent.

In the first step, the two active ingredients' antibacterial activity was measured individually and combined against *E. coli* and *S. aureus*. It can be concluded from the results that the antibacterial activity of zinc sulfate was higher than that of copper sulfate against the tested microorganisms (Figure 3). Results also confirmed that copper sulfate and zinc sulfate have a synergistic activity, as shown by their larger zone of inhibition against tested microorganisms ($p = 0.05$).

In the next step, the antibacterial activity of the selected cream (C1) and gels (G1 and G5) with varying amounts of active ingredients (0, 0.1, 0.25, 0.5, 1, 2, and 3%) was studied against *E. coli* and *S. aureus*. The results are shown in Table 5 and Figure 4. The blank formulation did not contain any active ingredients or any preservative. The formulation named paraben contained preservative but no active ingredients. Gentamicin 10 μg standard disc was used as the control in the study. No zone of inhibition was observed for the blank, paraben, and 0.1% strength formulations for either the cream or the gels. The zones of inhibition increased as the concentration of copper sulfate and zinc sulfate increased. This indicated that the antibacterial activity of copper sulfate and zinc sulfate increased against *E. coli* and *S. aureus* as the concentration of the actives was increased. As for the C1 formulation, the antibacterial activity of the sample containing 2% active ingredients was as good as that of the control (gentamicin) against *S. aureus*, while the antibacterial activity of the sample containing 3% active ingredients was statistically significantly higher than the control and the rest of the samples against both *E. coli* and *S. aureus* ($p = 0.05$). A visual representation of these results for C1 can be found in Figure 4. In the case of G1, similar results were seen. Samples containing 2% active ingredients had a similar antibacterial activity to that of the control, while the samples containing 3% active ingredients had statistically significantly higher activity against both microorganisms. As for G5, both the 2% and 3% samples had a similar antibacterial activity as the control against *E. coli*, while only the samples containing 3% of each active ingredient had an antibacterial activity comparable to the control against *S. aureus*. Based on the results, it can be concluded that both active ingredients have to be present in a concentration of at least 3% to achieve a similar or better antibacterial activity as the control against *E. coli* and *S. aureus*.

The final *in vitro* antimicrobial study was performed to compare the antibacterial activity of the selected formulations to those of marketed products against *E. coli* and *S. aureus*. As there is currently no marketed product available with

TABLE 5: Antimicrobial activity of the selected gel formulations in various dilutions against *Escherichia coli* and *Staphylococcus aureus* ($n = 3$).

	Zone of inhibition (mm) (mean ± SD)			
Concentration of each active (%)	G1		G5	
	E. coli	S. aureus	E. coli	S. aureus
0 (blank)	0	0	0	0
0 (paraben concentrate)	0	0	0	0
0.1	0	0	0	0
0.25	8.4 ± 0.2	9.1 ± 0.3	9.2 ± 0.5	9.2 ± 0.17
0.5	11.4 ± 0.1	11.9 ± 0.5	12.3 ± 0.6	11.3 ± 0.4
1	16.5 ± 0.1	18.1 ± 0.9	16.6 ± 1.3	13.9 ± 0.2
2	21.9 ± 0.6	23.1 ± 0.2	21.8 ± 0.2	17.6 ± 0.4
3	24.9 ± 0.3	26.3 ± 0.4	24.4 ± 0.4	19.7 ± 0.4
Gentamicin (control)	22.4 ± 0.15	23.5 ± 0.2	22.7 ± 1.8	21.3 ± 1.2

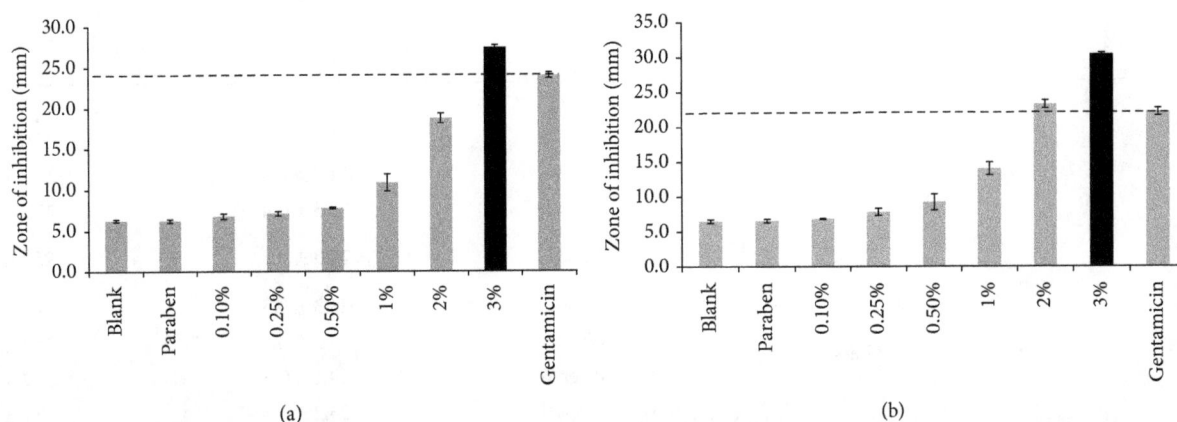

(a)

(b)

FIGURE 4: Antimicrobial activity of the selected cream (C1) containing copper sulfate and zinc sulfate in various concentrations against (a) *Escherichia coli* and (b) *Staphylococcus aureus* ($n = 3$, results are shown as mean ± SD) ($p = 0.05$).

zinc sulfate and copper sulfate, two commercially available cold sore gels and a diaper rash cream, Nexcare Cold Sore Treatment Cream, Campho-Phenique Cold Sore Treatment Gel, and Equate Diaper Rash Relief Cream, were used as comparators in the study. Nexcare Cold Sore Treatment Cream contains the following active ingredients: benzocaine as an external analgesic and allantoin as a skin protectant. The active ingredients in Campho-Phenique Cold Sore Treatment Gel are camphor and phenol as pain relievers or antiseptics, and, in Equate Diaper Rash Relief Cream, zinc oxide is a skin protectant. The results of this study are displayed in Figure 5. Results indicated that the antibacterial activity of C1, G1, and G5 was similar to that of the control (gentamicin), while the marketed products had a significantly lower activity against the two tested microorganisms. G1 and G5 had higher antibacterial activity against the tested bacteria than C1, which may be related to the composition of these products. The cream formulation contained oily components, which are immiscible with water and may slow down the diffusion of the drugs from the cream base.

3.2. Stability Study. All formulations maintained their blue color and intensity of color for 12 weeks in all storage conditions. Similarly, the physical appearance, homogeneity,

and texture of all formulations remained the same by the end of the storage period. None of the formulations showed signs of physical or chemical instability in any of the containers or at any of the temperatures. The antibacterial activity of all formulations was maintained for 12 weeks in both containers and at both temperatures. Results are shown in Figure 6 for G5 as well as in Table 6 for C1 and G1.

4. Discussion

Twenty different cream bases (C1–C20) were formulated using different ingredients in varying concentrations. After incorporating the active ingredients into the bases, the physical stability of a number of bases was affected negatively by the metal ions, leading to creaming and breaking of the emulsions. Formulations C5–C20 suffered from such issues; therefore, they were discontinued from further characterization. Formulations C1–C4 were formulated with the same ingredients, but with varied concentrations of the emulsifiers and thickeners. These four creams had similar consistency, and no apparent change in their physical appearance was observed after adding the metal salts. Based on the overall evaluation for physical appearance and immediate skin feel, C1 was selected as the final formulation for further testing.

TABLE 6: Antimicrobial activity during the stability study.

Product	Type of storage container	Testing period	Zone of inhibition (mm) (mean ± SD) Temperature	
			4°C	25°C
C1	Plastic jar	Day 1	22.7 ± 0.4	23.9 ± 0.2
		Week 3	23.4 ± 0.6	22.4 ± 0.7
		Week 6	23.1 ± 0.4	22.2 ± 0.5
		Week 9	22.8 ± 0.5	21.4 ± 0.1
		Week 12	22.1 ± 0.3	21.7 ± 0.4
	Glass jar	Day 1	23.6 ± 0.1	24.1 ± 0.8
		Week 3	21.9 ± 0.2	21.9 ± 0.2
		Week 6	22.1 ± 0.2	21.7 ± 0.5
		Week 9	22.1 ± 0.5	21.6 ± 0.3
		Week 12	21.9 ± 0.2	21.2 ± 0.2
G1	Plastic jar	Day 1	25.3 ± 0.3	24.8 ± 0.4
		Week 3	25.5 ± 0.4	25.0 ± 0.2
		Week 6	24.2 ± 0.3	24.2 ± 0.6
		Week 9	25.5 ± 0.4	25.6 ± 0.5
		Week 12	24.3 ± 0.6	25.1 ± 0.1
	Glass jar	Day 1	25.3 ± 0.3	24.7 ± 0.7
		Week 3	25.6 ± 0.3	25.1 ± 0.2
		Week 6	24.1 ± 0.3	24.2 ± 0.2
		Week 9	25.2 ± 0.3	25.7 ± 0.2
		Week 12	24.4 ± 0.2	24.7 ± 0.4
Control (gentamicin)			22.4 ± 0.8	

In addition to the creams, eighteen different gels (G1–G18) were formulated using eight different gelling agents. Only two polymers, namely, carrageenan and HPMC, proved to be optimal gelling agents for the metallic active ingredients used. G1 and G2 were formulated using carrageenan. These gels incorporated the active ingredients well. They had similar texture, consistency, and viscosity. The appearance, viscosity, and skin feel provided by G1 was considered better for a topical gel; therefore, it was selected for further testing. G3–G6 were formulated using different concentrations of HPMC. Out of these four samples, only G5 provided an optimal gel. To be considered optimal in this study, a gel (1) had to be homogenous without showing signs of physical or chemical instability; (2) had to be able to dissolve and keep the active ingredients in a dissolved form without precipitating or aggregating; and (3) had to have a high enough viscosity not to flow off the skin during/after application. In the case of G3 and G4, precipitation or aggregation of the polymers was observed when the active ingredients were added to the 5% HPMC gel. The explanation for this is that the amount of water used in these gels was not enough to dissolve the crystalline actives and keep the gelling agent dispersed. G4 contained more water compared to G3; however, even that higher amount did not prove to be enough for a stable

formulation. G5 met all our requirements; therefore this formulation was selected for further testing. G6 had a too low viscosity, which was not deemed appropriate for a topical gel. As for the other polymers used, including xanthan gum, guar gum, poloxamer 407, Kollidon 90F, FlexiThix, and Carbomer 940, the gels' physical stability was compromised when the active ingredients were added to the gel bases.

The three selected formulations were optimal in terms of their appearance, homogeneity, and viscosity. Previous studies [6–9] indicated that both active ingredients had antibacterial activity, which this study confirmed. The two metal salts had a synergistic activity when combined in the creams and gels, which was also confirmed by our study. The second antibacterial study indicated that both zinc sulfate and copper sulfate have to be present in at least a 3% concentration in order to achieve similar or better results against the tested microorganisms than gentamicin, which was used as the control. As there are no marketed products available today with copper sulfate and/or zinc sulfate, commercial products for the treatment/prevention of cold sores and diaper rash with active ingredients other than copper sulfate and zinc sulfate were used as comparators in the final antibacterial study. This limited study showed that the formulated creams and gels had a significantly higher antibacterial activity

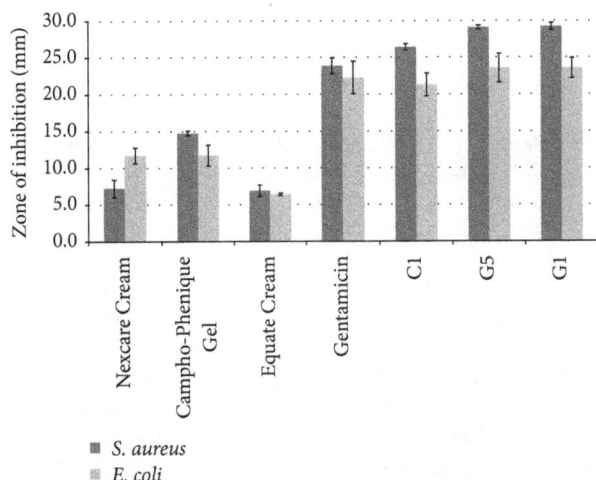

FIGURE 5: Antimicrobial activity of the selected cream (C1), gels (G1 and G5), and three marketed products (Nexcare Cold Sore Treatment Cream, Campho-Phenique Cold Sore Treatment Gel, and Equate Diaper Rash Relief Cream) against *Escherichia coli* and *Staphylococcus aureus* ($n = 3$, results shown as mean ± SD).

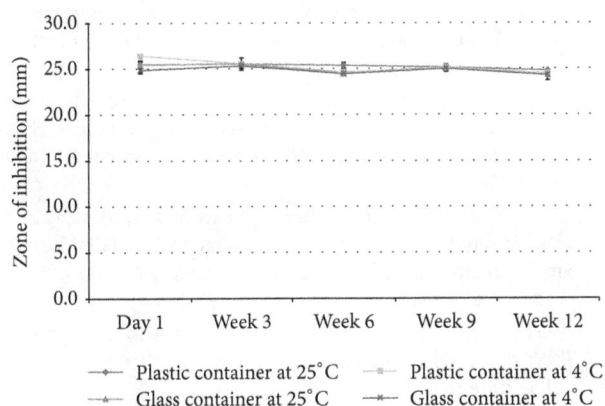

FIGURE 6: Antimicrobial activity of one of the selected gels (G5) during the stability testing compared to the control (gentamicin) against *Escherichia coli* ($n = 3$, results shown as mean ± SD).

against the two tested microorganisms than the marketed products. With a properly planned and conducted follow-up study using additional microorganisms—preferably fungi, bacteria, and viruses—the true antimicrobial activity of the products could be evaluated, and a more realistic comparison could be made.

The stability study indicated that both gels and the cream were able to maintain their integrity for 12 weeks without showing signs of instability. Additionally, the main function, that is, antibacterial activity of all formulations, remained stable for the tested time period, which is promising. As discussed in the introduction, incorporating metal salts into emulsions and gels can be a challenging task for formulators due to the high reactivity of these salts. Many of our formulations were affected by the metal ions, which resulted in precipitation, phase separation, color change, and other forms of instability. Only a few formulations, that is, the

selected creams and gels, were able to remain stable after incorporating the active ingredients into them.

5. Conclusions

In this study, various creams and gels were formulated with copper sulfate and zinc sulfate, which act as antimicrobial agents. During the formulation process, the quality, appearance, and stability of many creams and gels were affected by the highly reactive metal ions. A cream and two gels were found to be optimal for our purpose, and these were selected for further evaluation based on their physical properties, *in vitro* antibacterial activity, and product stability. Although only a small fraction of the formulated products were deemed optimal, a great achievement is that the integrity, pH values, texture, appearance, and antibacterial activity of these selected products were maintained for 12 weeks.

A major finding of this study is that copper sulfate and zinc sulfate have a synergistic antibacterial activity in creams and gels. The minimum effective concentration *in vitro* was found to be 3% for both active ingredients. A properly planned and conducted *in vitro* follow-up study could confirm the antimicrobial activity of the formulations against other microorganisms, and a more realistic comparison could be made between our products and marketed products for various skin conditions.

Competing Interests

The authors report no conflict of interests.

Acknowledgments

The authors would like to thank the various suppliers for providing samples of ingredients used in the study.

References

[1] H. W. Boucher, G. H. Talbot, J. S. Bradley et al., "Bad bugs, no drugs: no ESKAPE! An update from the Infectious Diseases Society of America," *Clinical Infectious Diseases*, vol. 48, no. 1, pp. 1–12, 2009.

[2] R. S. Sellar and K. S. Peggs, "Management of multidrug-resistant viruses in the immunocompromised host," *British Journal of Haematology*, vol. 156, no. 5, pp. 559–572, 2012.

[3] E. van der Vries, F. F. Stelma, and C. A. B. Boucher, "Emergence of a multidrug-resistant pandemic influenza A (H1N1) virus," *New England Journal of Medicine*, vol. 363, no. 14, pp. 1381–1382, 2010.

[4] K. Gulshan and W. S. Moye-Rowley, "Multidrug resistance in fungi," *Eukaryotic Cell*, vol. 6, no. 11, pp. 1933–1942, 2007.

[5] G. S. Liptak, "Diaper rash," in *Pediatric Primary Care*, R. Hoekelman, H. M. Adam, N. M. Nelson et al., Eds., Mosby, Maryland Heights, Mo, USA, 2001.

[6] D. B. Ward, A. B. Fleischer Jr., S. R. Feldman, and D. P. Krowchuk, "Characterization of diaper dermatitis in the United States," *Archives of Pediatrics and Adolescent Medicine*, vol. 154, no. 9, pp. 943–946, 2000.

[7] L. S. Nield and D. Kamat, "Prevention, diagnosis, and management of diaper dermatitis," *Clinical Pediatrics*, vol. 46, no. 6, pp. 480–486, 2007.

[8] J. J. Zeelie and T. J. McCarthy, "Effects of copper and zinc ions on the germicidal properties of two popular pharmaceutical antiseptic agents cetylpyridinium chloride and povidone-iodine," *Analyst*, vol. 123, no. 3, pp. 503–507, 1998.

[9] C. R. Pringle, Herpes Simplex Virus Infections. Merck and the Merck Manuals, https://www.merckmanuals.com/home/infections/viral-infections/herpes-simplex-virus-infections#resourcesInArticle.

[10] M. Arens and S. Travis, "Zinc salts inactivate clinical isolates of herpes simplex virus in vitro," *Journal of Clinical Microbiology*, vol. 38, no. 5, pp. 1758–1762, 2000.

[11] J. A. Fernández-Romero, C. J. Abraham, A. Rodriguez et al., "Zinc acetate/carrageenan gels exhibit potent activity in vivo against high-dose herpes simplex virus 2 vaginal and rectal challenge," *Antimicrobial Agents and Chemotherapy*, vol. 56, no. 1, pp. 358–368, 2012.

[12] J.-L. Sagripanti, L. B. Routson, A. C. Bonifacino, and C. D. Lytle, "Mechanism of copper-mediated inactivation of herpes simplex virus," *Antimicrobial Agents and Chemotherapy*, vol. 41, no. 4, pp. 812–817, 1997.

[13] A. Clewell, M. Barnes, J. R. Endres, M. Ahmed, and D. K. S. Ghambeer, "Efficacy and tolerability assessment of a topical formulation containing copper sulfate and *Hypericum perforatum* on patients with herpes skin lesions: a comparative, randomized controlled trial," *Journal of Drugs in Dermatology*, vol. 11, no. 2, pp. 209–215, 2012.

[14] W. Kneist, B. Hempel, and S. Borelli, "Clinical double-blind trial of topical zinc sulfate for herpes labialis recidivans," *Arzneimittel-Forschung*, vol. 45, no. 5, pp. 624–626, 1995.

[15] G. Kumel, S. Schrader, H. Zentgraf, H. Daus, and M. Brendel, "The mechanism of the antiherpetic activity of zinc sulphate," *Journal of General Virology*, vol. 71, no. 12, pp. 2989–2997, 1990.

[16] Z. Zarrab, M. Zanardelli, A. Pietrzak et al., *European Handbook of Dermatological Treatments: Tine Versicolor*, Springer, Berlin, Germany, 2015.

[17] G. H. Jameel, W. M. Al-Shamery, R. O. Hussain et al., "Treatment of Pityriasis versicolor by 2% solution of Copper sulfate," *Diyala Journal for Pure Sciences*, vol. 10, no. 1, pp. 129–134, 2014.

[18] K. E. Sharquie, R. K. Hayani, W. S. Al-Dori et al., "Treatment of pityriasis versicolor with topical 15% zinc sulfate solution," *Iraqi Journal of Community Medicine*, vol. 21, no. 1, pp. 61–63, 2008.

[19] Q. L. Feng, J. Wu, G. Q. Chen, F. Z. Cui, T. N. Kim, and J. O. Kim, "A mechanistic study of the antibacterial effect of silver ions on Escherichia coli and Staphylococcus aureus," *Journal of Biomedical Materials Research*, vol. 52, no. 4, pp. 662–668, 2000.

[20] G. Ren, D. Hu, E. W. C. Cheng, M. A. Vargas-Reus, P. Reip, and R. P. Allaker, "Characterisation of copper oxide nanoparticles for antimicrobial applications," *International Journal of Antimicrobial Agents*, vol. 33, no. 6, pp. 587–590, 2009.

[21] N. Padmavathy and R. Vijayaraghavan, "Enhanced bioactivity of ZnO nanoparticles—an antimicrobial study," *Science and Technology of Advanced Materials*, vol. 9, no. 3, Article ID 035004, 2008.

[22] M. J. Miller and F. Malouin, "Microbial iron chelators as drug delivery agents: the rational design and synthesis of siderophore-drug conjugates," *Accounts of Chemical Research*, vol. 26, no. 5, pp. 241–249, 1993.

[23] X. Pan, Y. Wang, Z. Chen et al., "Investigation of antibacterial activity and related mechanism of a series of Nano-Mg(OH)$_2$," *ACS Applied Materials and Interfaces*, vol. 5, no. 3, pp. 1137–1142, 2013.

[24] A. Besinis, T. De Peralta, and R. D. Handy, "The antibacterial effects of silver, titanium dioxide and silica dioxide nanoparticles compared to the dental disinfectant chlorhexidine on *Streptococcus mutans* using a suite of bioassays," *Nanotoxicology*, vol. 8, no. 1, pp. 1–16, 2014.

[25] K. E. Sharquie, A. A. Khorsheed, and A. A. Al-Nuaimy, "Topical zinc sulphate solution for treatment of viral warts," *Saudi Medical Journal*, vol. 28, no. 9, pp. 1418–1421, 2007.

[26] B. B. Mahajan, M. Dhawan, and R. Singh, "Herpes genitalis—topical an alternative therapeutic modality," *Indian Journal of Sexually Transmitted Diseases*, vol. 34, no. 1, pp. 32–34, 2013.

[27] K. E. Sharquie, A. A. Noaimi, and M. M. Al-Salih, "Topical therapy of acne vulgaris using 2% tea lotion in comparison with 5% zinc sulphate solution," *Saudi Medical Journal*, vol. 29, no. 12, pp. 1757–1761, 2008.

[28] M. Sierra, A. Sanhueza, R. Alcántara, and G. Sánchez, "Antimicrobial evaluation of copper sulfate (II) on strains of *Enterococcus faecalis*. In vitro study," *Journal Oral Of Research*, vol. 2, no. 3, pp. 114–118, 2013.

[29] G. Grass, C. Rensing, and M. Solioz, "Metallic copper as an antimicrobial surface," *Applied and Environmental Microbiology*, vol. 77, no. 5, pp. 1541–1547, 2011.

[30] R. Gyawali and S. A. Ibrahim, "Synergistic effect of copper and lactic acid against Salmonella and Escherichia coli O157: H7: a review," *Emirates Journal of Food and Agriculture*, vol. 24, no. 1, pp. 1–11, 2012.

[31] S. J. S. Flora, "Structural, chemical and biological aspects of antioxidants for strategies against metal and metalloid exposure," *Oxidative Medicine and Cellular Longevity*, vol. 2, no. 4, pp. 191–206, 2009.

[32] *2015 Performance Standards for Antimicrobial Disk Susceptibility Tests; Approved Standard*, M02 -A12, CLSI, Wayne, Pa, USA, 12th edition, 2015.

14

Functional Performance of Chitosan/Carbopol 974P NF Matrices in Captopril Tablets

Yuritze Alejandra Aguilar-López and Leopoldo Villafuerte-Robles

Departamento de Farmacia, Escuela Nacional de Ciencias Biológicas, Instituto Politécnico Nacional de México, Ciudad de México, Mexico

Correspondence should be addressed to Leopoldo Villafuerte-Robles; lvillarolvillaro@hotmail.com

Academic Editor: Anthony A. Attama

Chitosan and Carbopol have been used to form a complex through an electrostatic interaction between the protonated amine ($NH3^+$) group of chitosan and the carboxylate (COO^-) group of Carbopol. In situ polyelectrolyte complexes formations based on the physical mixture of chitosan and sodium alginate were found and could be used as an oral controlled release matrix. The aim of this work is the assessment of a possible interaction between the particles of chitosan and Carbopol 974P NF that could modify their technological performance in captopril tablets. The drug and excipients were evaluated as mixtures of powders and tablets. The mixtures with captopril contained Carbopol 974P NF, chitosan, or a 1:1 mixture thereof with polymer proportions of 10%, 20%, and 30%. The evaluated parameters were the powder flow rate, the powder compressibility index, and the compactibility and release behavior of the tablets. The observed technological behavior points out to a greater interaction between the particles of polymers with different charge than between particles of the individual polymers. This produces more coherent matrices restricting more efficiently the drug dissolution, more coherent tablets with higher compactibility, and less flowing powder mixtures. All this, however, requires additional investigation to confirm the current results.

1. Introduction

Characterization of the functional performance of pharmaceutical excipients can not only be considered as a requirement but also provide data that can be predictive in nature regarding the performance of final dosage forms. This data may provide insight into how a material will behave in a given process or dosage form. The characterization of the components of the formulations may be beneficial in developing a design space or control strategies [1].

Controlled release formulations are used to overcome the drawbacks of immediate release formulations. Matrix system is the most widely used method for development of controlled release formulations due to its easy of manufacture. Different natural and synthetic polymers are used for controlled release matrix systems which have the property to extend the release of the drug from the matrix system [2].

Chitosan is a partially deacetylated form of chitin and has received attention as a new excipient or functional material of potential in the pharmaceutical industry. Chitosan displays good excipient properties as well as chemical and physical stability [3].

Chitosan exhibits properties such as biocompatibility, biodegradability, and low immunogenicity. Its high positive charge density confers mucoadhesive properties. Mucoadhesivity is a desired property for the delivery of drugs to mucosal tissues. Chitosan also has a very low toxicity [4].

The release of drugs from chitosan particulate systems involves three different mechanisms: erosion, by diffusion and release from the surface of the particle. The release of drug mostly follows more than one type of mechanism. In the case of release from the surface, particulate and adsorbed drug dissolves rapidly and it leads to burst effect when it comes in contact with the release medium [5].

Carbopol polymers and Noveon AA1 polycarbophil have been included in a variety of different tablet forms such as swallowable (peroral), chewable, buccal, and sublingual tablets, providing controlled release properties, bioadhesion, and good binding characteristics [6].

Carbopol 974P NF polymer is highly crosslinked and produces highly viscous gels with short flow. Carbopol 974P NF is an oral pharmaceutical grade of carbomers. It readily hydrates, absorbs water, and swells. These properties make it a potential candidate for use in controlled release systems.

An increasing amount of Carbopol 974P NF in tablets formulations results in a reduced rate of drug release and a linearization of the drug release curve. The release kinetics from carbomer matrix tablets can display a zero-order drug release. However, added excipients can have a dramatic effect on in vitro drug release profiles, commonly, an increased drug release rate [7].

Carbopol is a polyacrylic acid polymer, which shows a sol to gel transition in aqueous solution as the pH raises above its pKa (5.5). Chitosan is an amine-polysaccharide that is also pH dependent. At pH exceeding 6.2 it forms a hydrated gel like precipitate. When these two polymers are combined, the gel strength could be significantly enhanced. The application of this principle to a timolol ophthalmic solution produced an in situ gelling drug solution. The Carbopol/chitosan mixture was found to be more efficient in retaining the drug as compared to Carbopol solution alone [8].

Chitosan and Carbopol have been used to form a complex through an electrostatic interaction between the protonated amine ($NH3^+$) group of chitosan and the carboxylate (COO^-) group of Carbopol. The formed complex showed a similar release pattern to that of HPMC when compacted as theophylline matrix tablets. The main release mechanism was diffusional. The complex showed as advantage a reduced pH dependency of Carbopol [9].

Polyelectrolyte complexes are the association complexes formed due to electrostatic interaction between oppositely charged polycations and polyanions, avoiding the use of chemical crosslinking agents, thereby reducing the toxicity and the unwanted effects of the reagents [10].

In the same way, it was reported that chitosan-sodium alginate polyelectrolyte complexes could be used as an oral controlled release matrix. In previous reports, in situ polyelectrolyte complexes formations based on the physical mixture of chitosan and sodium alginate were found, avoiding the process of preparing polyelectrolyte complexes. In this sense, physical mixtures of chitosan-sodium alginate were studied as extended release matrices. Using trimetazidine hydrochloride as a model drug, it was found that sodium alginate alone produced a drug release after 2 h of 52%; once sodium alginate was mixed with chitosan the drug release decreased significantly, to 43% after 2 h [11].

The aim of this work is the assessment of a possible interaction between the particles of chitosan and Carbopol that could modify the technological performance of these polymers in a controlled release matrix, using as a model drug captopril.

2. Materials and Methods

2.1. Materials.
The materials used in this study were Carbopol 974P NF obtained from Lubrizol Mexico, chitosan mesh 100 obtained from Pronaquim, Mexico, and captopril obtained from Química Alkano, Mexico.

2.2. Mixtures to Be Evaluated.
The drug and excipients were evaluated as mixtures. Corresponding amounts of captopril and Carbopol 974P NF, chitosan, and a 1 : 1 mixture thereof were weighed to obtain 60 g of mixtures of captopril with polymer proportions of 10%, 20%, and 30%. The powders were transferred into a small V-type powder mixer and mixed for 30 min.

2.3. Compressibility Index: Bulk and Tapped Density.
The equipment used to assess the powders densities is of our own fabrication and similar to that used to determine the tap density of powders, described in the Handbook of Pharmaceutical Excipients [12, 13]. The tapper was adjusted at a rate of 50 taps per minute and the graduated cylinder was elevated up to a height of 15 mm. This device uses a 100 mL graduated cylinder joined to a glass funnel with an orifice of 8.2 mm. The bulk (ρb) and tapped density (ρt) of powders were determined using the above-mentioned tapping machine ($n = 5$). The 100 mL measuring cylinder was filled with 30 g of sample. The volumes were recorded at the beginning (bulk volume) and after 10 taps. The process continued until three successive volume measurements remained constant (tapped volume). The bulk density was calculated as the ratio of mass and bulk volume while the tapped density was calculated as the ratio of mass and tapped volume. The registered results are the average of five repetitions with the same sample. The powders were sieved through a mesh number 20 after each repetition. Carr's Index or compressibility index (CI-%) was calculated according to the following equation [14]:

$$\text{Compressibility Index} = \frac{(\rho t - \rho b)}{\rho t * 100}. \qquad (1)$$

2.4. Powders Flow Rate.
The material is weighed (approximately 30 g) and its flow rate assessed using the equipment described to assess the powders densities. The sample is gently poured into the funnel whose bottom opening was blocked. While unlocked, the tapper starts the movement. The powder flows through the orifice of the funnel, falling to the bottom of the cylinder. The time it takes to move the total powder poured through the funnel is registered. The flow rate is calculated by dividing the sample mass by the time. The assay is repeated 5 times, sieving the powder through a mesh number 20 after each measurement. The average of the repetitions is taken as the flow rate.

2.5. Compactibility.
Tablets weighing 200 mg were compacted for 20 s in a hydraulic press, at a series of compaction pressures from 27 MPa to 163 MPa and using 8 mm circular flat-shaped punch and die. Tablet crushing strength was measured in triplicate, registering the results as an average. For this purpose, a tablet hardness tester Erweka TBH30 was used. The procedure involved placing each tablet diametrically between two flat surfaces and applying pressure until the tablet breaks down.

2.6. Dissolution Test.
Tablets obtained as described in the subtitle compactibility and compacted at a compaction pressure of 109 MPa were used to determine the dissolution

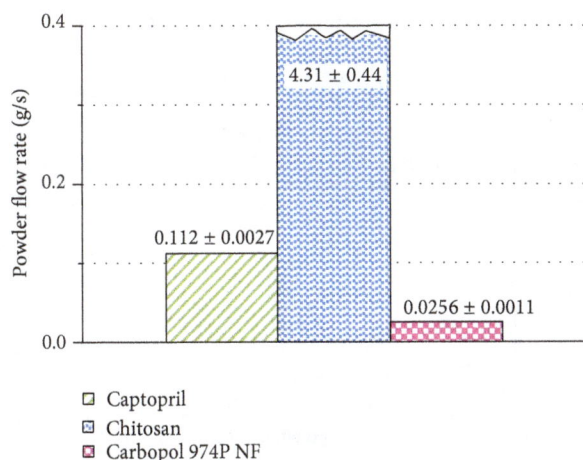

FIGURE 1: Powder flow rate through an orifice of 8.2 mm of captopril, Carbopol 974P NF, and chitosan.

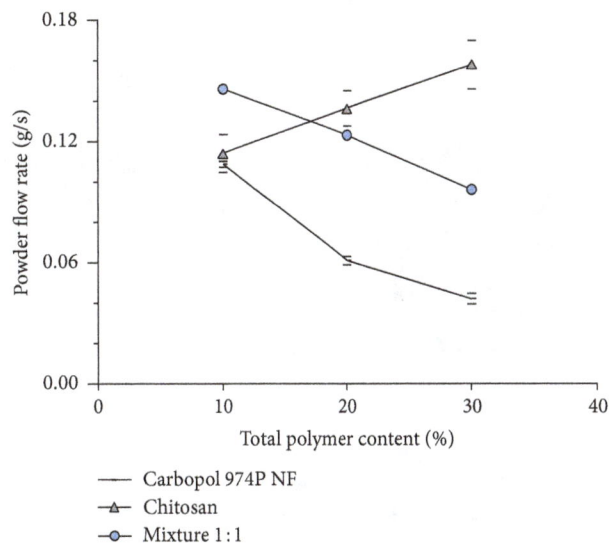

FIGURE 2: Effect of polymer proportion on the powder flow rate of admixtures with captopril, through a funnel with an opening of 8.2 mm (± St. Dev.).

behavior. The dissolution profile was carried out in a Hanson Research SR6 under sink conditions, for a period of 6 hours using a paddle apparatus at 50 rpm. 900 mL of HCL 0.1N was used as the dissolution medium. For each composition, a dissolution test was performed with three repetitions at 37°C. Each tablet was placed in a coil of stainless steel wire, to prevent sticking or floating. At predetermined time intervals samples were removed, filtered, and evaluated with a spectrophotometer (Beckman DU 650, λ = 208 nm). After each sample was removed, the same amount of liquid was replaced, thus maintaining the volume in the vessel. The dissolution profile was expressed as the percentage of drug released, based on the total tablet content after dissolution in a magnetic stirring device.

3. Results and Discussion

3.1. Effect of Carbopol 974P NF and Chitosan on Flowability of Captopril Powder Blends. Powder flow is critical during tableting, as powders must flow easily and uniformly into the tablet dies to ensure tablet weight uniformity and tablets with consistent and reproducible properties.

Propiconazole formulations containing 20% Carbopol have shown a poor powder flowability, indicating the need of glidants to make them processable. Carbopol was considered dysfunctional in this respect [15]. Contrasting, it has been observed that the fluidity of combined powders of lactose or potato starch with chitosan was greater than that of powder mixtures containing microcrystalline cellulose [16].

Figure 1 shows the powder flow rate of captopril and the individual polymers, through a glass funnel with an opening of 8.2 mm and using a tapper as the driving force. The powder flowability of chitosan is quite superior when compared to captopril and Carbopol 974P NF. Chitosan is, according to Figure 1, a material hundred times more fluid than Carbopol 974P NF.

Figure 2 depicts the effect of Carbopol 974P NF, chitosan, and the mixture thereof on the powder flow rate of captopril mixtures containing different polymer proportions.

The results in Figure 2 confirm the in literature mentioned effect of chitosan. Chitosan increases the powder flowability of the mixtures as the proportion of this polymer increases.

Contrasting, increasing proportions of Carbopol 974P NF in the powder mixtures decrease their flowability. Powder blends containing the combination of chitosan and Carbopol 974P NF display powder flow rates with the same tendency to decrease the flowability as that shown by Carbopol 974P NF alone. However, the powder flow rates are higher. Chitosan improves the flowability of captopril blends with Carbopol 974P NF. So far, a special interaction between the polymers with different charge cannot be observed.

Figure 3 shows the effect of adding Carbopol 974P NF on the powder flow rate of mixtures of captopril with chitosan. Powder mixtures with a total polymer content of 20% and 30% display a slight decrease in powder flow rate, when including 5% Carbopol 974P NF. Dilution of chitosan with captopril reduces drastically its powder flow rate. The subsequent addition of Carbopol 974P NF does not reduce further, in an important manner, the powder flow rate.

Bulk and tapped densities can provide information on flowability of powders when used to calculate the Carr Index. The lower the Carr Index is, the better the flowability of the powder is. According to the powder compressibility index, chitosans have been observed to display an average poor flowability (CI = 28) when compared to Avicel PH 200 (CI = 15) [17].

Figure 4 shows the powder compressibility index of captopril and individual polymers. As observed before by the powder flow rate (Figure 1), chitosan displays a lower compressibility index standing for a higher powder flowability. However, the difference in flowability between Carbopol 974P NF and chitosan is much smaller than that observed by the powder flow rate measurement (Figure 1). The powder flow rate of chitosan is more than one hundred times faster

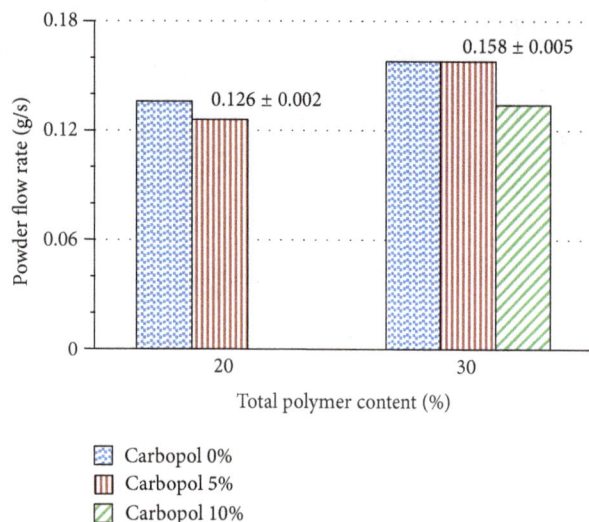

FIGURE 3: Effect of addition of Carbopol 974P NF on the powder flow rate of captopril/chitosan powder mixtures with a total polymer content of 20% and 30%.

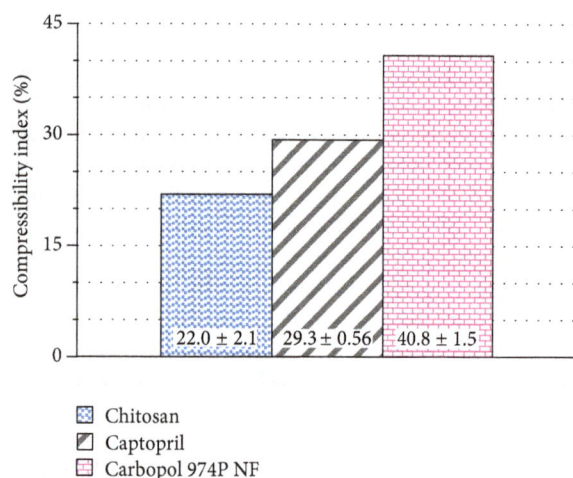

FIGURE 5: Effect of polymer proportion on the powder compressibility index of admixtures with captopril (± St. Dev.).

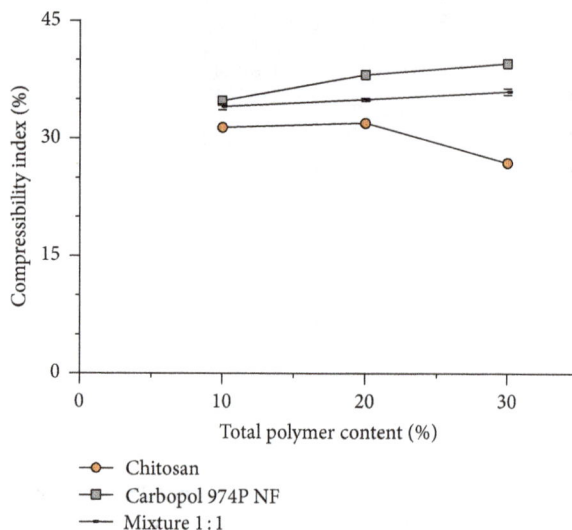

FIGURE 4: Compressibility index displayed by captopril, Carbopol 974P NF, and chitosan.

with different proportions of the blend of equal parts of both polymers display an average compressibility index laying in between (35%).

The results observed in Figure 5 show the same trends observed earlier by the flow rate of the powders. The increase in proportion of Carbopol 974P NF in mixtures with captopril shows an increase in the compressibility index values, indicating a decrease of powder flowability. This occurs in the same way as observed before in a direct measurement of the powder flow rate (Figure 2). On the other hand, the increase in the proportion of chitosan in mixtures with captopril shows a decrease of compressibility index values, indicating an increase in flowability.

Captopril mixtures containing different proportions of the combination of the two polymers show a similar trend to that observed before by the measurement of the powder flow rate of mixtures containing only Carbopol 974P NF. The increase in the proportion of the polymer mixture increases the compressibility index values, indicating less fluidity. However, the compressibility index values of the mixtures of captopril with the combination of the two polymers are lower, indicating more fluid mixtures than those containing only Carbopol 974P NF.

The average value of the compressibility index of captopril mixtures containing individual polymers (33.8%) is less than the result observed with captopril mixtures with the combination of the two polymers (35.0%). This could indicate a higher adhesiveness between the particles of the polymer blend than between the particles of the individual polymers. However this would not be free of questioning given such a small difference.

Figure 6 shows the effect of adding Carbopol 974P NF on the compressibility index of powder mixtures of captopril with chitosan. The powder mixtures with a total polymer content of 20% and 30% show a slight increase in the compressibility index of the powders when Carbopol 974P NF is included in the mixture. This indicates a slight decrease

than that of Carbopol 974P NF. However, the compressibility index of Carbopol 974P NF is only twice that of chitosan. The compressibility index values stand for a chitosan powder flowability only two times greater than that of Carbopol 974P NF. The powder flow rate assessment expands the scale of powder flowability, making the differences between different powders more visible.

Figure 5 shows the compressibility index of captopril powder mixtures with different proportions of chitosan, Carbopol 974P NF, and the mixture thereof. Mixtures of captopril with chitosan show an average compressibility index of 30%, indicating a poor flowability. The original passable flowability of chitosan (Figure 4) decreases after mixing with captopril. However, mixtures with Carbopol 974P NF show an average compressibility index of 37.5%, which means a worse flowability than blends with chitosan. In addition, captopril mixtures

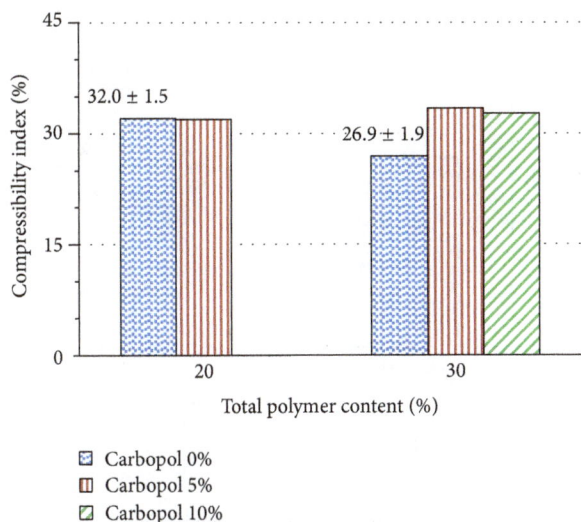

FIGURE 6: Effect of addition of Carbopol 974P NF on the powder compressibility index of captopril/chitosan mixtures with a total polymer content of 20% and 30%.

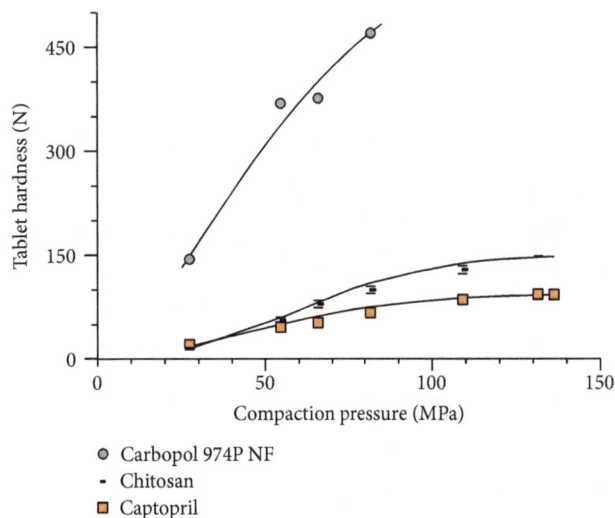

FIGURE 7: Compactibility curves of individual materials, captopril, Carbopol 974P NF, and chitosan (± St. Dev.).

of fluidity, in the same manner previously observed in determining the flow rate of the powder (Figure 3).

3.2. Effect of Carbopol 974P NF and Chitosan on Compactibility of Captopril Tablets.

Chitosan is known to reduce friction during tableting. The ejection force of lactose/chitosan tablets has been observed to be significantly smaller than that of lactose/microcrystalline cellulose [16].

Chitosans display deformation during compression combined with high elasticity after tableting. Chitosan shows tableting properties similar to those of microcrystalline cellulose (Avicel PH 200), although approximately 25% lower [17], even if the compactibility of chitosan has been reported to be less than a half of that of Avicel PH 102 [3]. The main difference with microcrystalline cellulose is that chitosan exhibits a high elastic recovery.

Figure 7 depicts the compactibility of individual materials. Carbopol 974P NF shows a quite superior compactibility followed by chitosan and captopril. Considering the tablet hardness at a compaction pressure of 66 MPa, the compactibility of chitosan is 20% of that of Carbopol 974P NF while that of captopril is only 13%.

The points in Figure 7 are experimental and the lines are the calculated regressions with (2) [18–21].

$$\ln\left(-\ln\left(1 - \frac{D}{D_{\max}}\right)\right) = n * \ln Pc + I, \qquad (2)$$

where D is the hardness or crushing strength of the tablets, $D_{\max}$ is the maximum hardness attained by the tablets, Pc is the compaction pressure, n is the slope of the curve, and I is the intercept of the curve.

The compactibility of captopril admixed with different proportions of chitosan can be seen in Figure 8. The points are experimental and the curve for compatibility is that calculated for tablets containing a proportion of chitosan of 30%.

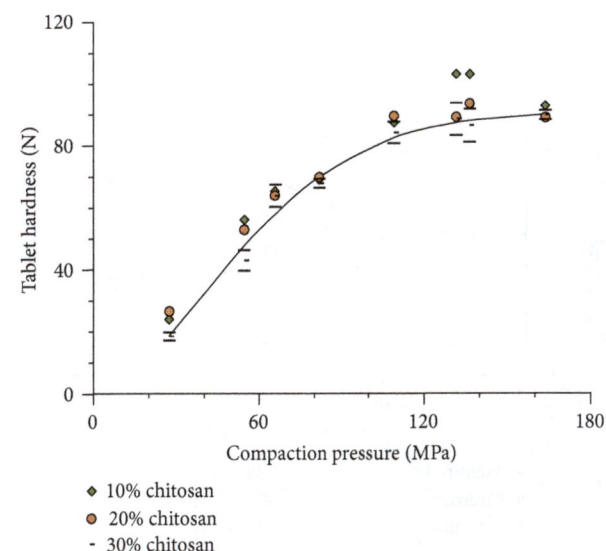

FIGURE 8: Effect of different proportions of chitosan on the compactibility profile of admixtures with captopril (± St. Dev.).

The experimental data depicted in Figure 8 do not allow the perception of different compactibility in captopril admixtures containing different proportions of chitosan. The influence of different proportions of chitosan on captopril compactibility is not appreciable. This can be ascribed to a small difference in compactibility between captopril and chitosan (Figure 7).

It has been observed that Carbopol forms tablets with higher hardness and lower friability than the known aggluti nant PVP-K30 [6]. Carbopol produces metronidazole tablets with a crushing strength 3 times greater than tablets with the same proportion of hydroxypropyl methylcellulose [22].

As can be seen in Figure 9, increasing proportions of Carbopol 974P NF produce tablets with an increasing tablet

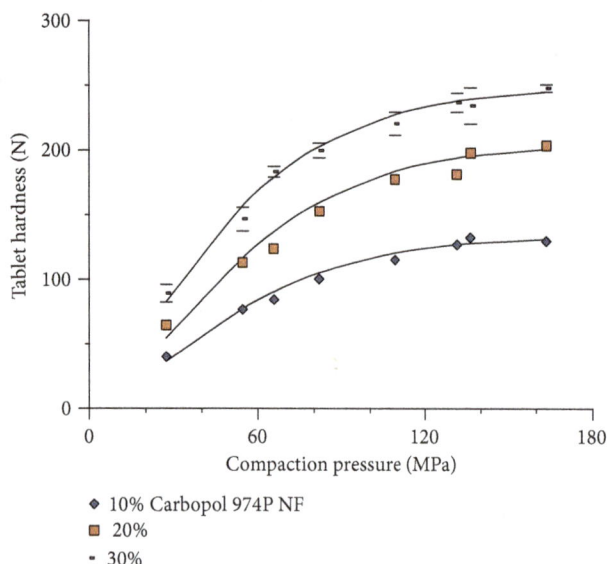

FIGURE 9: Effect of different proportions of Carbopol 974P NF on the compactibility profile of captopril tablets (± St. Dev.).

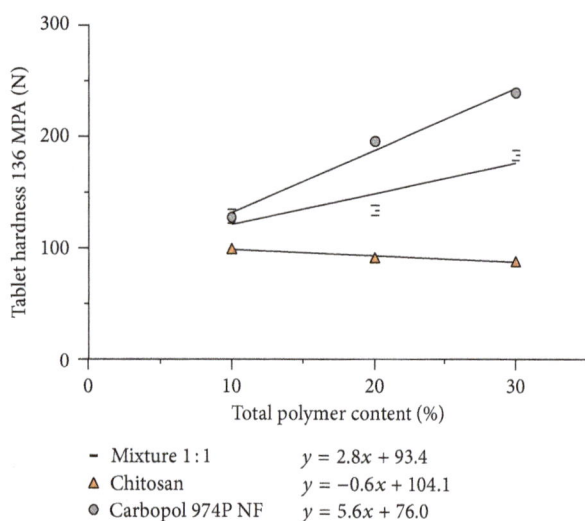

FIGURE 10: Effect of different polymer proportions on compactibility of captopril tablets calculated by regression at compaction pressure of 136 MPa (± St. Dev.).

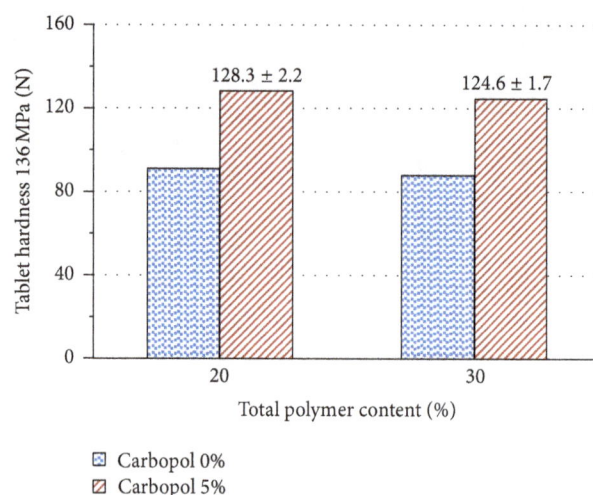

FIGURE 11: Effect of addition of 5% Carbopol 974P NF on the tablet hardness of captopril/chitosan tablets with a total polymer content of 20% and 30%.

hardness. This significant progressive increase in compatibility is attributed to the high binding capacity previously shown by Carbopol (Figure 7). The increase in compactibility of captopril tablets occurs at the expense of losing compactibility of Carbopol.

The greater compactibility of Carbopol 974P NF over that of chitosan observed in Figure 7 is maintained after dilution of the two polymers with captopril, although the difference in compatibility is lesser. This can be seen in Figure 10. As can be seen in the figure, the effect of the polymer proportion on the tablet hardness of captopril tablets obtained at 136 MPa can be described with a linear relationship. Tablets containing chitosan exhibit a tablet hardness of 99 N at a polymer proportion of 10%. The tablet hardness decreases 0.6 N per unit percentage of chitosan added, as shown by the slope of the calculated regression line displayed in the figure.

On the other hand, captopril tablets containing Carbopol 974P NF begin with a higher tablet hardness (128 N) and display a slope indicating an increase in 5.6 N per unit percentage of the added excipient. The addition of Carbopol 974P NF and chitosan admixture increases captopril tablet hardness in the same way as does the Carbopol 974P NF, although less, 2.8 N per unit of percentage of added polymer mixture (Figure 10).

The hardness of tablets depicted in Figure 10 shows an average for captopril/Carbopol 974P NF admixtures of 189 N. This value can be taken as reference for the binding or agglutinant ability of the polymer. This binding ability is about twice that exhibited by chitosan admixtures (93 N). As could be expected, the use of a mixture of chitosan and Carbopol 974P NF produces tablets with a hardness in between (149 N). This last average value of the tablet hardness (149 N) is somewhat higher than the average hardness of the tablets obtained with the individual polymers (141 N). This result would be indicative of a special interaction between Carbopol 974P NF and chitosan that could be attributed to increased adhesiveness between these polymers because they have different charges.

Figure 11 shows the influence of addition of Carbopol 974P NF on compatibility of captopril/chitosan tablets, calculated by regression for a compaction pressure of 136 MPa. Tablets with a total polymer content of 20% and 30% display an increase in compatibility of approximately 40%, after inclusion of 5% Carbopol 974P NF.

3.3. Effect of Carbopol 974P NF and Chitosan on the Release Profile of Captopril Tablets. Drug dissolution from solid dosage forms is described with kinetic models in which the amount of drug dissolved is a function of time. In most cases, there is not necessarily a theoretical concept behind the mathematical models and empirical equations can be used to properly describe the behavior of drug release [23].

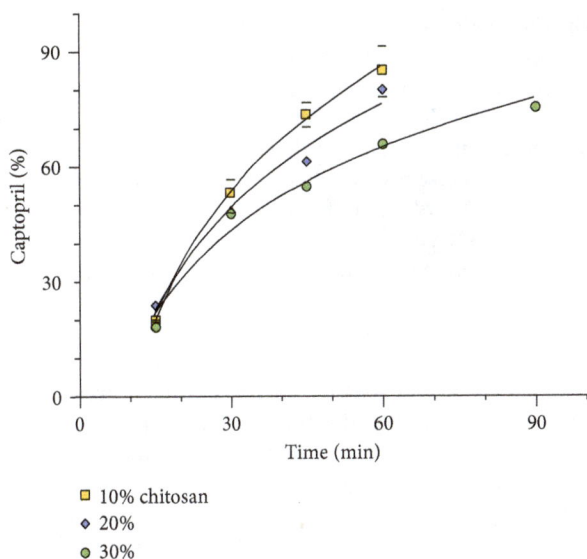

FIGURE 12: Effect of different proportions of chitosan in the dissolution profile of tablets of captopril (± St. Dev.).

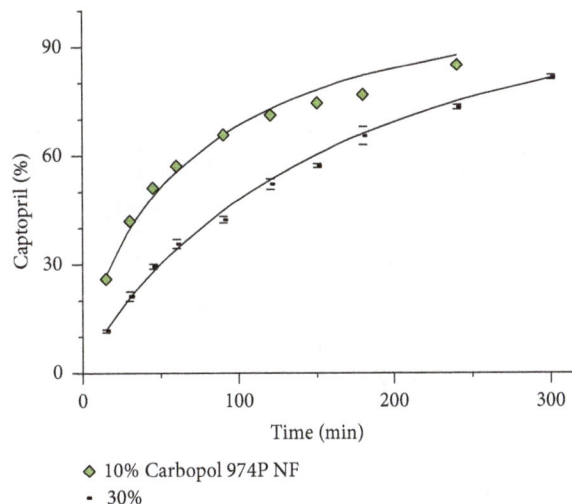

FIGURE 13: Effect of different proportions of Carbopol 974P NF on the dissolution profile of captopril tablets (± St. Dev.).

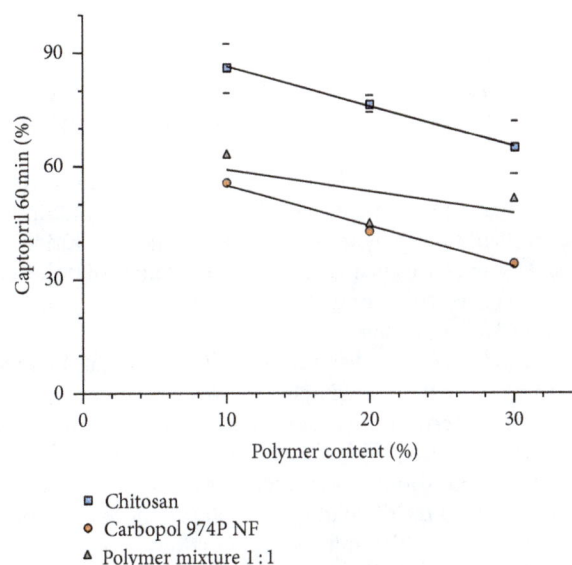

FIGURE 14: Effect of different proportions of Carbopol 974P NF, chitosan, and their 1:1 admixture on the calculated captopril dissolution at 60 min (± St. Dev.).

Figure 12 depicts the release profile of captopril from chitosan matrices containing different polymer proportions. The figure represents the experimental points and the calculated regressions with a logarithmic model. The effect of chitosan is an increasing restriction of drug release as the polymer proportion in the tablets increases. The restriction of drug dissolution produced by chitosan, even if significant, cannot be considered sufficient for a controlled release formulation.

Carbopols produce in many cases a linear release kinetics; however, the release kinetics is also dependent of the polymer proportion and added excipients. It has been observed that different proportions of Carbopol 974P between 10% and 30% produce drug release profiles with different degrees of curvature. Moreover, the addition of coexcipients changed the release profile towards higher degrees of curvature, away from a desired zero-order or linear release [7].

Figure 13 depicts the effect of different proportions of Carbopol 974P NF on the release profile of the tablets of captopril. As mentioned above, the degree of curvature of the release profile is dependent of the polymer proportion. Higher polymer proportions produce release profiles with a greater restriction of drug release and a lesser degree of curvature.

The release curves shown in Figure 13 are the result of a faster drug dissolution compared to hydration of the polymer and the subsequent binding of its particles. Once the gel layer has been established the release rate decreases [22]. The use of larger proportions of polymer increases the number of particles in the matrix, which facilitates their interaction and binding. This circumstance decreases the free drug dissolution.

Among the technological variables that influence the release from hydrophilic matrices, the use of polymer blends is a potential way of achieving the desired release properties [24]. Mixtures of different proportions of polymers with different permeation characteristics could provide a wide variety of release rates of a drug, due to changes in diffusivity of the drug through the polymeric barrier [25].

Figure 14 depicts the effect of different proportions of the polymers Carbopol 974P NF, chitosan, and a mixture thereof on the amount of captopril dissolved at 60 min. The admixture of Carbopol 974P NF with chitosan results in an intermediate release rate, when compared with release from matrices with individual polymers.

As shown in Figure 14, the use of the polymer blend does not allow a clear perception of additional interaction between polymers because they have different charges, even if the restriction of the dissolution of captopril, produced by the use of the polymer blend, is somewhat greater than the average release produced by individual polymers.

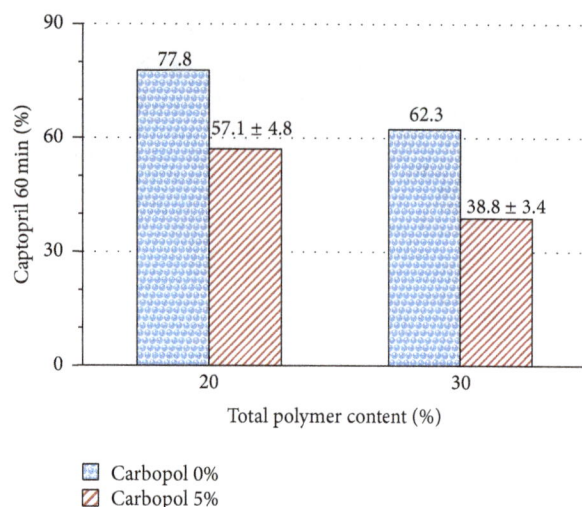

FIGURE 15: Effect of containing 5% Carbopol 974P NF on captopril dissolved in 60 min, from chitosan matrices with a total polymer content of 20% and 30%.

Taking the dissolution data of Figure 14 as a whole, matrices with chitosan display an average dissolution of 75.6% at 60 min. In the same way, the matrices with Carbopol 974P NF have an average dissolution of 44.2%. Taking these data as reference it might be expected that matrices containing equal parts of both polymers show an average dissolution of 59.9%. However, this is not the case. The average dissolution of the matrices containing the polymer mixture is 53.3%. This is 6.6% less dissolved captopril than might be expected. This means that the observed dissolution might include something more than the simple average of the two polymers with different permeation characteristics, possibly, a stronger interaction between polymer particles with a different charge. This interaction would produce matrices with greater coherence that restrict the dissolution of captopril more efficiently.

Figure 15 shows the influence of the addition of Carbopol 974P NF on captopril dissolved at 60 minutes, from matrices with chitosan. Matrices having a total polymer content of 20% and 30% show a reduction of captopril dissolved after 60 minutes of about 20%, when its content in Carbopol 974P NF is 5%.

4. Conclusion

Chitosan matrices exhibit about 40% higher captopril dissolution than Carbopol 974P NF matrices while the dissolution allowed by the polymer blend is approximately 6% lesser than the calculated average of dissolution of individual polymers. This can be possibly ascribed to a stronger interaction between particles with different charges producing more coherent matrices that restrict more efficiently the captopril dissolution.

The compactibility or agglutinant properties of Carbopol are twofold greater than those of chitosan. The compactibility obtained with the polymer mixture is something greater than the average compactibility of the tablets containing the

individual polymers, pointing out to a greater adhesiveness between particles of polymers with different charge.

The compressibility index of captopril mixtures with Carbopol 974P NF is about 20% higher than that of mixtures containing chitosan. Captopril containing the polymer mixture displays a compressibility index higher than the average observed by powders containing the individual polymers. This indicates a possible greater adhesion between particles of different polymers than cohesion between the particles of single polymers.

The observed technological behavior of mixtures of Carbopol 974P NF with chitosan points out to a greater interaction between the particles of polymers with different charge than between particles of the individual polymers. This produces more coherent matrices restricting more efficiently the drug dissolution, more coherent tablets with higher compactibility, and less flowing powder mixtures. All this, however, require additional investigation to confirm the current results.

Competing Interests

The authors declare that there is no conflict of interests regarding the publication of this paper.

References

[1] "Expanding the Material Characterization 'Toolbox' for Excipient and Active Pharmaceutical Ingredient (API) Vendor Qualification," Application Note 163, http://www.micromeritics.com/.

[2] A. Rehman, G. M. Khan, K. U. Shah, S. U. Shah, and K. A. Khan, "Formulation and evaluation of tramadol HCL matrix tablets using carbopol 974P and 934 as rate-controlling agents," Tropical Journal of Pharmaceutical Research, vol. 12, no. 2, pp. 169–172, 2013.

[3] V. G. Mir, J. Heinämäki, O. Antikainen et al., "Direct compression properties of chitin and chitosan," European Journal of Pharmaceutics and Biopharmaceutics, vol. 69, no. 3, pp. 964–968, 2008.

[4] E. Nagarajana, P. Shanmugasundarama, V. Ravichandirana, A. Vijayalakshmia, B. Senthilnathanb, and K. Masilamanib, "Development and evaluation of chitosan based polymeric nanoparticles of an antiulcer drug lansoprazole," Journal of Applied Pharmaceutical Science, vol. 5, no. 4, pp. 20–25, 2015.

[5] V. Bansal, P. K. Sharma, N. Sharma, O. P. Pal, and R. Malviya, "Applications of chitosan and chitosan derivatives in drug delivery," Advances in Biological Research, vol. 5, no. 1, pp. 28–37, 2011.

[6] Pharmaceutical Bulletin, Formulating Controlled Release Tablets and Capsules with Carbopol Polymers, Lubrizol, Wickliffe, Ohio, USA, 31st edition, 2011.

[7] G. M. Khan and Z. Jiabi, "Formulation and in vitro evaluation of ibuprofen-carbopol® 974P-NF controlled release matrix tablets III: influence of co-excipients on release rate of the drug," Journal of Controlled Release, vol. 54, no. 2, pp. 185–190, 1998.

[8] S. Gupta and S. P. Vyas, "Carbopol/chitosan based pH triggered in situ gelling system for ocular delivery of timolol maleate," Scientia Pharmaceutica, vol. 78, no. 4, pp. 959–976, 2010.

[9] S.-H. Park, M.-K. Chun, and H.-K. Choi, "Preparation of an extended-release matrix tablet using chitosan/Carbopol inter-polymer complex," *International Journal of Pharmaceutics*, vol. 347, no. 1-2, pp. 39–44, 2008.

[10] D. V. Gowda, A. Srivastava, G. Sebastian, and M. Prerana, "Fab-rication and characterization of chitosan-carbopol-71G poly-electrolyte complex-based mucoadhesive pellets of miconazole nitrate for vaginal candidiasis," *Journal of Chemical and Phar-maceutical Research*, vol. 7, no. 7, pp. 577–591, 2015.

[11] L. Li, J. Li, S. Si et al., "Effect of formulation variables on in vitro release of a water-soluble drug from chitosan-sodium alginate matrix tablets," *Asian Journal of Pharmaceutical Sciences*, vol. 10, no. 4, pp. 314–321, 2015.

[12] A. H. Kibbe, Ed., *Handbook of Pharmaceutical Excipients*, Pharmaceutical Press, London, UK, 3rd edition, 2000.

[13] L. Villafuerte Robles, "Propiedades reológicas de los polvos far-macéuticos: un nuevo equipo," *Revista Mexicana de Ciencias Farmacéuticas*, vol. 32, no. 1, pp. 11–15, 2001.

[14] S. Mehta, T. De Beer, J. P. Remon, and C. Vervaet, "Effect of disintegrants on the properties of multiparticulate tablets comprising starch pellets and excipient granules," *International Journal of Pharmaceutics*, vol. 422, no. 1-2, pp. 310–317, 2012.

[15] A. Stanescu, L. Ochiuz, I. Cojocaru, I. Popovici, and D. Lupu-leasa, "The influence of different polymers on the pharmaco-technological characteristics of propiconazole nitrate bioadhe-sive oromucosal tablets," *Farmacia*, vol. 58, no. 3, pp. 279–289, 2010.

[16] K. C. Gupta and M. N. Ravi Kumar, "Trends in controlled drug release formulations using chitin and chitosan," *Journal of Sci-entific & Industrial Research*, vol. 59, pp. 201–213, 2000.

[17] K. M. Picker-Freyer and D. Brink, "Evaluation of powder and tableting properties of chitosan," *AAPS PharmSciTech*, vol. 7, no. 3, article 75, 2006.

[18] S. Castillo-Rubio and L. Villafuerte-Robles, "Compactibility of binary mixtures of pharmaceutical powders," *European Journal of Pharmaceutics and Biopharmaceutics*, vol. 41, no. 5, pp. 309–314, 1995.

[19] S. Castillo and L. Villafuerte, "Compactibility of ternary mix-tures of pharmaceutical powders," *Pharmaceutica Acta Helve-tiae*, vol. 70, no. 4, pp. 329–337, 1995.

[20] C. C. Díaz Ramírez and L. Villafuerte Robles, "Surrogate func-tionality of celluloses as tablet excipients," *Drug Development and Industrial Pharmacy*, vol. 36, no. 12, pp. 1422–1435, 2010.

[21] L. Samayoa-Sandoval and L. Villafuerte-Robles, "Compactibil-ity as a functionality parameter of the excipient GalenIQ 720," *Revista Mexicana de Ciencias Farmaceuticas*, vol. 44, no. 3, pp. 34–45, 2013.

[22] Z. M. Aguilar-Hernández and L. Villafuerte-Robles, "Function-ality of Benecel/Carbopol matrices in direct compression tablets for controlled release," *Journal of Applied Pharmaceutical Sci-ence*, vol. 6, no. 9, pp. 001–008, 2016.

[23] P. Costa and J. M. Sousa Lobo, "Modeling and comparison of dissolution profiles," *European Journal of Pharmaceutical Sci-ences*, vol. 13, no. 2, pp. 123–133, 2001.

[24] N. Traconis, R. Rodríguez, M. E. Campos, and L. Villafuerte, "Influence of admixed polymers on the metronidazole release from hydroxypropyl methylcellulose matrix tablets," *Pharma-ceutica Acta Helvetiae*, vol. 72, no. 3, pp. 131–138, 1997.

[25] Y. W. Chien, *Novel Drug Delivery Systems*, Marcel Dekker, New York, NY, USA, 1982.

15

Antioxidant and Antibacterial Potential of Silver Nanoparticles: Biogenic Synthesis Utilizing Apple Extract

Upendra Nagaich, Neha Gulati, and Swati Chauhan

Department of Pharmaceutics, Amity Institute of Pharmacy, Amity University, Noida, Uttar Pradesh, India

Correspondence should be addressed to Swati Chauhan; 91chauhanswati@gmail.com

Academic Editor: Amnon Sintov

The advancement of the biological production of nanoparticles using herbal extracts performs a significant role in nanotechnology discipline as it is green and does not engage harsh chemicals. The objective of the present investigation was to extract flavonoids in the mode of apple extract and synthesize its silver nanoparticles and ultimately nanoparticles loading into hydrogels. The presence of flavonoids in apple extract was characterized by preliminary testing like dil. ammonia test and confirmatory test by magnesium ribbon test. The synthesized silver nanoparticles were characterized using UV spectroscopy, particle size and surface morphology, and zeta potential. Silver nanoparticles loaded hydrogels were evaluated for physical appearance, pH, viscosity, spreadability, porosity, *in vitro* release, *ex vivo* permeation, and antibacterial (*E. coli* and *S. aureus*) and antioxidant studies (DPPH radical scavenging assay). Well dispersed silver nanoparticles below were observed in scanning electron microscope image. Hydrogels displayed *in vitro* release of 98.01% ± 0.37% up to 24 h and *ex vivo* permeation of 98.81 ± 0.24% up to 24 h. Hydrogel effectively inhibited the growth of both microorganism indicating good antibacterial properties. The value of percent radical inhibition was 75.16% ± 0.04 revealing its high antioxidant properties. As an outcome, it can be concluded that antioxidant and antiageing traits of flavonoids in apple extract plus biocidal feature of silver nanoparticles can be synergistically and successfully utilized in the form of hydrogel.

1. Introduction

Nanotechnology is an emerging tool as drug delivery system in variety of serious disorders. It is an innovative technique which includes the design, characterization, production, and application of structures, devices, and systems by controlling shape and size at the nanometer scale. It covers the size range of 1 nm to 100 nm [1]. Nanoparticles are the materials with the overall size of 100 nm [2]. Nanoparticles can be classified as polymeric (natural and synthetic), lipoidal (biodegradable), and metal nanoparticles (iron oxide, gold nanoparticles, and silver nanoparticles) [3]. Metal nanoparticles using plant or plant extract are a way ahead towards greener approach for application as drug delivery system. Silver nanoparticles show good anti bacterial properties as silver has been widely used as healing and antibacterial agent for many years [4]. Silver nanoparticles (AgNPs) also possess antifungal, anti-inflammatory, antiviral, and antiplatelet activity [5]. Silver

nanoparticles can be synthesized by using any of the following methods [6], namely, physical methods, chemical reduction (thermal reduction, polyol process, microemulsion techniques), and photochemical reduction (microwave reduction, photoreduction, and X-ray radiolysis).

Malus domestica (Rosaceae) commonly known as apple is full of high levels of triterpenoids, anthocyanins, and phenolic compounds. Apple polyphenols and oligomeric proanthocyanidins are primarily responsible for its antioxidant activity [7]. Flavonoids, quercetin, and hesperetin present in apple contribute to its antiageing effects [8]. The utilization of natural compounds in protection of skin especially topical application of antioxidants indicates that they usefully decrease skin aging [9, 10].

Basically, premature skin ageing is a vast biological phenomenon that mainly occur by the combination of endogenous or intrinsic (genetics, cellular metabolism, hormone, and metabolic processes) and exogenous or extrinsic (chronic light exposure, pollution, ionizing radiation, chemicals, and toxins) factors [11]. Photosensitized skin is characterized by dry, rough, pigmented, and abraded skin. This is due to high exposure to direct sunlight [8]. Biological systems are damaged by the presence of free radicals. The responsible free radicals are oxygen free radicals or generally known as reactive oxygen species (ROS) [12].

Studies show that apple decreases the presence of ROS generated by hydrogen peroxide exposure in lymphocytes [13].

In present investigation, we have tried to investigate the synergistic effect of AgNPs and flavonoids in apple extract by loading apple extract AgNPs into hydrogel and characterizing it for antibacterial and antioxidant properties in a unit dose formulation. Apple extract was utilized for the green synthesis of silver nanoparticles via chemical reduction technique. Furthermore Apple extract acts as both reducing and capping agent. Moreover, optimized silver nanoparticles were selected and loaded to hydrogel to deliver actives via topical route for the therapy of premature skin ageing.

2. Materials and Methods

2.1. Materials. *Malus domestica*, family Rosaceae (apple), was purchased from local market. Methanol, formic acid, silver nitrate, carbopol-934, triethanolamine, glycerine, potassium dihydrogen phosphate, sodium hydroxide, 2,2-diphenyl-2-picrylhydrazyl hydrate (DPPH), agar, and nutrient medium were purchased from CDH Pvt. Ltd., New Delhi. All solvents used were of analytical grade.

2.2. Methodology

2.2.1. Preparation of Apple Extract. Phenolic compounds from apple were extracted using solvent mixture of methanol : formic acid : water in the ratio of 70 : 2 : 28. Weighed quantity of freshly cut apple pieces was added to the solution of methanol : formic acid : water (MFW) and homogenized in a blender (Polytron PT 1600E, kinematica AG) for 2 min. The mixture was transferred to a beaker, covered with parafilm, and held for 24 h at 4°C. Then the mixture was washed with 20 mL of MFW. Extract was collected and then evaporated for dryness at 45°C under vacuum with a rotary evaporator [14].

2.2.2. Synthesis of Silver Nanoparticles. 1 M silver nitrate solution was prepared by adding 1.699 g of AgNO3 to 1 L distilled water. 30 mL of apple extract was taken in a 100 mL conical flask. 20 mL of freshly prepared 0.1 M AgNO3 solution was added (drop-wise) to the flask. The flask was incubated in dark for 24 hrs at room temperature [15].

2.2.3. Preparation of Apple Extract Loaded Silver Nanoparticles Based Hydrogel. Apple extract loaded silver nanoparticles were then incorporated into a hydrogel base as given in Table 1. Accurately weighed quantity of carbopol-934 (poly (acrylic) acid or carbomer) was gradually dispersed in distilled water under mild stirring (Remi, Mumbai) for 30 min and kept for two hours for the proper swelling of polymer.

TABLE 1: Formulation table for apple extract loaded silver nanoparticles based hydrogels.

S. number	Ingredients	Formulations		
		F1	F2	F3
(1)	Apple AgNPs	8 mL	4 mL	4 mL
(2)	Carbopol-934	4%	4%	8%
(3)	Glycerine	2 mL	2 mL	2 mL
(4)	Triethanolamine	1 mL	1 mL	1 mL
(5)	Distilled water	q.s. to 100 mL	q.s. to 100 mL	q.s. to 100 mL

Glycerin was then added as viscosity enhancer and emollient. The glycerin-polymeric solution was then neutralized with triethanolamine to form a transparent gel as basic nature of triethanolamine helps in increasing the cross-linking of acidic polymer. Apple extract loaded silver nanoparticulate suspension (equivalent to 3–10% of apple extract) was then incorporated in hydrogel using slow mechanical mixing (Remi RQ121/D, Mumbai) for 10 min so as to avoid entry of air bubbles.

2.2.4. Characterization of Apple Extract Loaded Silver Nanoparticles

(1) Characterization of Apple Extract

Preliminary Screening for the Presence of Flavonoids and Polyphenols in Extract. The prepared apple extract was subjected to ultravoilet-visible spectrophotometry (Perkin Elmer, Waltham, MA) for detecting the presence of flavonoids. The extract was scanned in the region of 200 nm–800 nm against solvent mixture (MFW) as blank and peaks were obtained [16].

Few drops of dilute sodium hydroxide were added to 1 mL of apple extract to observe the yellow color which on further addition of few drops of dilute hydrochloric acid makes the solution colorless which confirms the presence of flavonoids.

Confirmatory Testing (Magnesium Ribbon Test) [17]. Magnesium ribbon test is known because of the use of magnesium ribbon in the testing of flavonoids. Concentrated hydrochloric acid and magnesium ribbon were added to 1 mL of apple extract which in turn gives pink-red color for the presence of flavonoids.

(2) Characterization of Apple Extract Loaded Silver Nanoparticles

Ultravoilet-Visible Spectrophotometry. The optical property of prepared AgNPs was analyzed via UV-visible absorption spectrophotometer with a deuterium and tungsten iodine lamp in range of 200–800 nm at room temperature (RT). UV-visible spectrophotometer monitors the formation of AgNPs with the color change. To analyze formation of AgNPs, samples were withdrawn with the help of pipette at different time intervals, that is, 5, 10, 15, 20, 30, and 60 minutes [18].

Shape and Surface Morphology of Silver Nanoparticles. Scanning electron microscopic (SEM) analysis was done for analyzing particle shape and morphology. The shape and surface morphology of the silver nanoparticles was visualized by scanning electron microscopy (Cart Zeiss EV018). The samples were prepared by lightly sprinkling nanoparticles on double-sided adhesive tape on an aluminum stub. The stubs were then coated with gold to a thickness of 200 to 500 Å under an argon atmosphere using a gold sputter module in a high vacuum evaporator. The samples were then randomly scanned and photomicrographs were taken at different magnifications with SEM [19].

Particle Size and Zeta Potential Measurement. Particle size was measured with the help of dynamic light scattering technique. For the determination of particle size, samples were prepared by tenfold dilution of 1 mL of the nanoparticulate suspension with distilled water. The analysis was carried out in triplicate. The average particle size was measured by photon correlation spectroscopy. Zeta potential was determined by the electrophoretic mobility of nanoparticles in U-type tube at 25°C, using a zetasizer (3000HS Malvern Instruments, UK) [19].

(3) Characterization of Apple Extract Loaded Silver Nanoparticles Based Hydrogels

pH. pH of prepared hydrogel was measured by dissolving 1 gm of hydrogel in 10 mL of distilled water. pH meter (Systronics, 361-micro pH meter) was used to evaluate the pH of hydrogel. The readings were taken in triplicate and the average pH was calculated.

Porosity Measurement. For porosity measurement, the solvent replacement technique was employed. Accurately weighed 1 gm of dried hydrogels was immersed in absolute ethanol and soaked overnight. Afterwards, excess ethanol on the surface of hydrogels was blotted and weighed again [20]. The porosity can be calculated from the following equation.

$$\text{Porosity} = \frac{(M2 - M1)}{\rho V}. \tag{1}$$

Here, $M1$ and $M2$ are the mass of hydrogel before and after the immersion in absolute ethanol, respectively; ρ is the density of absolute ethanol and V is the volume of the hydrogel.

Viscosity. To analyze the rheological properties, all the formulated gels were taken in beakers and placed beneath the spindle, and the spindle (RV-7) was rotated at 10 rpm at room temperature (25–27°C) in Brookfield viscometer.

Spreadability. The Spreadability measurements of the apple extract loaded silver nanoparticle gel were made in triplicate by using glass slide method. One gram per meter of gel was kept between the two slides. The preweighted plate was kept

above the gel, and more weights were added on the plate until the gel stop spreading. Final cumulative weight and the total time taken by the gel to spread were measured and noted. Then total weight applied and mass of the gel were compared by the time.

$$S = M \times \frac{L}{T}, \tag{2}$$

where S = spreadability, M = weight tide to upper slide, L = length of glass slide, and T = time taken to separate the slides completely from each other.

2.2.5. In Vitro Drug Diffusion Studies. The *in vitro* drug release was evaluated using Keshary-Chien (K-C) diffusion cell to evaluate the diffusion of nanoparticles across the dialysis membrane. The diffusion cells were thermoregulated with a water jacket at 37 ± 2°C. Dialysis membrane 70 (Hi-Media, Mumbai, India) having a pore size of 2.4 nm and a molecular weight cutoff between 12,000 and 14,000 Da was used and mounted on K-C cells. The surface area of the release membrane was 3.14 cm². Phosphate buffer saline (PBS; pH 6.8) was used as the receptor medium (10 mL) being stirred at 100 rpm. 0.5 gm of apple extract loaded silver nanoparticulate based hydrogel (equivalent to 3–10% of apple extract) was placed in the donor compartment. During the experiments, the solution in receptor side was maintained at 37 ± 0.5°C. At predetermined time intervals, 5 mL of the samples was withdrawn from the receiver compartment and replaced by the same volume of freshly prepared PBS (pH 6.8). The withdrawn samples were analyzed by the UV-visible spectrophotometer at 420 nm [21].

2.2.6. Ex Vivo Skin Permeation Studies. The *ex vivo* drug release studies were carried out with the help of K-C diffusion cell. Rat abdominal skin was used to study permeation. The subcutaneous tissue was removed surgically and the dermis side was wiped with isopropyl alcohol to remove adhering fat. The cleaned skin was washed with distilled water and stored at −18°C until further use. The skin was mounted between the donor and receiver compartments of the K-C cell where the stratum corneum side was facing the donor compartment and the dermal side was facing the receiver compartment. One gram (equivalent to 3–10% apple extract) of each gel was placed in a donor compartment. The receptor compartment was filled with 10 mL PBS (pH 6.8), thermoregulated at 37°C, and magnetically stirred at 400 rpm. Two milliliters of receptor fluid was withdrawn at an interval of 1, 2, 3, 5, 7, 12, 18, and 24 h. An equal volume of PBS was simultaneously added to the receptor compartment after each sampling to maintain sink conditions. Each sample was filtered and then determined for apple extract content by UV spectrophotometer at 420 nm. The concentrations of all the formulations in withdrawn samples were calculated and then the percent drug release was determined [22].

2.2.7. Antioxidant Activity of Silver Nanoparticulate Hydrogel (DPPH Radical Scavenging Assay). The antioxidant activity

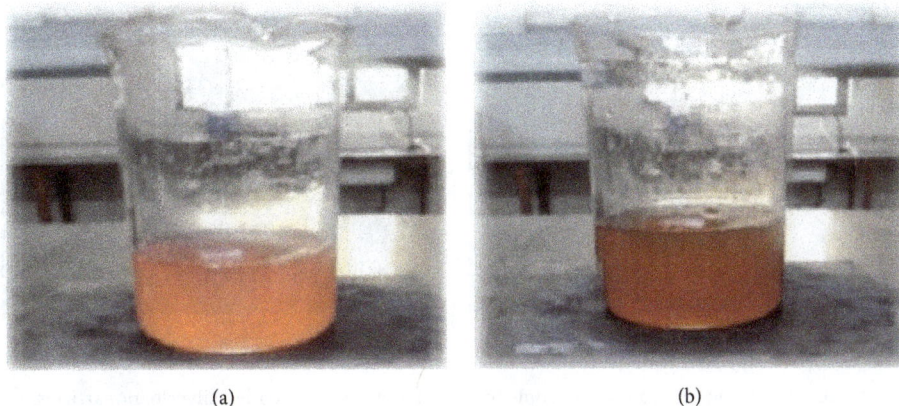

(a)   (b)

FIGURE 1: Formation of silver nanoparticles. (a) Color before initiation of reduction of silver ions; (b) color change after reduction.

was characterized utilizing DPPH (2,2-diphenyl-2-picrylhydrazyl hydrate) assay. A stock solution of DPPH in methanol was prepared. 1 mL of this stock solution was added to 3 mL of hydrogel solution (1 gm of prepared hydrogel in 10 mL of distilled water). The mixture was shaken vigorously and allowed to stand at room temperature for 30 min. Then the absorbance was measured at 517 nm by using a UV-visible spectrophotometer. Antioxidant activity was estimated by calculating the % inhibition by following formula [23]:

$$\text{DPPH scavenging effect (\%)} = \frac{(\text{control absorbance} - \text{sample absorbance})}{\text{control absorbance}} \times 100. \tag{3}$$

2.2.8. Antimicrobial Activity of Silver Nanoparticulate Hydrogel.
Antimicrobial activity was performed using well-diffusion technique employing agar and nutrient broth as media. Media was constituted by mixing agar and nutrient broth and then autoclaved at 121°C at 15 lbsi for 60 min for sterilization. Sterilized liquid media were then poured into two different petri plates and inoculated with *E. coli* and *S. aureus*, respectively. The petri plates were kept for 5 min till solidification is complete. The entire work was carried out in laminar air flow unit. Sterilized cork borer was used to create well of 1 cm diameter in the solidified media. Samples were poured in the well of prepared petri plates and then incubated at 37 ± 5°C for 24 h for inhibition to the growth of *E. coli* and *S. aureus* [24].

3. Results and Discussion

Apple extract was successfully prepared using MFW solution as explained in literature [14]. Extract obtained by the process was found to be pinkish red in color; the extract was further screened for the presence of flavonoids and phenols by preliminary screening and confirmatory testing. The phytochemical analysis of apple extract confirms the presence of phenols and flavonoids.

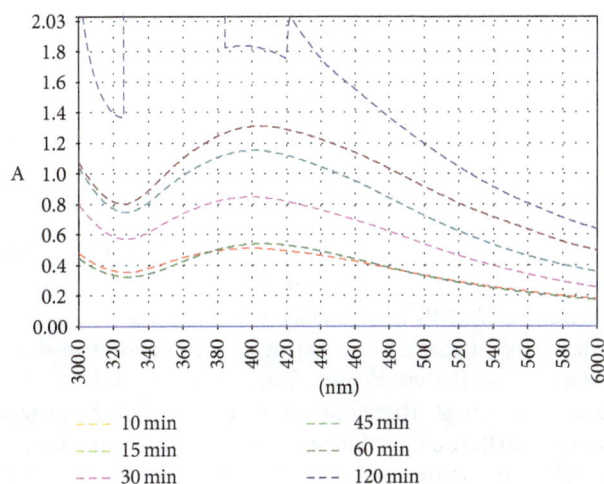

FIGURE 2: UV-visible spectra for apple extract loaded silver nanoparticles.

Silver nanoparticles prepared from apple extract showed the color change after 120 minutes of preparation giving the evidence for the reduction of silver ions and, eventually, formation of silver nanoparticles. The color change of the solution is clearly depicted in Figures 1(a) and 1(b).

The color change was recorded by visual observation in beaker which contains silver nitrate solution with apple extract. The color of AgNPS apple extract solution changes from colorless to light brown after 5 min and eventually to dark brown as shown in Figures 1(a) and 1(b). This color change indicates formation of AgNPs in solution [25, 26]. The synthesis of AgNPs was furthermore confirmed by UV-visible spectroscopy and scanning electron microscopy [24]. The UV-Vis spectrum of silver nanoparticles was recorded as a function of a reaction time. Aliquots of samples were withdrawn at different time intervals, that is, 10, 15, 30, 45, 60, and 120 min, to monitor the bioreduction of Ag+ ions. The graph obtained by UV spectrophotometer contains significant bell shaped peak indicating the formation of silver nanoparticles as shown in Figure 2.

Figure 2 shows UV-visible absorption spectrum of synthesized AgNPs. AgNPs have free electrons which give

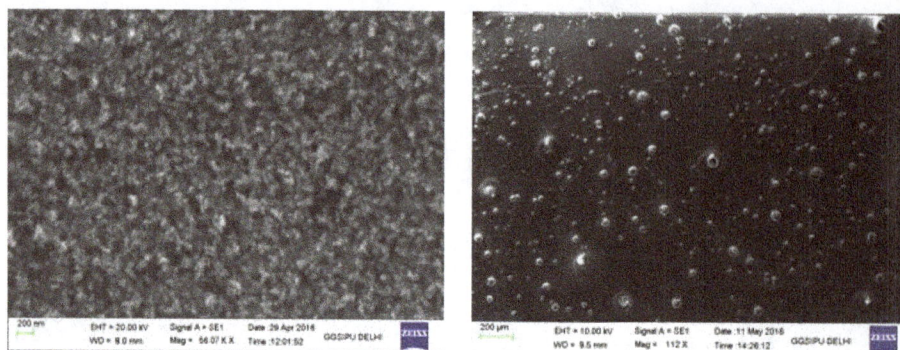

FIGURE 3: Scanning electron microscopic images of apple extract loaded silver nanoparticles.

TABLE 2: Evaluation parameters of apple extract loaded silver nanoparticles based hydrogels.

S. number	Parameters	F1	F2	F3
(1)	pH	6.11 ± 0.1	6.36 ± 0.15	6.66 ± 0.2
(2)	Viscosity	40000 cps	42000 cps	43000 cps
(3)	Spreadability	4.83 ± 0.3 g·cm/sec	5.56 ± 0.15 g·cm/sec	5.63 ± 0.15 g·cm/sec
(4)	Porosity	55.4%	61.2%	63.9%

surface plasmon resonance (SPR) absorption band. This SPR absorption band may be attributed to combined variation of electrons of AgNPs in resonance with light wave. It is very much familiar that silver nanoparticles in nanorange show absorption at the wavelength from 390 nm to 420 nm due to Mie scattering. Therefore, a broad absorption band was observed in the range of 400 nm–440 nm which is the characteristic of Mie scattering [27, 28]. No other peak was recorded in spectrum which confirms that synthesized nanoparticles are silver particles only. SEM technique was employed to evaluate AgNPs size, shape, and surface morphology. The average size of the particles was found to be below 200 nm and the particles formed were spherical in shape, as shown in Figure 3.

From Figure 3, it can be illustrated that morphology of AgNPs is spherical and particles are well dispersed without any aggregation. The particle size of the silver nanoparticles was found to be in the range of 100 nm indicating best suitability for topical delivery as particles on nanoscale can easily permeate through skin. The zeta potential was found to be very negative on higher scale revealing good stability of AgNps in dispersion form. The prepared hydrogel was evaluated for pH, viscosity, spreadability, and porosity. The pH of all formulated hydrogel was found in the range of 5.5–7.5, which mimics the pH of skin; therefore, formulation shows no sign of irritation on skin. The results of rheological studies, namely, viscosity and spreadability of the formulation, were found to be 42000 cps and 5.56 ± 0.15 g·cm/sec, respectively, which clearly signify that the hydrogel is easy to spread on skin. The results of all the three batches formulated are mentioned in Table 2. Furthermore, hydrogel formulations were then subject to *in vitro* drug release to compute the rate and extent of drug release.

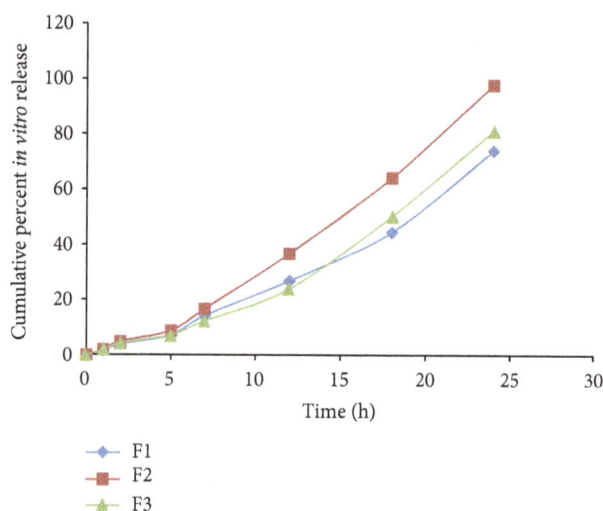

FIGURE 4: Cumulative percent *in vitro* release of apple extract loaded silver nanoparticles.

3.1. In-Vitro Release.

The results of *in vitro* drug release of all three formulations were in the range of 74.1% ± 0.28 to 98.01% ± 0.37 up to 24 h concluding the maximum release was shown by F2 hydrogel formulation as shown in Figure 4. On the basis of results in Table 2, optimized hydrogel formulation was selected. Primary focus was laid on particle size as this will play significant role in nanoparticle permeation from skin. The smaller the particle size is, the easier the permeation will be. Additionally, to confirm the permeation of nanoparticle across the membrane, rat abdominal skin was selected. F2 hydrogel formulation displayed the maximum release.

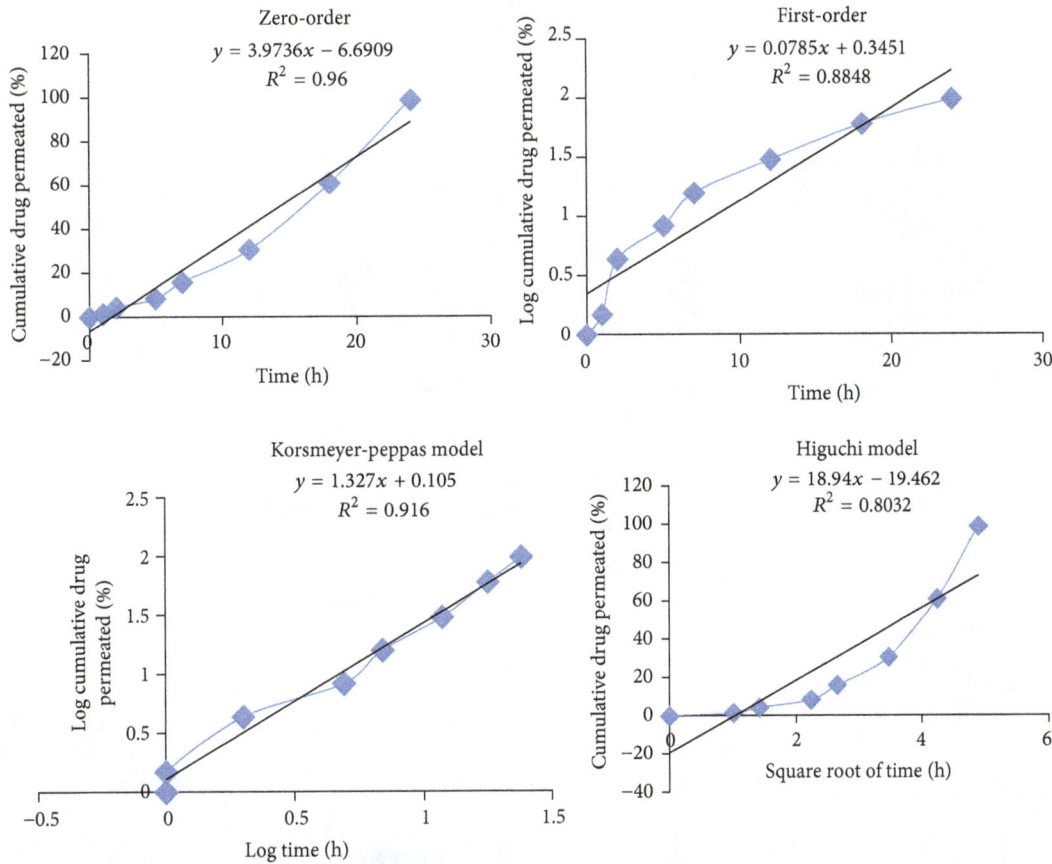

FIGURE 5: *Ex vivo* drug permeation kinetics of apple extract loaded silver nanoparticles based hydrogels.

TABLE 3: Release kinetics and permeation parameters for apple extract loaded silver nanoparticles based hydrogels.

Apple extract loaded AgNPs based hydrogel (F2)										
Zero-order		1st-order equation		Korsmeyer-Peppas equation		Higuchi equation		Flux $(\mu g/cm^2/h)$	Permeability coefficient (P) (cm/h)	Lag time (h)
k	R^2	k	R^2	n	R^2	k	R^2			
3.973	0.96	0.078	0.884	0.105	0.916	19.46	0.803	0.0124	0.315	1.763

3.2. Ex Vivo Permeation Studies and Release Kinetics. Ex vivo permeation studies were only conducted for batch F2 as smaller particle size and maximum *in vitro* release was shown by this formulation. Cumulative percent permeation was found to be 98.81% ± 0.24 up to 24 h. The permeation studies were best explained by zero-order kinetics (R^2 = 0.96), followed by first-order kinetics (R^2 = 0.884) and Higuchi equation (R^2 = 0.803). *Ex vivo* permeation kinetics through zero-order, first-order, Korsmeyer-Peppas model, and Higuchi model have been explained in Figure 5. The values of R^2 and k for all release kinetics models are tabulated in Table 3. Zero-order process is a constant rate process that is independent of drug concentration [29]. This perfectly highlights apple extract silver nanoparticles loaded hydrogels as sustained release dosage form. Permeation parameters like flux, permeability coefficient, and lag time are summarized in Table 3.

3.3. Antioxidant Activity of Apple Extract Loaded Silver Nanoparticles Loaded Hydrogels. DPPH radical scavenging assay was investigated for the evaluation of antioxidant potential of the prepared hydrogel formulations. The purple solution containing DPPH turns yellow on addition of formulation, which indicates the scavenging of free radicals and presence of antioxidant activity [30]. The results are compiled in Table 4 and showed that the ratio of AgNPs with carbopol (2 : 1), that is, F1, demonstrated maximum inhibition with a value of 75.16 ± 0.04. At the same time, the value differs with other ratios, namely, AgNPs with carbopol (1 : 1) F2 and AgNPs with carbopol (1 : 2) F3. Thus, it can be concluded that maximum concentration of apple extract revealed maximum percent inhibition.

3.4. Antimicrobial Activity of Silver Nanoparticulate Hydrogel. Apple extract loaded silver nanoparticles based hydrogels

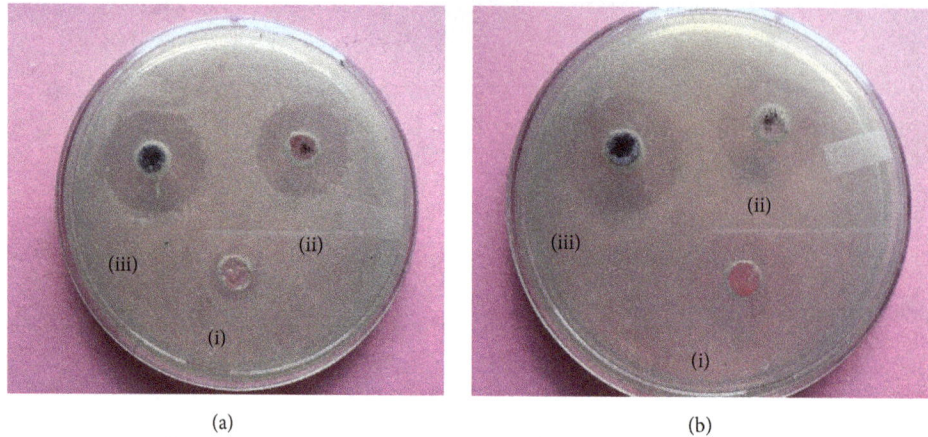

(a)   (b)

FIGURE 6: Antibacterial activity of silver nanoparticles (a) inhibition against *E. coli* and (b) inhibition against *S. aureus*. (i) Plain extract containing hydrogel, (ii) silver nanoparticles containing apple extract, and (iii) apple AgNPs loaded hydrogel.

TABLE 4: Antioxidant activity of apple extract silver nanoparticles loaded hydrogels (DPPH radical scavenging assay).

S. number	Formulations	Percent DPPH scavenging effect
(1)	F1	75.16% ± 0.04
(2)	F2	69.22% ± 0.02
(3)	F3	68.18% ± 0.03

showed higher antimicrobial properties against the bacterial species of *E. coli* and *S. aureus*. Well-diffusion method was opted to evaluate the antibacterial activity. The inhibitory action of silver compounds may be attributed to the strong interaction of silver with thiol groups present in key respiratory enzymes in bacteria [31].

The samples shows good zone of inhibition. Figures 6(a) and 6(b) show the zone of inhibition obtained against *E. coli* and *S. aureus,* respectively. A good inhibition was shown by silver nanoparticles based hydrogel contrary to plain hydrogel containing apple extract where no zone of inhibition was seen against *E. coli* as well as for *S. aureus*.

4. Conclusion

In the present research, green synthesis of apple extract loaded Ag-NPs was successfully achieved by treatment of silver nitrate with extract of *Malus domestica* (apple). This technique revealed that the apple extracts can be used as an effective stabilizing reducing and capping agent for the synthesis of AgNPs. This method of reduction utilized here is very simple, easy to perform, inexpensive, eco-friendly, and superior substitute to chemical synthesis. The finally fashioned AgNPs based hydrogels were highly stable formulations, showing strong antibacterial and antioxidant activity.

Competing Interests

The authors report no competing interests.

Acknowledgments

The authors wish to thank Founder President Dr. Ashok K. Chauhan, Amity University, for their kind support during research. The authors also like to acknowledge Professor A. K Narula Director C.E.P.S, Guru Gobind Singh Indraprasth University, for providing facility of SEM.

References

[1] S. Raj, S. Jose, U. S. Sumod, and M. Sabitha, "Nanotechnology in cosmetics: opportunities and challenges," *Journal of Pharmacy and Bioallied Sciences*, vol. 4, no. 3, pp. 186–193, 2012.

[2] U. Nagaich, "Nanocosmeceuticals: a boon to personal care products," *Journal of Advanced Pharmaceutical Technology and Research*, vol. 7, article 1, 2016.

[3] D. Kumar, N. Jain, N. Gulati, and U. Nagaich, "Nanoparticles laden in situ gelling system for ocular drug targeting," *Journal of Advanced Pharmaceutical Technology and Research*, vol. 4, no. 1, pp. 9–17, 2013.

[4] S. Ghosh, S. Patil, M. Ahire et al., "Synthesis of silver nanoparticles using Dioscorea bulbifera tuber extract and evaluation of its synergistic potential in combination with antimicrobial agents," *International Journal of Nanomedicine*, vol. 7, pp. 483–496, 2012.

[5] L. Ge, Q. Li, M. Wang, J. Ouyang, X. Li, and M. M. Q. Xing, "Nanosilver particles in medical applications: synthesis, performance, and toxicity," *International Journal of Nanomedicine*, vol. 9, no. 1, pp. 2399–2407, 2014.

[6] S. Iravani, H. Korbekandi, S. V. Mirmohammadi, and B. Zolfaghari, "Synthesis of silver nanoparticles: chemical, physical and biological methods," *Research in Pharmaceutical Sciences*, vol. 9, no. 6, pp. 385–406, 2014.

[7] V. Palermo, F. Mattivi, R. Silvestri, G. La Regina, C. Falcone, and C. Mazzoni, "Apple can act as anti-aging on yeast cells," *Oxidative Medicine and Cellular Longevity*, vol. 2012, Article ID 491759, 8 pages, 2012.

[8] S. Jadoon, S. Karim, M. H. H. B. Asad et al., "Anti-aging potential of phytoextract loaded-pharmaceutical creams for human skin cell longevity," *Oxidative Medicine and Cellular Longevity*, vol. 2015, Article ID 709628, 17 pages, 2015.

[9] A. Rasul and N. Akhtar, "Formulation and in vivo evaluation for anti-aging effects of an emulsion containing basil extract using non-invasive biophysical techniques," *Journal of Faculty of Pharmacy, Tehran University of Medical Sciences*, vol. 19, no. 5, pp. 344–350, 2011.

[10] D. L. Bissett, R. Chatterjee, and D. P. Hannon, "Photoprotective effect of super-oxide scavenging antioxidants against ultraviolet radiation-induced chronic skin damage in the hairless mouse," *Photodermatology Photoimmunology and Photomedicine*, vol. 7, no. 2, pp. 56–62, 1990.

[11] R. Ganceviciene, A. I. Liakou, A. Theodoridis, E. Makrantonaki, and C. C. Zouboulis, "Skin anti-aging strategies," *Dermato-Endocrinology*, vol. 4, no. 3, pp. 308–319, 2012.

[12] K. Rahman, "Studies on free radicals, antioxidants, and cofactors," *Clinical Interventions in Aging*, vol. 2, no. 2, pp. 219–236, 2007.

[13] D. A. Hyson, "A comprehensive review of apples and apple components and their relationship to human health," *Advances in Nutrition*, vol. 2, no. 5, pp. 408–420, 2011.

[14] N. Akhtar, H. M. S. Khan, F. Gulfishan Rasool, M. Ahmad, and T. Saeed, "Formulation and in vitro evaluation of a cosmetic emulsion containing apple juice extract," *Asian Journal of Chemistry*, vol. 22, pp. 7235–7242, 2010.

[15] R. R. Banala, V. B. Nagati, and P. R. Karnati, "Green synthesis and characterization of *Carica papaya* leaf extract coated silver nanoparticles through X-ray diffraction, electron microscopy and evaluation of bactericidal properties," *Saudi Journal of Biological Sciences*, vol. 22, no. 5, pp. 637–644, 2015.

[16] G. Giomaro, A. Karioti, A. R. Bilia et al., "Polyphenols profile and antioxidant activity of skin and pulp of a rare apple from Marche region (Italy)," *Chemistry Central Journal*, vol. 8, no. 1, article 45, 2014.

[17] P. S. Pavithra, N. Sreevidya, and R. S. Verma, "Antibacterial and antioxidant activity of methanol extract of *Evolvulus nummularius*," *Indian Journal of Pharmacology*, vol. 41, no. 5, pp. 233–236, 2009.

[18] G. Marslin, R. K. Selvakesavan, G. Franklin, B. Sarmento, and A. C. P. Dias, "Antimicrobial activity of cream incorporated with silver nanoparticles biosynthesized from *Withania somnifera*," *International Journal of Nanomedicine*, vol. 10, pp. 5955–5963, 2015.

[19] N. Gulati, U. Nagaich, and S. A. Saraf, "Intranasal delivery of chitosan nanoparticles for migraine therapy," *Scientia Pharmaceutica*, vol. 81, no. 3, pp. 843–854, 2013.

[20] N. Vishal Gupta and H. G. Shivakumar, "Preparation and characterization of superporous hydrogels as gastroretentive drug delivery system for rosiglitazone maleate," *DARU, Journal of Pharmaceutical Sciences*, vol. 18, no. 3, pp. 200–210, 2010.

[21] A. Chatterjee, B. B. Bhowmik, and Y. S. Thakur, "Formulation, in vitro and in vivo pharmacokinetics of anti-HIV vaginal bioadhesive gel," *Journal of Young Pharmacists*, vol. 3, no. 2, pp. 83–89, 2011.

[22] I. Özcan, E. Azizoğlu, T. Şenyiğit, M. Özyazici, and Ö. Özer, "Enhanced dermal delivery of diflucortolone valerate using lecithin/chitosan nanoparticles: in-vitro and in-vivo evaluations," *International Journal of Nanomedicine*, vol. 8, pp. 461–475, 2013.

[23] M. Biswas, P. K. Haldar, and A. K. Ghosh, "Antioxidant and free-radical-scavenging effects of fruits of *Dregea volubilis*," *Journal of Natural Science, Biology and Medicine*, vol. 1, no. 1, pp. 29–34, 2010.

[24] T. N. V. K. V. Prasad and E. K. Elumalai, "Biofabrication of Ag nanoparticles using *Moringa oleifera* leaf extract and their antimicrobial activity," *Asian Pacific Journal of Tropical Biomedicine*, vol. 1, no. 6, pp. 439–442, 2011.

[25] R. Geethalakshmi and D. V. L. Sarada, "Gold and silver nanoparticles from *Trianthema decandra*: synthesis, characterization, and antimicrobial properties," *International Journal of Nanomedicine*, vol. 7, pp. 5375–5384, 2012.

[26] K. S. Mukunthan, E. K. Elumalai, T. N. Patel, and V. R. Murty, "*Catharanthus roseus*: a natural source for the synthesis of silver nanoparticles," *Asian Pacific Journal of Tropical Biomedicine*, vol. 1, no. 4, pp. 270–274, 2011.

[27] R. Singh, P. Wagh, S. Wadhwani et al., "Synthesis, optimization, and characterization of silver nanoparticles from Acinetobacter calcoaceticus and their enhanced antibacterial activity when combined with antibiotics," *International Journal of Nanomedicine*, vol. 8, pp. 4277–4290, 2013.

[28] P. Balashanmugam and P. T. Kalaichelvan, "Biosynthesis characterization of silver nanoparticles using Cassia roxburghii DC. aqueous extract, and coated on cotton cloth for effective antibacterial activity," *International Journal of Nanomedicine*, vol. 10, supplement 1, pp. 87–97, 2015.

[29] V. Senthil, R. S. Kumar, C. V. V. Nagaraju, N. Jawahar, G. N. K. Ganesh, and K. Gowthamarajan, "Design and development of hydrogel nanoparticles for mercaptopurine," *Journal of Advanced Pharmaceutical Technology & Research*, vol. 1, no. 3, pp. 334–337, 2010.

[30] S. Jelodarian, A. Haghir Ebrahimabadi, A. Khalighi, and H. Batooli, "Evaluation of antioxidant activity of Malus domestica fruit extract from Kashan area," *Avicenna Journal of Phytomedicine*, vol. 2, no. 3, pp. 139–145, 2012.

[31] K. Singh, M. Panghal, S. Kadyan, U. Chaudhary, and J. P. Yadav, "Antibacterial activity of synthesized silver nanoparticles from Tinospora cordifolia against multi drug resistant strains of Pseudomonas aeruginosa isolated from burn patients," *Journal of Nanomedicine and Nanotechnology*, vol. 5, article 192, 2014.

16

Formulation and Evaluation of New Glimepiride Sublingual Tablets

Wafa Al-Madhagi,[1,2] **Ahmed Abdulbari Albarakani,**[2] **Abobakr Khaled Alhag,**[2] **Zakaria Ahmed Saeed,**[2] **Nahlah Mansour Noman,**[3] **and Khaldon Mohamed**[4]

[1]*Department of Pharmaceutical Chemistry, Faculty of Pharmacy, Sana'a University, Sana'a, Yemen*
[2]*Department of Pharmacy, Faculty of Medicine and Health Sciences, Yemeni Jordanian University, Sana'a, Yemen*
[3]*Department of Pharmacy, Faculty of Medicine and Health Sciences, Thamar University, Dhamar, Yemen*
[4]*Department of Biomedical Science, Sana'a University, Sana'a, Yemen*

Correspondence should be addressed to Wafa Al-Madhagi; w_almadhaji@hotmail.com

Academic Editor: Francisco Javier Flores-Murrieta

Oral mucosal delivery of drugs promotes rapid absorption and high bioavailability, with a subsequent immediate onset of pharmacological effect. However, many oral mucosal deliveries are compromised by the possibility of the patient swallowing the active substance before it has been released and absorbed locally into the systemic circulation. The aim of this research was to introduce a new glimepiride formula for sublingual administration and rapid drug absorption that can be used in an emergency. The new sublingual formulation was prepared after five trials to prepare the suitable formulation. Two accepted formulations of the new sublingual product were prepared, but one of them with disintegration time of 1.45 min and searching for preferred formulation, the binder, is changed with Flulac and starch slurry to prepare formula with disintegration time of 21 seconds that supports the aim of research to be used in an emergency. The five formulations were done, after adjusting to the binder as Flulac and aerosil with disintegration time of 21 seconds and accepted hardness as well as the weight variation. The assay of a new product (subglimepiride) is 103% which is a promising result, confirming that the formula succeeded. The new product (subglimepiride) is accepted in most quality control tests and it is ready for marketing.

1. Introduction

Glimepiride is an orally active hypoglycemic substance belonging to the sulphonylurea group [1, 2]. It acts at ATP-sensitive potassium channels (KATP) on pancreatic β-cells to promote insulin release. It binds to 65 kD protein on β-cells, which appears to be a part of the same sulphonyl urea receptor that binds Glibenclamide. Glimepiride after oral administration lowers blood glucose 3.5 times more potently than Glibenclamide. Glimepiride is classified under class II according to biopharmaceutical classification system [3]. The drug shows low, pH dependent solubility. In acidic and neutral aqueous media, glimepiride exhibits very poor solubility at 37°C (<0.004 mg/mL). In media with pH > 7, the solubility of drug is slightly increased to 0.02 mg/mL [4]. This poor solubility may cause poor dissolution and unpredicted

bioavailability [2, 3]. The very poor aqueous solubility and wettability of glimepiride give rise to difficulties in the design of pharmaceutical formulations and led to variable oral bioavailability so it is beneficial to prepare it into a new dosage form [5]. A novel fast-disintegrating tablet (FDT) can be done based on three-dimensional printing (3DP) technology that can control the material composition, microstructure, and surface texture during its layer-by-layer manufacturing process to provide the products with special properties. In addition, the in vitro release rate can reflect the combined effect of several physical and chemical parameters, including solubility and particle size of the active ingredient and rheological properties of the dosage form. The sublingual (SL) cavity is characterized by unique anatomical and physiological conditions compared with other segments of the GIT such as the stomach and small intestine. A tablet that is swallowed will be subjected to GIT peristalsis in the presence of relatively large volumes of digestive fluids secreted throughout the GIT, facilitating tablet disintegration and drug dissolution. In the SL cavity, tablets are exposed to minimal physiological agitation; moreover, a limited volume of saliva, 0.3 mL/min resting flow rate up to 1 mL/min stimulated flow rate [6], is available to facilitate tablet disintegration and drug dissolution. The sublingual route usually produces a faster onset of action than orally ingested tablets and the portion absorbed through the sublingual blood vessels bypasses the hepatic first-pass metabolic processes [7–10]. Various techniques can be used to formulate rapidly disintegrating or dissolving tablets [11, 12]. This research was aimed at formulating glimepiride into a new fast-disintegrating tablets for sublingual administration as potential emergency to prevent hyperglycemia coma using direct compression technique.

2. Material and Methods

2.1. Materials. Glimepiride RS and acetonitrile were obtained from Alpha Chemika, India; sodium dihydrogen phosphate, phosphoric acid, and methanol obtained were from Merck.

2.2. Methods

2.2.1. Procedure of Formulation. Sublingual tablets of glimepiride were prepared by the method of direct compression. The excipients used were lactose, pregelatinized starch, sodium starch glycolate, croscarmellose sodium, maize starch, sucralose, and lemon flavor. The accurate amount of the active ingredient and all additives were homogenously blended using geometric dilution after passing through sieve number 60 (standard sieve size) and finally magnesium stearate was added for lubrication and triturated well [13]. Different quantities of excipients were used to prepare various formulations of sublingual tablets as shown in Table 1. The blended material was compressed on 8 mm standard concave punch using a mini press tablet punching machine (RIMEK, India). The total weight of formulation was made up to 150 mg [14, 15].

Preparation of Formula 1 (F1). All ingredients were weighed separately and then mixed except for Mg-stearate and glimepiride by geometric mixing. Finally the Mg-stearate was added to the final mixture and compressed.

Preparation of Formula 2 (F2). All ingredients were weighed separately and then mixed together except for Mg-stearate and glimepiride by geometric mixing. After that, he glimepiride was added to mixture according to geometric mixing. The mixture was granulated by distilled water and dried in oven at 50°C.

After drying, the mixture was passed through sieve (0.5 mm). Finally, the Mg-stearate was added to the final mixture and compressed.

Preparation of Formula 3 (F3). All ingredients were weighed separately. The pregelatinized starch was mixed with distilled water until a paste was formed. Then, the glimepiride, maize starch, 2/3 sodium starch glycolate, and 2/3 croscarmellose sodium were mixed together and then the mixture was granulated by paste and dried in oven 50°C. The granulated mixture passed through sieve 35 (0.5 mm). After that, 1/3 sodium starch glycolate and 1/3 croscarmellose sodium were added to mixture and mixed. Finally, the Mg-stearate was added to the final mixture and compressed.

Preparation of Formula 4 (F4). All ingredients were weighed separately and then the pregelatinized starch was mixed with distilled water until a paste was formed. After that, the glimepiride, maize starch, 2/3 sodium starch glycolate, 2/3 croscarmellose sodium, and povidone were mixed together and then the mixture was granulated by paste and dried in oven at 50°C. After that, the mixture granules were sieved by sieve 35 (0.5 mm). Then, 1/3 sodium starch glycolate and 1/3 croscarmellose sodium were added to the mixture and mixed. Finally, the Mg-stearate was added to the final mixture and compressed.

Preparation of Formula 5 (F5). All ingredients were weighed separately. The glimepiride, maize starch, aerosil 200, and dicalcium phosphate were mixed together. After binder was prepared (starch paste), the mixture was granulated by starch paste and dried at 45°C. After that, the aerosil and Flulac were mixed; then sucralose and lemon flavor were added to this mixture. Finally, the Mg-stearate was added and compressed.

Preparation of Starch Paste (the Binder). The maize starch was dissolved in 3 L of distilled water (40–45°C) and was checked for being free of lumps. This slurry was charged into 10 mL of water (95°C) into vessels until complete gelatinization. Finally, the mixture cooled to 50°C.

2.2.2. Procedure of Evaluation of the Best Formula

(1) Chemical Test. Assay test was done using HPLC method as follows.

Mobile Phase Preparation. Sodium di-hydrogen phosphate 0.5 gm was dissolved in 500 mL of distilled water. Adjust pH to 2.4 with H_3PO_4 and add 500 mL of acetonitrile; mix it well and filter it through 0.45 μm micromembrane filter.

HPLC Conditions. The conditions were as follows: column: ODS1 (C18) 15 * 0.45 cm; flow rate: 1.0 mL/min; wavelength: 220 nm; sensitivity: 1; pressure: 28 Mpa.

Preparation of Standard Solution. Weigh accurately equivalent to 21 mg of glimepiride RS into 100 VF and dissolve and then dilute it with acetonitrile solution 80% and mix well to get concentration at 0.21 mg/mL.

Preparation of Sample Solution. Transfer 7 tablets (equivalent to 21 mg of glimepiride) into 100 VF and dilute them to with acetonitrile solution 80% and mix well to get concentration. Sonicate the solution for 10 minutes and filter to get 0.21 mg/mL [16].

TABLE 1: The table illustrates the materials and their quantities which used to formulate new glymipride subligual tablet formulations (F1, F2, F3, F4, and F5).

Number	Material	F1		F2		F3		F4		F5	
		Amount/unit	Actual amount	Amount/unit	Actual amount	Amount/unit	Actual amount	Amount/unit	Actual amount	Amount/unit	Actual amount
1	Glimepiride	0.003 g	0.9 g	0.003 g	0.9 g	0.002 g	0.6 g	0.003 g	0.9 g	3 mg	0.9 g
2	Lactose	0.05 g	16.5 g	0.069 g	20.7 g	—	—	—	—	—	—
3	Croscarmellose sodium	0.01 g	3 g	0.026 g	7.8 g	—	—	—	—	—	—
4	Pregelatinized starch	0.02 g	6 g	0.02 g	6 g	0.002 g	0.6 g	0.0033 g	1 g	—	—
5	Mg-stearate	0.002 g	0.6 g	0.002 g	0.6 g	0.002 g	0.6 g	0.002 g	0.6 g	0.5 mg	0.15 g
6	Mais starch	—	—	—	—	0.002 g	0.6 g	0.06 g	18 g	61 mg	18.3 g
7	Na starch glycolate	—	—	—	—	0.002 g	0.6 g	0.02 g	6 g	—	—
8	Croscarmellose Na	—	—	—	—	0.002 g	0.6 g	0.02 g	6 g	—	—
9	Sucralose	—	—	—	—	0.002 g	0.6 g	0.003 g	0.9 g	3 mg	0.9 g
10	Lemon flavor	—	—	—	—	0.002 g	0.6 g	0.002 g	0.6 g	2 mg	0.6 g
11	Povidone	—	—	—	—	—	—	0.002 g	0.6 g	—	—
12	Aerosil 200	—	—	—	—	—	—	—	—	1 mg	0.3 g
13	Aerosil	—	—	—	—	—	—	—	—	1 mg	0.3 g
14	Flulac	—	—	—	—	—	—	—	—	10 mg	3 g
15	Dicalcium phosphate	—	—	—	—	—	—	—	—	40 mg	12 g
Total		0.09 g	27 g	0.12 g	36 g	0.1133 g	34 g	0.1153 g	34.6 g	107.5 mg	36.45 g

TABLE 2: The table shows the reading and results of glimepiride sublingual tablet formulation.

Name of the test		Reading			Comments
		Amaryl	F5 (new glimepiride)		
Assay		100.5%	103%		Conformed
Friability		0.02%	0.40%		Conformed
Weight variation	1	0.1669	0.116		Conformed
	2	0.168	0.116		
	3	0.1676	0.116		
	4	0.167	0.115		
	5	0.1687	0.115		
	6	0.1673	0.115		
	7	0.168	0.113		
	8	0.1688	0.115		
	9	0.1679	0.114		
	10	0.169	0.114		
	11	0.1672	0.113		
	12	0.169	0.115		
	13	0.1673	0.117		
	14	0.1684	0.117		
	15	0.169	0.115		
	16	0.1685	0.111		
	17	0.1669	0.111		
	18	0.1674	0.111		
	19	0.1678	0.115		
	20	0.1678	0.114		
	Average	0.167925	0.1141		
	Number	Reading	Number	Reading	
Hardness	1	5.35	1	3.8	Not conformed
	2	4.28	2	4.5	Conformed
	3	4.06	3	4.3	Conformed
	4	3.81	4	4.3	Conformed
	5	5.3	5	3.5	Not conformed
Disintegration time		1.15 minutes	21 seconds		Conformed

(2) Physical Test: Micrometrics. The thickness and diameter of 10 tablets were measured using micrometres. Limits: diameter should be less than 13 mm.

Weight Variation. 20 tablets of the product were weighed; then the higher limit (HL) and lower limit (LL) were calculated as follows:

Average wt = total wt/20

Average wt × 5% = n

HL = Av. wt + n

LL = Av. wt − n [16, 17]

Friability Test. The tablets of this product were weighed ($w1$), then put in the instrument for 4 minutes, and then weighed again ($w2$). After that, the following were calculated:

Friability = [($w2$)/($w1$)] ∗ 100

Limit for compression tabs: not more than 1% [16]

Hardness Test. Ten tablets were put in specific place and fixed; then turn it on and wait until the fraction occurs. The limit is 4–8 kg/cm^2 [16].

Disintegration Time Test. The disintegration time is calculated using disintegrator using water as media and the limit of tablet is 5–30 minutes [16].

2.3. *Statistical Analysis.* Data were presented as means ± standard deviation (SD). SPSS version 12 was used for statistical analysis. A t-test and the one-way ANOVA were performed to examine the differences among the groups. A P value of <0.05 was considered to be statistically significant.

3. Results and Discussion

In formula 1 (F1), the tablets were very friable and cannot be compressed because the hardness was weak due to the presence of high amount of croscarmellose as disintegrant agent and, therefore, the binder would increase in formula 2. Formula 2 (F2) showed disintegration time of about 1.45 min, but while searching for a preferred formula with fast disintegration, low croscarmellose sodium was used as disintegrant agent and therefore add super disintegrant, flavoring agent, and sweetening agent and change the diluent in formula 3. Formula 3 (F3) showed the high friability of tablet due to the fact that the binder is not suitable and, therefore, add new binder in formula 4. In formula 4 (F4), the hardness is strong due to the fact that the binder is high and not suitable and therefore change the formula. Formula 5 showed the best result as shown in Table 2.

The new sublingual formula showed good disintegration with 21 seconds which is more preferred than formula 2, as the assay gives good result compared to Amaryl as the standard drug as well as the hardness and friability.

4. Conclusion

The five formulations were done and after adjusting to the binder as Flulac and aerosil with disintegration time of 21 seconds and accepted hardness as well as the weight variation. The assay of new sublingual glimepiride is 103% which is a promising result and confirms that the formula succeeded and is accepted in most quality control tests and it is ready for marketing. The sublingual glimepiride has fast dissolving time that would be more targeted in emergency DM.

Competing Interests

There are no competing interests regarding the publication of this paper.

Acknowledgments

The authors are grateful for the Department of Pharmacy, Faculty of Medical Sciences, Yemeni Jordanian University, for supplying of all the basic requirements of this search.

References

[1] M. Massi-Benedetti, "Glimepiride in type 2 diabetes mellitus: a review of the worldwide therapeutic experience," *Clinical Therapeutics*, vol. 25, no. 3, pp. 799–816, 2003.

[2] S. N. Davis, "The role of glimepiride in the effective management of Type 2 diabetes," *Journal of Diabetes and its Complications*, vol. 18, no. 6, pp. 367–376, 2004.

[3] A. Frick, H. Moller, and E. Wirbitzki, "Biopharmaceutical characterization of oral immediate release drug products. In vitro/in vivo comparison of phenoxymethylpenicillin potassium, glimepiride and levofloxacin," *European Journal of Pharmaceutics and Biopharmaceutics*, vol. 46, no. 3, pp. 305–311, 1998.

[4] S. Vidyadhara, J. R. Babu, R. Sasidhar et al., "Formulation and evaluation of glimepiride solid dispersions and their tablet formulations for enhanced bioavailability," *Pharmanest*, vol. 2, no. 1, pp. 15–20, 2011, http://www.pharmanest.net.

[5] S. Vidyadhara, J. R. Babu, R. L. C. Sasidhar, A. Ramu, S. Siva Prasad, and M. Tejasree, "Formulation and evaluation of glimepiride solid dispersions and their tablet formulations for enhanced bioavailability," *Pharmanest-An International Journal of Advances in Pharmaceutical Sciences*, vol. 2, pp. 15–20, 2011.

[6] O. Rachid, M. Rawas-Qalaji, F. E. R. Simons, and K. J. Simons, "Dissolution testing of sublingual tablets: a novel in vitro method," *AAPS PharmSciTech*, vol. 12, no. 2, pp. 544–552, 2011.

[7] R. Birudaraj, B. Berner, S. Shen, and X. Li, "Buccal permeation of buspirone: mechanistic studies on transport pathways," *Journal of Pharmaceutical Sciences*, vol. 94, no. 1, pp. 70–78, 2005.

[8] T. Ishikawa, N. Koizumi, B. Mukai et al., "Pharmacokinetics of acetaminophen from rapidly disintegrating compressed tablet prepared using microcrystalline cellulose (PH-M-06) and spherical sugar granules," *Chemical and Pharmaceutical Bulletin*, vol. 49, no. 2, pp. 230–232, 2001.

[9] T. M. Price, K. L. Blauer, M. Hansen, F. Stanczyk, R. Lobo, and G. W. Bates, "Single-dose pharmacokinetics of sublingual versus oral administration of micronized 17β-estradiol," *Obstetrics and Gynecology*, vol. 89, no. 3, pp. 340–345, 1997.

[10] S. C. Sweetman Martindale, *The Complete Drug Reference*, vol. 34, Pharmaceutical Press, 2005.

[11] L. V. Allen, "Rapid-dissolve technology: an interview with Loyd V. Allen," *International Journal of Pharmacy and Technology*, vol. 7, pp. 449–450, 2003.

[12] Y. Fu, S. Yang, S. H. Jeong, S. Kimura, and K. Park, "Orally fast disintegrating tablets: developments, technologies, taste-masking and clinical studies," *Critical Reviews in Therapeutic Drug Carrier Systems*, vol. 21, no. 6, pp. 433–476, 2004.

[13] S. S. Biradar, S. T. Bhagavati, and I. J. Kuppasad, "Fast dissolving drug delivery systems: a brief overview," *The Internet Journal of Pharmacology*, vol. 4, no. 2, 2006.

[14] R. V. Keny, C. Desouza, and C. F. Lourenco, "Formulation and evaluation of rizatriptan Benzoate mouth disintegrating tablets," *Indian Journal of Pharmaceutical Sciences*, vol. 72, no. 1, pp. 79–85, 2010.

[15] C. Wayne, R. Dipan, and D. Ann, Selecting super disintegrants for Orally Disintegrating Tablet Formulations in Pharmaceutical Technology, 2006.

[16] *British Pharmacopeia*, 2011.

[17] United States pharmacopeia, 2007.

Cellulose Acetate 398-10 Asymmetric Membrane Capsules for Osmotically Regulated Delivery of Acyclovir

Alka Sonkar, Anil Kumar, and Kamla Pathak

Department of Pharmaceutics, Rajiv Academy for Pharmacy, Mathura, Uttar Pradesh 281001, India

Correspondence should be addressed to Kamla Pathak; kamlapathak5@gmail.com

Academic Editor: Giuseppina De Simone

The study was aimed at developing cellulose acetate asymmetric membrane capsules (AMCs) of acyclovir for its controlled delivery at the absorption site. The AMCs were prepared by phase inversion technique using wet process. A 2^3 full factorial design assessed the effect of independent variables (level(s) of polymer, pore former, and osmogen) on the cumulative drug release from AMCs. The buoyant optimized formulation F7 (low level of cellulose acetate; high levels of both glycerol and sodium lauryl sulphate) displayed maximum drug release of 97.88 ± 0.77% in 8 h that was independent of variation in agitational intensity and intentional defect on the cellulose acetate AMC. The *in vitro* data best fitted zero-order kinetics (r^2 = 0.9898). SEM micrograph of the transverse section confirmed the asymmetric nature of the cellulose acetate capsular membrane. Statistical analysis by Design Expert software indicated no interaction between the independent variables confirming the efficiency of the design in estimating the effects of variables on drug release. The optimized formulation F7 (desirability = 0.871) displayed sustenance of drug release over the drug packed in AMC in pure state proving the superiority of osmotically active formulation. Conclusively the AMCs have potential for controlled release of acyclovir at its absorption site.

1. Introduction

Asymmetric membrane capsule is a controlled drug delivery device which consists of a drug core surrounded by a membrane of asymmetric structure (relatively thin, dense region supported on a thicker, porous region). Similar to a conventional hard gelatin capsule, the asymmetric membrane capsule (AMC) consists of a cap and a body that snugly fit into each other. The cap is shorter in length and has a slightly larger diameter than the body which is longer and has a smaller diameter. In contrast to gelatin capsules, however, the walls of AMCs are made from water-insoluble polymer(s) such as cellulose acetate, ethyl cellulose, cellulose acetate butyrate, and their mixtures [1]. Thus, the capsule shell does not dissolve to instantly release the drug filled in it. Instead, the drug is released over a prolonged duration by diffusion through the capsule walls and/or via osmotic pumping by convection through pores in the capsule walls [2]. The use of asymmetric membranes as rate controlling membrane of drug delivery devices is being widely explored. The basic mechanism of drug release from asymmetric membrane capsule is osmosis. When the capsule comes into contact with water, water imbibes into it and dissolves the soluble component in the core, forming the solution of the drug. The hydrostatic pressure was generated within the core which acts as a driving force to deliver the drug through preexisting pores, after all components are depleted and asymmetric membrane coating remains intact [3].

Asymmetric membrane capsules have been proven to be efficient gastroretentive systems carriers for osmotically regulated delivery of highly water-soluble drug, ranitidine hydrochloride, by a report published from our lab [4]. This concept is being extrapolated for a poorly water-soluble drug, acyclovir, based on the literature support of suitability of AMCs for delivery of poor water-soluble drug due to high water flux capability [5–7].

Acyclovir is an antiviral agent used for the treatment of *Herpes simplex* virus types I and II and *Varicella zoster* virus. It has an oral bioavailability of 10–20% with a very short biological half-life of 2–4 h, so high frequent dosing is required [8]. The absorption of acyclovir from the gastrointestinal tract is variable and incomplete; 10–30% of an oral dose may be absorbed [9]. Because of its high hydrophilic nature, absorption of acyclovir occurs mainly by passive diffusion mechanism and is slow, variable, and incomplete [10]. Food does not appear to affect gastrointestinal absorption [11]. The absorption window of the drug is in the stomach and upper part of the intestine that can result in incomplete drug release from the drug delivery system leading to reduced efficacy of the administered dose. Hence designing a gastroretentive formulation that would provide controlled release of the drug may offer reduction in total dose and frequency of administration and enhanced absorption and hence bioavailability.

Thus, the aim of the project was to optimize cellulose acetate AMCs for osmotically controlled gastroretentive delivery of acyclovir using 2^3 factorial design. Acyclovir was selected as an active agent as it met the desired criteria for being the potential candidate for asymmetric membrane technology controlled drug delivery system: (i) poor aqueous solubility (2.5 mg/mL), (ii) short plasma half-life (2–4 h), and (iii) absorption that is unaffected by presence of food in stomach. Prior to developing AMCs, the solubility of acyclovir was modulated for achieving a controlled release formulation.

2. Materials and Methods

2.1. Materials. Acyclovir was a kind gift from Zen Lab & Preet Remedies Pvt. Ltd., Baddi, India.

Cellulose acetate 398-10 was brought from Sigma Aldrich Chemical, Germany; glycerol was brought from S. D. Fine Chemicals, Mumbai, India; sodium lauryl sulphate was brought from Ranbaxy Fine Chemicals Ltd., New Delhi, India. Acetone, ethanol 95% v/v, potassium dihydrogen orthophosphate, and methylene blue were obtained from S. D. Fine Chemicals, Mumbai, India.

2.2. Equilibrium Solubility and Its Modulation. An excess amount of acyclovir was suspended in 10 mL each of double distilled water and phosphate buffer, pH 4.5, and maintained at $37 \pm 0.5°C$. The flasks were then shaken for 72 h in water bath shaker (Hicon Enterprises, New Delhi, India). The suspension was filtered through $0.2 \mu m$ size filter paper and the temperature was maintained at $37 \pm 0.5°C$ using lab fabricated temperature regulating boxes. The solution was analyzed spectrophotometrically at 252 nm in a double-beam UV spectrophotometer (Shimadzu Pharmaspec-1700, Kyoto, Japan) after appropriate dilution. The solubility was determined using validated calibration curve. The solubility of acyclovir was modulated by sodium lauryl sulphate. To solutions of sodium lauryl sulphate of varying molar strength (0.25, 0.50, 0.75, 1.00, 1.25, 1.50, and 1.75 M) in double distilled water and in phosphate buffer, pH 4.5, excess drug was added and solubility determination was carried out as described in the preceding text.

2.3. Differential Scanning Calorimetry. The differential scanning thermograms profiles of pure drug, excipients, and physical mixtures thereof were recorded on DSC-60 controlled by TA-60 WS software (Shimadzu, Kyoto, Japan). The samples were weighed and transferred to the equipment for analysis in hermetically sealed aluminium pans. An indium standard was used to calibrate the differential scanning calorimeter temperature. The samples were heated, over a temperature range of $0–300°C$. An inert atmosphere was maintained by purging with nitrogen at the flow rate of 20 mL/min.

2.4. Determination of Controlled Release Dose. The controlled release dose was calculated using the following equation [12]:

$$D_t = D_i \left(1 + 0.693 \times \frac{t}{t_{1/2}} \right), \tag{1}$$

where D_t is total dose required for the dosage form, t is time for drug release (8 h), $t_{1/2}$ is half-life of the drug (4 h), and D_i is immediate release dose (200 mg). Thus D_t was calculated as 477.2 mg and for the experimental purpose it was rounded off to 480 mg.

2.5. Experimental Design. A 2^3 full factorial design [13] was utilized for the formulation and optimization of AMCs. The independent variables in the study were concentration of cellulose acetate 398-10 (A), concentration of glycerol (B), and content of sodium lauryl sulphate (C). For each of these variables, an experimental range in terms of levels was selected based on the results of preliminary experiments. Each factor was taken at two levels ($+1$, -1), which were coded as high or low levels, respectively. The response was percent cumulative drug release (% CDR) in 8 h. The composition of all the formulations ($n = 8$) with coded values was given (Table 1).

2.6. Fabrication of AMCs. Asymmetric membrane capsules were made by dip coating (phase inversion) process [14] wherein the polymeric membrane was precipitated on fabricated glass mould pins of diameters 7.30 ± 0.05 mm and 7.73 ± 0.02 mm for the body and the cap, respectively. The glass mould pins were dipped into polymeric solution of cellulose acetate 398-10 in acetone (50% v/v) and mixed with a mixture of glycerol in ethanol (25% v/v). The polymeric membrane precipitated on the pins was air-dried for 15 s, followed by dipping in aqueous quenching solution of glycerol for 10 min. Thereafter the pins were withdrawn manually and allowed to air-dry for at least 8 h. The capsules were stripped off the pins, trimmed to size, and kept in desiccators until use. The AMC's body was manually filled with a constant drug load mixed with sodium lauryl sulphate in accordance with the design. The body of the AMCs was then capped and sealed with 10% w/v sealing solution of cellulose acetate 398-10 in a mixture of acetone and ethanol (1 : 1).

2.7. Physical Characterization. The AMCs were characterized for surface, appearance, and dimensions and compared visually for transparency and opacity. Dimensions of AMCs were determined using vernier calliper. The results were statistically compared with conventional hard gelatin capsule of "zero" size at $p < 0.05$. A multiple of three determinants was used for measurement of each dimension.

2.8. Evaluation

2.8.1. Uniformity of Weight. The weight of the capsule content was measured as a difference between the weight of intact

TABLE 1: Actual and coded values of independent variables used for fabrication of AMCs of acyclovir in 2^3 full factorial design.

Formulation code	Cellulose acetate 398-10 (% w/v) (A)	Glycerol (% v/v) (B)	Sodium lauryl sulphate (mg) (C)	Dependent variable
F1	10 (−1)	10 (−1)	215 (−1)	
F2	15 (+1)	10 (−1)	215 (−1)	
F3	10 (−1)	18 (+1)	215 (−1)	
F4	15 (+1)	18 (+1)	215 (−1)	
F5	10 (−1)	10 (−1)	290 (+1)	% CDR_{8h}[b] (Y1)
F6	15 (+1)	10 (−1)	290 (+1)	
F7	10 (−1)	18 (+1)	290 (+1)	
F8	15 (+1)	18 (+1)	290 (+1)	
F9[a]	12	(14)	(250)	

[a]Extra design checkpoint; [b]cumulative drug release.

capsule and that of the shell after removing the contents of the capsule. A total of twenty capsules were used for performing test and compared with the limit mentioned in Indian Pharmacopoeia, 2007 [15].

2.8.2. Content of Active Ingredient.
The amount of active ingredient in each capsule was determined as per method mentioned in Indian Pharmacopoeia, 2007. Five capsules from each formulation were used for the study.

2.8.3. In Vitro Release.
In vitro drug release test of the formulations was performed using USP paddle type II apparatus (Hicon Enterprises, New Delhi, India). The in vitro drug release was assessed in 900 mL of phosphate buffer, pH 4.5, stirred at 75 rpm, and maintained at a temperature of 37 ± 0.5°C for 8 h. Five milliliters of sample was withdrawn on hourly basis and the release medium was replenished with fresh dissolution media. The samples were suitably diluted with fresh media and analyzed spectrophotometrically at 252 nm. The studies were conducted in triplicate and the drug released at each time point was calculated as mean ± SE and plotted against time. The release data was modeled for zero-order, first-order, Higuchi square root, and Hixson-Crowell models [12] using PCP Disso Version 2.08 software, Pune, India. The criterion for selecting the most appropriate model was chosen on the basis of maximum linearity of the data to fit with the model. Additionally, each AMC formulation was monitored for its floating ability during in vitro drug release study and data was recorded every hour.

2.9. Statistical Analysis.
The effect of independent variables on the responses was analyzed using Design Expert software version 9 (Stat-Ease, Inc., Minneapolis, USA). The polynomial equation was generated after omitting the insignificant coefficients at 95% confidence level using Pareto chart. The values of effects of coefficients were interpreted with the help of bar graph of coefficients obtained between the Bonferroni line and t-limit line. The generated polynomial equation for response parameter was used for validation of design. The 3D response surface graphs were used to analyze the influence of different levels of the variables on the response parameter (% CDR_{8h}).

2.10. Selection of Optimized Formulation and Validation of Experimental Design.
The optimized formulation was selected on the basis of maximum % CDR_{8h}. The extra design checkpoint formulation (F9) was prepared by taking mean value of two levels for all three factors. The predicted value determined using polynomial equation was compared with experimental value at 95% confidence interval ($p < 0.05$).

2.11. Scanning Electron Microscopy.
The asymmetric membrane was sputter-coated for 5–10 min with gold using fine coat ion sputter and examined under scanning electron microscope Ultra Plus, Carl Zeiss, Germany. The samples examined include (i) both sides of asymmetric membrane before and after in vitro release test, (ii) membrane with intentional defect before and after the in vitro release test, and (iii) transverse section of the membrane. On completion of the in vitro release study, asymmetric membrane structures were air-dried at 45°C for 12 h and stored between sheets of wax paper in desiccator until use.

2.12. Effect of Variables on Drug Release.
In order to study the effect of variables on the drug release, the in vitro release test of optimized formulation was conducted under varied conditions. The effect of agitational intensity was studied by varying the rotational speeds (50, 100, and 150 rpm) of paddle (USP-II apparatus). Another factor studied was effect of intentional defect on the release of acyclovir.

A defect was intentionally incurred in the AMC using a needle so that a hole of 2 mm dia was made and the defective optimized formulation was subjected to in vitro release test.

The presence/absence of osmogen and its concentration in the formulation plays a vital role in deciding the release of drug from the AMC. In order to demonstrate this, four different experimental systems were used. The study was carried out by dye test wherein methylene blue was selected as color producing agent. The release of dye from the AMC was monitored in variable molar environment created by sodium lauryl

TABLE 2: Various osmotic conditions used for studying the effect of osmotic pressure on drug release from asymmetric membrane capsule of acyclovir.

AMC code	SLS in AMC (mg)	SLS outside AMC (mg)	Osmotic condition	Result
F7A	0	0	Absent	Dye release intensified with time
F7B	290	0	Perfect osmotic gradient	Controlled release
F7C	290	145	Hypoosmotic	Slight release
F7D	290	430	Hyperosmotic	No release

sulphate inside and outside the capsule. Various osmotic conditions used for the study are documented in Table 2. The experimental setup(s) were stationed on lab shelf and the release of methylene blue was observed visually and interpreted. The release of the dye was indicative of its osmotic expulsion from core of capsule. Additionally, the osmotically regulated release of the drug was monitored quantitatively. The optimized formulation was introduced in phosphate buffer, pH 4.5 (900 mL), and variation in osmotic pressure was accomplished by controlling the amount of SLS in the capsule and in the surrounding environment. Condition A represents F7 without osmogen inside and outside the capsule that represented zero osmotic gradient; condition B represents F7 containing 290 mg SLS inside the capsule and 0 mg outside the capsule for perfect osmotic gradient; condition C represents 290 mg SLS inside and 145 mg outside the capsule (hypoosmotic); condition D represents F7 containing 290 mg SLS inside and 430 mg in the media for hyperosmotic condition. Conditions C and D were intended to analyze the effect of increasing the osmotic pressure (28.46 and 115.28 mmHg, resp., for C and D) of the external media on drug release.

2.13. Stability. The optimized formulation was subjected to stability testing as per ICH Q1 A [16]. Formulation F7 was sealed in aluminium foil coated inside with polyethylene and kept in stability chamber maintained at $40 \pm 2°C$ and $75 \pm 5\%$ RH for 3 months. The samples were analyzed for any deterioration in terms of any changes in physical parameters (texture and color), the percent drug content, and *in vitro* drug release. The sampling intervals were 0, 1, 2, and 3 months.

3. Results and Discussion

3.1. Equilibrium Solubility and Its Modulation. The solubility studies data indicated that acyclovir was poorly soluble in both phosphate buffer, pH 4.5 (1.74 mg/mL), and double distilled water (1.36 mg/mL). The results are consistent with the literature report on acyclovir as "slightly soluble in water" at room temperature (22–25°C) and solubility values range from 1.2 to 1.6 mg/mL [17, 18]. The solubility is a prominent factor in governing the drug release from an osmotically controlled drug delivery system [19]. A poorly soluble drug (<10 mg/mL) will be governed by first-order release kinetics rather than zero-order kinetics. Hence, for achieving a controlled release formulation of acyclovir, its solubility was modulated using sodium lauryl sulphate. The target solubility range of 50–300 mg/mL [14] is presumed to be appropriate for controlled drug delivery from an osmotically regulated

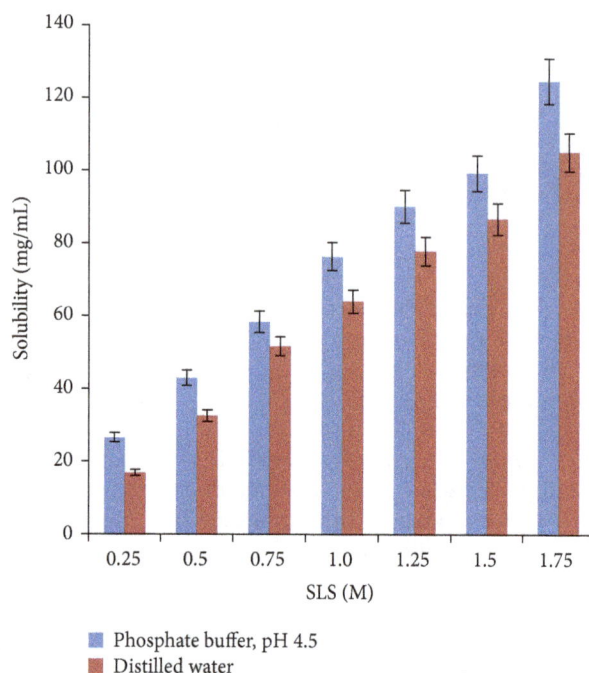

FIGURE 1: Bar chart for solubility modulation of acyclovir in the presence of sodium lauryl sulphate of varying molar strength.

system. In the solubility modulation experiment, the solubility of acyclovir was observed to increase almost linearly with increasing molarity of sodium lauryl sulphate (Figure 1) in both phosphate buffer, pH 4.5, and distilled water.

The solubility enhancement is attributable to the micellization of acyclovir by sodium lauryl sulphate. The anionic with high HLB value of 40 [20] surfactant was selected as the osmogen owing to its high water solubility and it is GRAS listed and recommended to be employed in a wide range of nonparenteral pharmaceutical formulations. The solubility enhancement in phosphate buffer, pH 4.5, was of higher magnitude than in water (though not significant) at all molar strengths of sodium lauryl sulphate. At 0.25 M and 0.5 M strengths the solubility values were <50 mg/mL. A strength of 0.75 M of sodium lauryl sulphate resulted in solubility value(s) of 58.39 mg/mL in phosphate buffer, pH 4.5, and of 51.72 mg/mL in distilled water. Further, increase in strength to 1.0 M resulted in a solubility of 76.43 mg/mL in phosphate buffer, pH 4.5, and of 64.05 mg/mL in distilled water. Beyond this strength of SLS, the solubility increased but was not taken into consideration because it may not help in achieving sustained effect of the drug in the given dose of the drug.

TABLE 3: Physical characterization of asymmetric membrane capsule (AMC) as compared to conventional hard gelatin capsule (HGC).

| Type of capsule | Appearance | Dimensions (mm) | | | | |
| | | Cap | | Body | | Lock length |
		Length	Diameter	Length	Diameter	
HGC	Transparent	10.88 ± 0.10	7.52 ± 0.02	18.60 ± 0.12	7.24 ± 0.04	21.32 ± 0.09
AMC	Opaque	10.89 ± 0.16	7.74 ± 0.01	18.74 ± 0.08	7.31 ± 0.09	21.58 ± 0.30

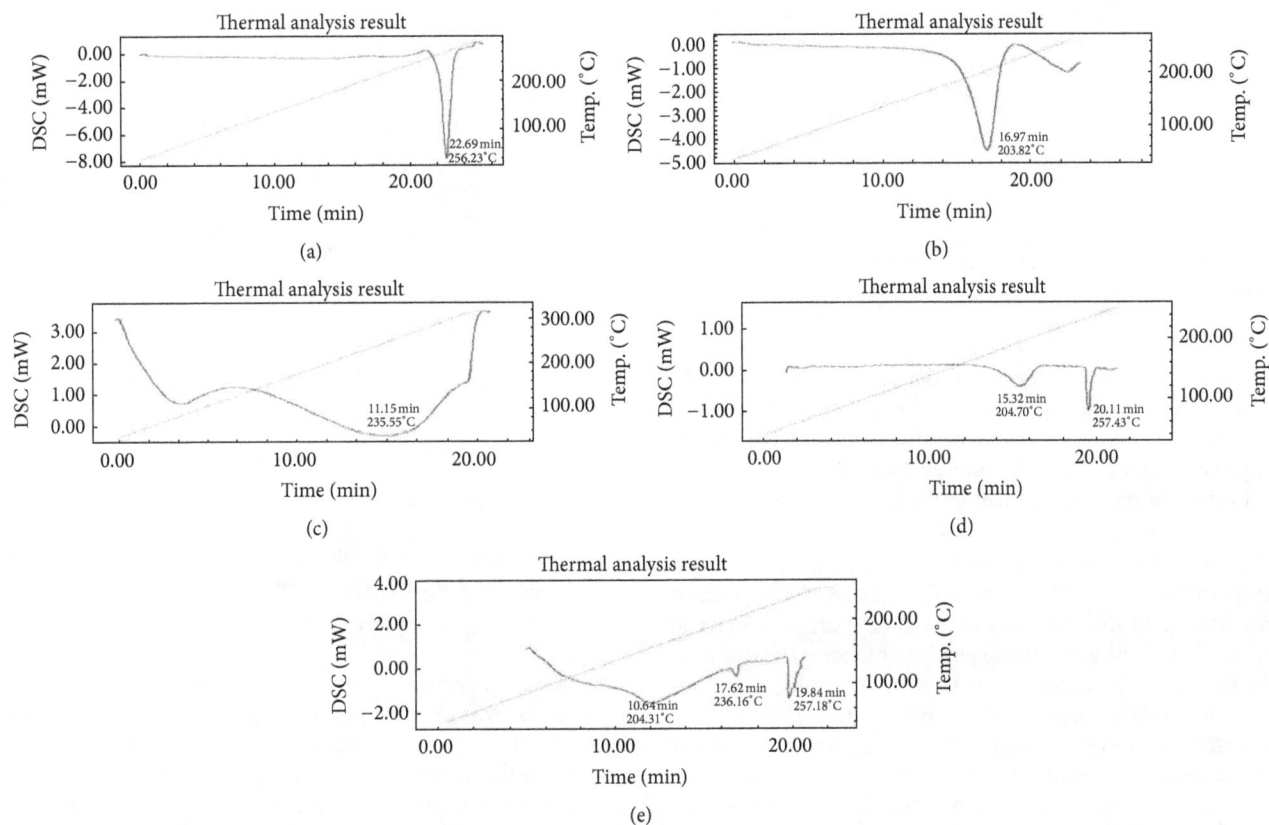

FIGURE 2: Differential scanning colorimetric thermographs of (a) acyclovir, (b) sodium lauryl sulphate, (c) cellulose acetate 398-10, (d) physical mixture of acyclovir and sodium lauryl sulphate, and (e) physical mixture of acyclovir, cellulose acetate 398-10, and sodium lauryl sulphate.

3.2. Drug Excipient Compatibility. The physical mixtures of drug and excipients did not show any physical incompatibility in terms of caking, discoloration, odour, and liquefaction. Investigation of thermal behaviour of the stored samples resulted in differential scanning calorimetric profiles (Figure 2).

The thermogram of pure acyclovir revealed a sharp endothermic peak at 256.23°C (Figure 2(a)) representing the melting point in crystalline state [21]. At 203.82°C, a sharp endothermic peak was recorded for crystalline sodium lauryl sulphate (Figure 2(b)) and a broad endothermic peak at 235°C was observed for cellulose acetate 398-10 that showed broad peak (Figure 2(c)) corresponding to the amorphous nature of cellulose acetate [22]. The endothermic peak of the drug was retained in the physical mixture (Figure 2(d)) of acyclovir and sodium lauryl sulphate (257.43°C and 204.70°C) suggesting compatibility between the two. Furthermore, the peaks retained in the physical mixture of acyclovir with cellulose acetate 398-10 and sodium lauryl were retained at

257.18°C, 236.16°C, and 204.31°C, respectively (Figure 2(e)), with no significant shift. Absence of any peak confirmed the compatibility of the drug with the excipients.

3.3. AMCs of Acyclovir

3.3.1. Appearance and Dimensions. The AMCs were opaque in appearance. The dimensions of the AMC capsule body and cap were significantly similar ($p = 0.00116$) to conventional hard gelatin capsules (Table 3). Furthermore, very low SE values around the mean suggest reproducibility of the method.

3.3.2. Uniformity of Weight. The weight of AMCs varied between 697.60 ± 1.18 and 769.35 ± 0.74 mg (Table 4). The average weight of AMCs formulations was in accordance with IP guidelines [15]. Not more than two of the individual weights deviated from the average weight by more than 5% and none deviated by more than twice that percentage. This indicated uniform filling of powder blend in the capsule body.

TABLE 4: Percent drug content, weight uniformity, and cumulative drug release data of the asymmetric membrane capsules of acyclovir.

Formulation code	Weight[#] (mg) ± S.D.	Drug content[##] (%) ± S.D.	CDR$_{8h}$ (%) ± S.D.
F1	697.60 ± 1.18	97.74 ± 0.55	70.07 ± 1.93
F2	697.80 ± 1.05	98.21 ± 0.60	70.04 ± 1.36
F3	697.95 ± 0.99	98.36 ± 0.54	91.16 ± 0.30
F4	698.40 ± 0.75	92.61 ± 1.44	84.11 ± 0.95
F5	769.10 ± 0.91	94.63 ± 1.08	80.59 ± 1.48
F6	768.75 ± 1.06	93.23 ± 1.33	74.63 ± 0.46
F7	769.35 ± 0.74	99.45 ± 0.37	97.88 ± 0.77
F8	769.00 ± 1.02	96.65 ± 1.51	86.86 ± 1.25
F9[*]	732.95 ± 1.09	97.12 ± 1.08	95.20 ± 0.75

[#]Average of 20 determinations; [##]average of five determinations.
[*]Extra design check point.

3.3.3. Content of Active Ingredient. The drug content of AMCs formulations was in accordance with IP guidelines. In all the eight formulations, the values for drug content closely ranged between 92.61 ± 1.44 and 99.45 ± 0.37% that ensured uniformity of the drug content in the capsules (Table 4).

3.3.4. In Vitro Release. Among the formulations, the lowest drug release was observed from F2 (70.04 ± 1.36%) which may be due to the low level of glycerol (pore former) and sodium lauryl sulphate (osmogen) and high level of cellulose 398-10 (film former), since low level of glycerol leads to the formation of less porous film that did not provide the channels for water to get entered within the system and the low level of osmogen decreased the water influx and the high level of cellulose acetate 398-10 also provided thicker film that hinders the water to get penetrated and initiate the osmogen to exhibit osmotic effect [22]. F6 showed higher release (74.63 ± 0.46%) than F2 due to higher amount of osmogen, which led to increased water influx. F1 with lowest level of cellulose acetate 398-10 showed better release (78.07 ± 1.93%) than F2 and F6. This may be the result of formation of thinner asymmetric film of F1 that did not hinder the penetration of water and initiated the osmogen to exhibit its osmotic effect. F5 had better tendency to release the drug (80.59 ± 1.48%) due to higher amount of osmogen as compared to F1 and F2 since it had lower level of cellulose acetate as compared to F6. F4 exhibited higher drug release (84.11 ± 0.95%) than all the above-discussed formulations because the amount of glycerol was higher in F4 which facilitated the pore formation. F8 had higher amount of glycerol and higher amount of sodium lauryl sulphate thus giving further higher release of 86.86 ± 1.25%, due to the combined effect of increased pores and hence higher water influx. Similarly, highly porous film of F3 made of lower level of cellulose acetate and higher level of glycerol provided channels for water to enter the system and facilitate drug release to the tune of 91.16%. Finally, F7 made with high levels of both glycerol and sodium lauryl sulphate and low level of cellulose acetate 398-10 showed highest drug release of 97.88 ± 0.77%. The superior effect of F7 was a result

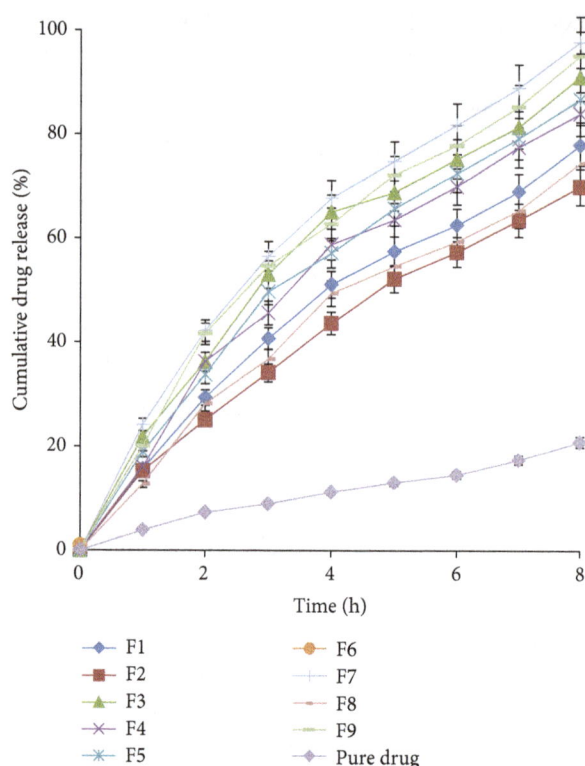

FIGURE 3: *In vitro* release profiles of acyclovir from cellulose acetate AMCs and pure drug in phosphate buffer, pH 4.5.

of formation of a highly porous film that facilitated high water uptake and was selected as the optimized formulation. Most of the resistance to mass transfer is exerted by the dense portion of the membrane while the porous substrate provides mechanical strength and durability to the membrane [23]. The results of effect of formulation variables on drug release are consistent with our previous reports on osmotically regulated systems of poorly water-soluble drugs from AMCs [24, 25].

The drug release pattern of F7 was compared with the release profile of the extra design checkpoint formulation, F9. The % CDR of 95.20 ± 0.75% and a release profile comparable to F7 proved the feasibility of the formulation design. The release profile of the optimized formulation (F7) was also compared with pure drug (PD). Comparative *in vitro* drug release profile of F7 and PD (Figure 3) displayed superior sustenance of drug release from the formulation F7 over the drug packed in AMC in pure state (20.94%) proving that osmotically active formulation has better performance characteristics. The developed formulation has the potential to offer patient compliance by reducing the frequency of administration.

3.4. Kinetics. The *in vitro* release profiles of F1–F8 were modeled and the results showed that the best fit model for most of formulations was the zero-order model. F7 identified as optimized formulation displayed controlled drug release owing to the fact that coefficient of determination (r^2) was 0.9898 (Table 5). Cellulose acetate membranes are reported to

TABLE 5: Kinetic modelling of *in vitro* release data of acyclovir from asymmetric membrane capsules.

Formulation code	r^2			
	Zero-order	First-order	Higuchi	Hixson-Crowell
F1	0.9768	0.5417	0.9667	0.6886
F2	0.9784	0.5501	0.9527	0.6983
F3	0.9845	0.5072	0.9408	0.6520
F4	0.9782	0.5350	0.9507	0.6761
F5	0.9780	0.5407	0.9594	0.6850
F6	0.9719	0.5499	0.9453	0.6853
F7	0.9898	0.4997	0.9448	0.6465
F8	0.9818	0.5270	0.9581	0.6741
F9*	0.9880	0.5141	0.9476	0.6606

*Extra design check point.

generate semipermeable membranes of controlled porosity that have been utilized for osmotic pump-based controlled release systems [26]. The results of the present work are closely correlated with those cited in the literature.

3.5. In Vitro Buoyancy. Visual monitoring of the formulations during *in vitro* drug release studies in phosphate buffer, pH 4.5, exhibited buoyancy till 8 h. The capsule shell was composed of cellulose acetate 398-10 that has a density of about $0.4\,g/cm^3$ [27], which is much lower than the density of gastric fluid ($1.004\,g/cm^3$), and hence assisted floating of the AMC. All the remaining excipients were water-soluble; therefore the floating ability is corelatable to cellulose acetate 398-10. To confirm the buoyant characteristics of the capsule, the true density of the optimized F7 was found to be $0.398\,g/cm^3$ when determined by liquid displacement method using ethanol 95% v/v as the displacement liquid. Accordingly, the AMCs floated in the release media for 8 h, thus affirming the use of AMCs as gastroretentive system for a poorly soluble drug.

3.6. Statistical Analysis. Statistical analysis was carried out using Design Expert software version 9 (Stat-Ease, Inc., Minneapolis, USA). The effect of independent variables can be described by polynomial equation generated by Pareto chart (Figure 4). Bonferroni limit line (*t*-value of effect = 5.06751) and *t*-limit line (*t*-value of effect = 2.77645) were generated by the software. The coefficients having *t*-value between Bonferroni lines were called certainly significant coefficient and, the *t*-value of effect between Bonferroni line and *t*-limit line was called likely to be significant coefficient, while the *t*-values below the *t*-limit line were called statistically insignificant coefficient [13] and were removed from the analysis.

The significant response polynomial equation generated for response parameter (CDR) was

$$\% \text{ CDR}_{8\,h} = 95.87 - 3.45\,(A) + 2.46\,(B) + 0.74\,(C). \quad (2)$$

The equation suggests the negative impact of cellulose acetate (A) on the *in vitro* drug release whereas glycerol (B) and sodium lauryl sulphate (C) contributed positively to the release of acyclovir from AMCs. In order to analyze the

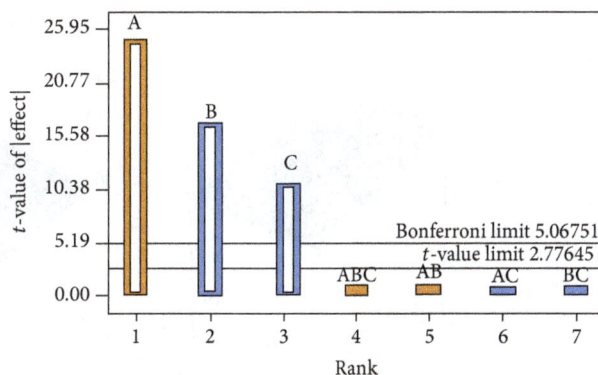

FIGURE 4: Pareto chart depicting significant coefficients above the Bonferroni line for the response cumulative drug release.

effect of varying levels of independent variables the response surface plots were analyzed. The 3D surface response graphs depict the simultaneous influence of independent variables on the dependent variables (Figure 5). On simultaneous increase of level of glycerol and cellulose acetate, the % CDR was increased (Figure 5(a)) whereas simultaneous increase in levels of SLS and glycerol did not influence the % CDR (Figure 5(b)). Whereas a concurrent increase in the levels of cellulose acetate and SLS influenced the CDR characteristically (Figure 5(c)). The positive effect of SLS was counteracted with cellulose acetate levels.

3.7. Interaction between Independent Factors. The possible interactions between independent variables AB, AC, and BC on the response parameter were studied by interaction plots (Figure 6). Graphically, interaction can be visualized by the lack of parallelism in the lines. In our case the parallel lines indicated no interaction between the two variables which indicated independency of variables. Thus the design has maximum efficiency in estimating effects of variables on drug release [28].

3.8. Selection of Optimized Formulation and Validation of Experimental Design. On the basis of the % CDR of 97.88% $\pm$ 0.77, r^2 = 0.9898, and maximum desirability of 0.871 F7 was selected as the optimized formulation. The experimental design was validated by preparing an extra design checkpoint formulation F9 (Table 1) and evaluated. The close resemblance between predicted and experimental value ascertained the validity of experimental design. The predicted value of %CDR$_{8\,h}$ was deduced as 95.87% and the experimental value was 95.20%. Low value (0.70%) of percentage error between predicted and experimental values affirmed the prognostic ability of the design. The *in vitro* release profile of acyclovir from F7 was statistically compared with the theoretical formulation (extra design checkpoint). The statistical significance was tested at $p < 0.05$. The formulation F7 displayed high similarity factor ($f2$) of 74.11.

3.9. Effect of Variables on Drug Release

3.9.1. Effect of Varying Speed. The *in vitro* release profiles at three different speeds 50, 100, and 150 rpm were compared

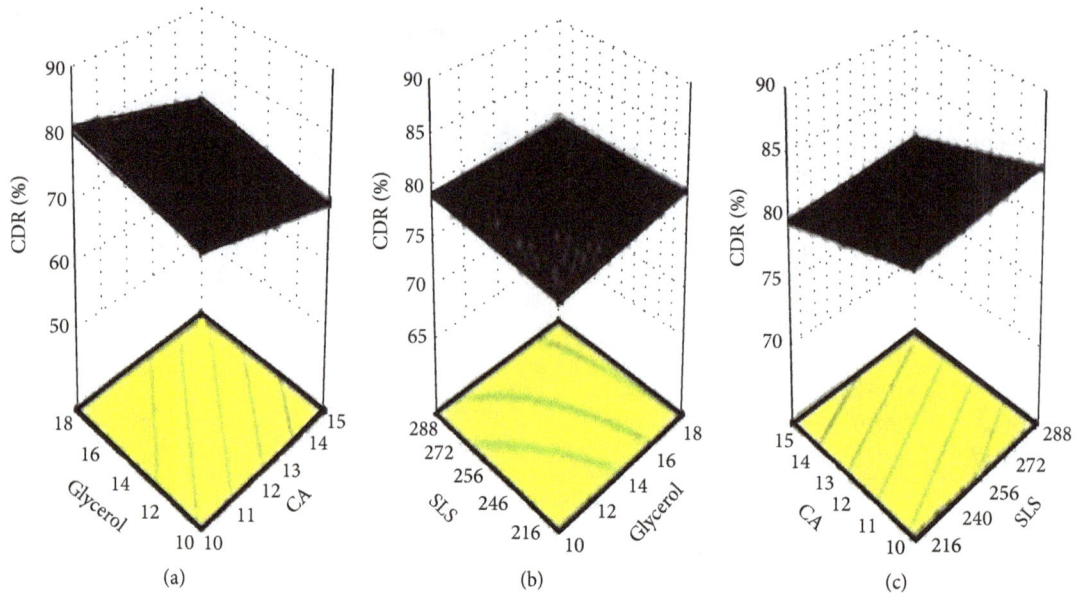

FIGURE 5: 3D response surface plots depicting the simultaneous effect of independent variables on the response (% CDR_{8h}).

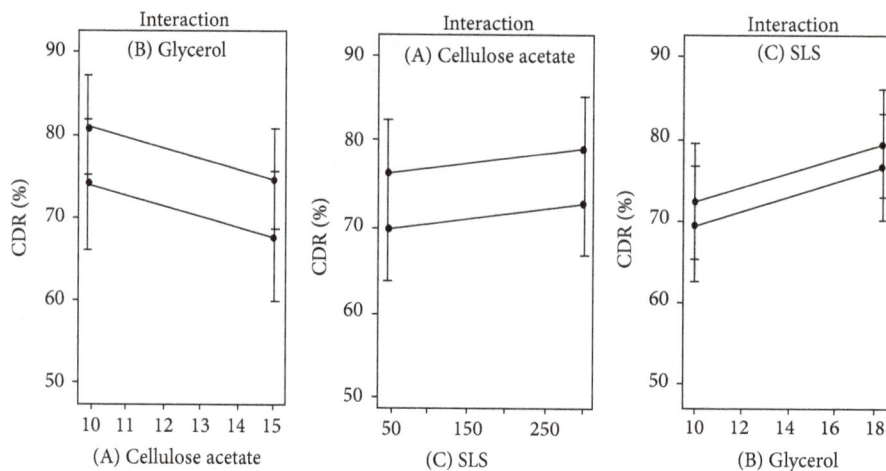

FIGURE 6: Interaction plots of independent variables.

using one-way ANOVA (Figure 7(a)). Rotation rates outside 25 to 150 rpm limits are usually inappropriate because of the inconsistency of hydrodynamics below 25 rpm and because of turbulence above 150 rpm [29]. The calculated F-value (0.02052) was found to be less than tabulated value (1.029), thus suggesting that the variation in agitational intensity did not affect the release profile of the drug from the AMC (Figure 7(a)). This effect describes the fact that the *in vitro* release from the AMCs is independent of the hydrodynamic conditions of the body because of semipermeable nature of the rate controlling membrane and design of delivery orifice used in osmotic systems. Thus, it can be stated that drug release from F7 was due to the controlled entry of dissolution medium across the cellulose acetate barrier and not due to turbulence in dissolution medium.

3.9.2. Effect of Intentional Defect. To establish that the defects in the asymmetric membrane on the release kinetics will not influence the release, intentional defect (pore of 2 mm dia) was introduced in capsular membrane and *in vitro* release studies were accomplished on F7 (Figure 7(b)). The release profile of intentionally defected F7 was compared with optimized F7 using one-way ANOVA. The calculated F-value (0.038) and t-value (0.5905) were found to be less than tabled F-value (4.60) and t-value (2.36). These results demonstrate that release kinetics from AMCs was independent of defects in the membrane, a unique property of osmotic devices [30].

3.9.3. Effect of Varying Osmotic Pressure. The capsules were visually studied for release of dye which indicates its osmotic expulsion from core of capsule. Figure 8 shows four plates,

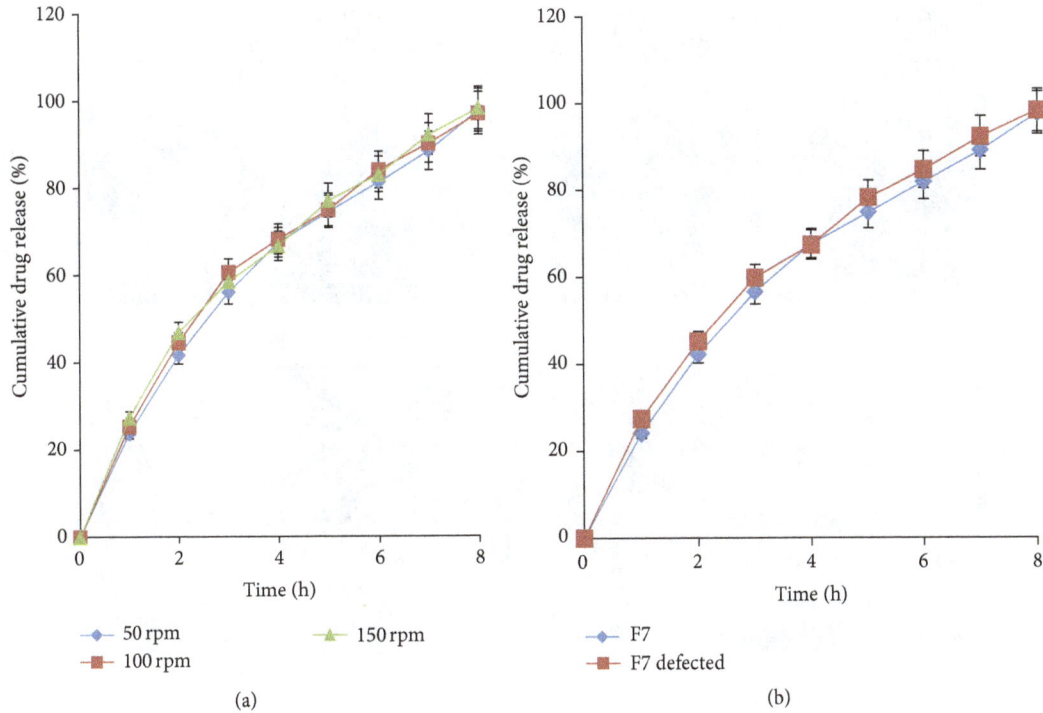

FIGURE 7: (a) Effect of agitational intensity on *in vitro* release and (b) effect of intentional defect on *in vitro* release of acyclovir from cellulose acetate AMC.

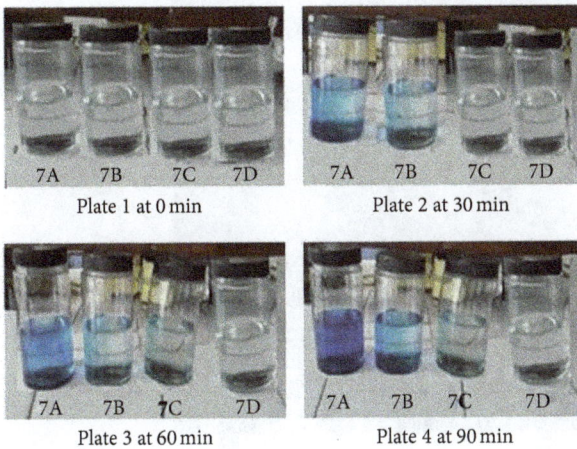

FIGURE 8: Images depicting the effect of varying osmotic conditions of dye release from AMC, plate 1 at 0 min, plate 2 after 30 min, plate 3 after 60 min, and plate 4 after 90 min.

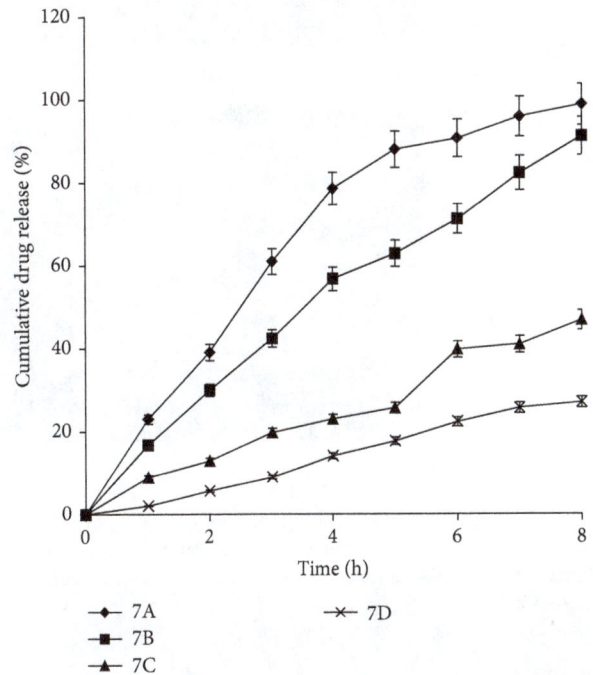

FIGURE 9: 7A: without osmogen inside and outside the capsule (zero osmotic gradient); 7B: 290 mg SLS inside the capsule and 0 mg outside the capsule (perfect osmotic gradient); 7C: 290 mg SLS inside and 145 mg outside the capsule (hypoosmotic); 7D: 290 mg SLS inside and 430 mg in the media (hyperosmotic).

1, 2, 3, and 4, showing release at 0 min, 30 min, 60 min, and 90 min, respectively. F7A showed solubility dependent release of methylene blue from the AMCs that intensified with time (plates 1–4). F7B comprising both the dye and the osmotic agent in the AMC showed gradual release suggesting an osmotic pressure gradient across the capsule membrane.

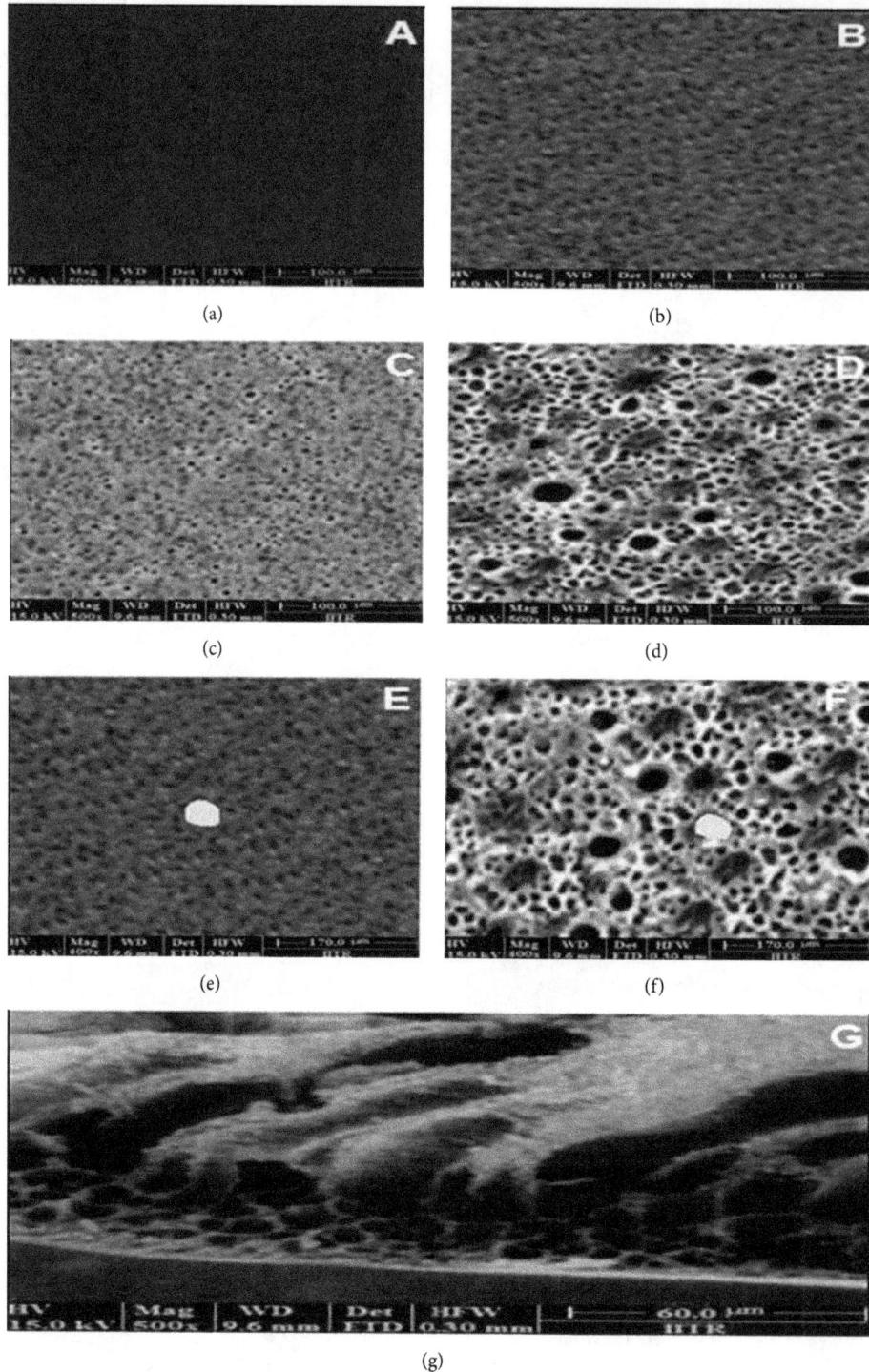

FIGURE 10: SEM of asymmetric membrane depicting (a) outer dense region and (b) inner porous region before drug release (original magnification at 500x), (c) outer dense region and (d) inner porous region after drug release (original magnification at 500x), (e) inner surface with intentional defect before dissolution and (f) inner surface with intentional defect after dissolution (400x), and (g) transverse section (500x).

The dye release was initiated after 30 min of immersion of the AMC in the solution due to the gradual build-up of osmotic gradient that facilitated the release of the dye in a sustained manner. F7C and F7D were kept in hypoosmotic and hyperosmotic conditions, respectively, to demonstrate that the principle mechanism of drug delivery was the property of osmogen incorporated into the formulation. As the osmotic gradient was reduced, delayed methylene blue release was seen in F7C. No color was observed for F7D in all the plates indicating zero release of methylene blue from the AMC

TABLE 6: Stability data cellulose acetate AMCs of acyclovir for 3 months.

Parameter	Time interval (months)			
	0	1	2	3
Appearance	White	White	White	White
Surface	Smooth	Smooth	Smooth	Smooth
Drug content (%)	99.45	99.14	98.83	98.52

under hyperosmotic conditions conforming to osmotic gradient as essential requirement for drug release. This confirmed that the mechanism of drug release from the developed AMCs was solely dependent on the osmotic pressure gradient across the AMCs and the surrounding environment drug release is inversely proportional to the osmotic pressure. Quantitative assessment of varying the osmotic pressure on the drug release was also analyzed. Figure 9 displays that the drug release is inversely proportional to the osmotic pressure. It is evident that the drug release decreased as the osmotic pressure of the release media increased. The release profiles, when compared using one-way ANOVA, led to a calculated F-value of 2.91, which was more than the tabulated F-value of 2.78. This confirmed that the mechanism of drug release from the developed AMC was solely dependent on the osmotic pressure gradient across the asymmetric membrane.

3.10. Scanning Electron Microscopy (SEM). The SEM images of asymmetric membrane obtained before dissolution clearly indicated an outer, dense, nonporous, and smooth membranous structure of cellulose acetate (Figure 10(a)) at 500x, while the inner surface was porous and rough (Figure 10(b)). Numerous pores on the outer surface of membrane (Figure 10(c)) and large pores (0.73 μm in diameter) in the inner layer of membrane (Figure 10(d)) were clearly seen. The pore enlargement is attributed to the dissolution of glycerol into the aqueous media during drug release. With *in vitro* release study the permselectivity of the outer membrane also increased. The original concept was to form an asymmetric membrane film consisting of a thick porous region to provide mechanical support and a thin dense region to provide permselectivity. Thus, a significant factor in determining the permeability of a given membrane is the porous nature of the membrane. The membrane structure is controlled by both the formulation and processing variables [23]. Intentionally defected asymmetric membrane showed a 2 mm hole (Figure 10(e)) which remained almost of the same size even after 8 h of dissolution (Figure 10(f)). Transversally sectioned micrograph of the capsule shell (Figure 10(g)) clearly shows the asymmetric nature of membrane with an outer thin dense region supported by an inner porous substructure with deep micropores.

3.11. Stability. The result showed that the formulation was stable at 40 ± 2.0°C/75 ± 5% RH. No change in the capsule texture and color was seen. The percent drug content profile showed comparable results, thus suggesting that there was no stability issue for AMCs (Table 6). The *in vitro* drug release in phosphate buffer, pH 4.5, showed insignificant changes in

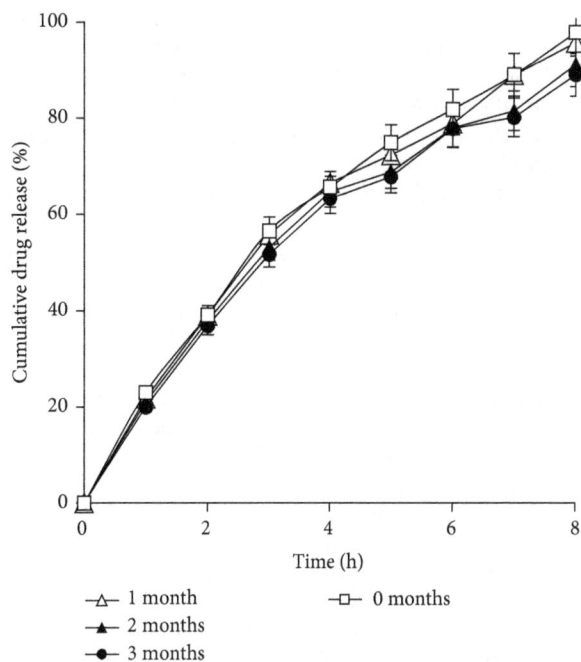

FIGURE 11: *In vitro* drug release profiles of fresh and aged F7 formulation.

the release profiles ($p > 0.05$), $f2 > 85$ confirming stability in the release of drug from AMCs even after storage (Figure 11).

4. Conclusion

The cellulose acetate AMCs of acyclovir were successfully developed that showed osmotically driven controlled release of the drug, independent of the agitational intensity and intentional defect on the membrane. Osmotic gradient was the primary mechanism for the release of poorly water-soluble drug acyclovir from the buoyant AMC. The levels of cellulose acetate influenced the performance characteristics of the AMCs but did not influence the buoyancy. Designing a system that can be retained at the site of absorption may resolve the poor permeability issues but this needs to be proved by experimental studies *in vivo*. However, the generated system has the potential to improve patient compliance by sustenance of drug release and to improve bioavailability by zero-order release of the drug.

Conflict of Interests

The authors declare that there is no conflict of interests regarding the publication of this paper.

References

[1] S. M. Herbig, J. R. Cardinal, R. W. Korsmeyer, and K. L. Smith, "Asymmetric-membrane tablet coatings for osmotic drug delivery," *Journal of Controlled Release*, vol. 35, no. 2-3, pp. 127–136, 1995.

[2] C.-Y. Wang, H.-O. Ho, L.-H. Lin, Y.-K. Lin, and M.-T. Sheu, "Asymmetric membrane capsules for delivery of poorly water-soluble drugs by osmotic effects," *International Journal of Pharmaceutics*, vol. 297, no. 1-2, pp. 89–97, 2005.

[3] A. G. Thombre, A. R. DeNoto, and D. C. Gibbes, "Delivery of glipizide from asymmetric membrane capsules using encapsulated excipients," *Journal of Controlled Release*, vol. 60, no. 2-3, pp. 333–341, 1999.

[4] M. S. Chauhan, A. Kumar, and K. Pathak, "Osmotically regulated floating asymmetric membrane capsule for controlled site-specific delivery of ranitidine hydrochloride: optimization by central composite design," *AAPS PharmSciTech*, vol. 13, no. 4, pp. 1492–1501, 2012.

[5] P. K. Choudhury, M. S. Ranawat, M. K. Pillai, and C. S. Chauhan, "Asymmetric membrane capsule for osmotic delivery of flurbiprofen," *Acta Pharmaceutica*, vol. 57, no. 3, pp. 343–350, 2007.

[6] A. Garg, M. Gupta, and H. N. Bhargava, "Effect of formulation parameters on the release characteristics of propranolol from asymmetric membrane coated tablets," *European Journal of Pharmaceutics and Biopharmaceutics*, vol. 67, no. 3, pp. 725–731, 2007.

[7] K. C. Waterman, G. S. Goeken, S. Konagurthu et al., "Osmotic capsules: a universal oral, controlled-release drug delivery dosage form," *Journal of Controlled Release*, vol. 152, no. 2, pp. 264–269, 2011.

[8] S. Dhaliwal, S. Jain, H. P. Singh, and A. K. Tiwary, "Osmotic capsules: a universal oral, controlled-release drug delivery dosage form," *The AAPS Journal*, vol. 10, pp. 322–330, 2008.

[9] A. Kristl, S. Srčič, F. Vrečer, B. Šuštar, and D. Vojnovic, "Polymorphism and pseudopolymorphism: influencing the dissolution properties of the guanine derivative acyclovir," *International Journal of Pharmaceutics*, vol. 139, no. 1-2, pp. 231–235, 1996.

[10] *AHFS Drug Information*, American Society of Hospital Pharmacists, Bethesda, Md, USA, 2004.

[11] C. Fletcher and B. Bean, "Evaluation of oral acyclovir therapy," *Drug Intelligence and Clinical Pharmacy*, vol. 19, no. 7-8, pp. 518–524, 1985.

[12] E. A. Rawlins, *Bentley's Textbook of Pharmaceutics*, Bailliere Tindall, London, UK, 2004.

[13] S. Bolton, *Pharmaceutical Statistics: Practical and Clinical Application*, Marcel Dekker, New York, NY, USA, 1990.

[14] R. Dev, A. Kumar, and K. Pathak, "Solubility-modulated asymmetric membrane tablets of triprolidine hydrochloride: statistical optimization and evaluation," *AAPS PharmSciTech*, vol. 13, no. 1, pp. 174–183, 2012.

[15] *Indian Pharmacopoeia, Government of India, Ministry of Health & Family Welfare*, vol. 2, Controller of Publication, New Delhi, India, 2007.

[16] Stability Testing of New Drug Substances and Products Q1A-Q1F, December 2014, http://www.ich.org/products/guidelines/quality/quality-single/article/stability-testing-of-new-drug-substances-and-products.html.

[17] A. Kristl, "Estimation of aqueous solubility for some guanine derivatives using partition coefficient and melting temperature," *Journal of Pharmaceutical Sciences*, vol. 88, no. 1, pp. 109–110, 1999.

[18] J. Luengo, T. Aránguiz, J. Sepúlveda, L. Hernández, and C. Von Plessing, "Preliminary pharmacokinetic study of different preparations of acyclovir with β-cyclodextrin," *Journal of Pharmaceutical Sciences*, vol. 91, no. 12, pp. 2593–2598, 2002.

[19] A. Kumar, A. K. Philip, and K. Pathak, "Asymmetric membrane capsules of phenylephrine hydrochloride: an osmotically controlled drug delivery system," *Current Drug Delivery*, vol. 8, no. 5, pp. 474–482, 2011.

[20] R. A. Keraliya, C. Patel, P. Patel et al., "Osmotic drug delivery system as a part of modified release dosage form," *ISRN Pharmaceutics*, vol. 2012, Article ID 528079, 9 pages, 2012.

[21] S. Budavari, *The Merck Index: An Encyclopedia of Chemicals, Drugs and Biological*, Merck Research Laboratories, Division of Merck and Co, 12th edition, 1996.

[22] L. Liu, G. Khang, J. M. Rhee, and H. B. Lee, "Preparation and characterization of cellulose acetate membrane for monolithic osmotic tablet," *Korea Polymer Journal*, vol. 7, no. 5, pp. 289–297, 1999.

[23] A. K. Philip and K. Pathak, "Osmotic flow through asymmetric membrane: a means for controlled delivery of drugs with varying solubility," *AAPS PharmSciTech*, vol. 7, no. 3, article 56, 2006.

[24] A. K. Philip and K. Pathak, "In situ-formed asymmetric membrane capsule for osmotic release of poorly water-soluble drug," *PDA Journal of Pharmaceutical Science and Technology*, vol. 61, no. 1, pp. 24–36, 2007.

[25] A. K. Philip, K. Pathak, and P. Shakya, "Asymmetric membrane in membrane capsules: a means for achieving delayed and osmotic flow of cefadroxil," *European Journal of Pharmaceutics and Biopharmaceutics*, vol. 69, no. 2, pp. 658–666, 2008.

[26] S. N. Makhija and P. R. Vavia, "Controlled porosity osmotic pump-based controlled release systems of pseudoephedrine: I. Cellulose acetate as a semipermeable membrane," *Journal of Controlled Release*, vol. 89, no. 1, pp. 5–18, 2003.

[27] R. C. Rowe, P. J. Shesky, and S. C. Owens, *Handbook of Pharmaceutical Excipients*, Pharmaceutical Press, London, UK, 5th edition, 2006.

[28] M. K. Shah and K. Pathak, "Development and statistical optimization of solid lipid nanoparticles of simvastatin by using 2^3 full-factorial design," *AAPS PharmSciTech*, vol. 11, no. 2, pp. 489–496, 2010.

[29] *United States Pharmacopoeia*, Asian Edition, US Pharmacopeial Convention, Rockville, Md, USA, 2004.

[30] L. W. Donald, *Handbook of Pharmaceutical Controlled Release Technology*, Marcel Dekker, New York, NY, USA, 2000.

18

Novel Concepts for Drug Hypersensitivity Based on the Use of Long-Time Scale Molecular Dynamic Simulation

Takahiro Murai,[1] Norihito Kawashita,[1,2] Yu-Shi Tian,[3] and Tatsuya Takagi[1,2]

[1]*Graduate School of Pharmaceutical Sciences, Osaka University, 1-6 Yamadaoka, Suita, Osaka 565-0871, Japan*
[2]*Research Institute for Microbial Diseases, Osaka University, 3-1 Yamadaoka, Suita, Osaka 565-0871, Japan*
[3]*Graduate School of Information Science and Technology, Osaka University, 1-5 Yamadaoka, Suita, Osaka 565-0871, Japan*

Correspondence should be addressed to Tatsuya Takagi; ttakagi@phs.osaka-u.ac.jp

Academic Editor: Giuseppina De Simone

The discovery that several drug hypersensitivity reactions (DHRs) are associated with specific human leukocyte antigen (HLA) alleles has attracted increasing research interest. However, the underlying mechanisms of these HLA-induced DHRs remain unclear, especially for drug-induced immediate activation of T-cell clones (TCCs). Recently, a novel hypothesis involving partial detachment between self-peptide(s) and the HLA molecule (altered peptide-HLA (pHLA) model) has been proposed to explain these phenomena. In order to clarify this hypothesis, we performed long-timescale molecular dynamics (MD) simulations. We focused on HLA-B∗57:01-restricted abacavir hypersensitivity reactions (AHRs), one of the most famous DHRs. One of the simulation results showed that this altered-pHLA model might be driven by an increase in the distance not only between HLA and self-peptides but also between the α_1 and α_2 helices of HLA. Our findings provide novel insights into abacavir-induced immediate activation of TCCs and these findings might also be applied to other DHRs, such as HLA-B∗58:01-restricted allopurinol hypersensitivity reactions.

1. Introduction

Administration of particular drugs sometimes causes drug hypersensitivity reactions (DHRs). Abacavir, a nucleoside reverse transcriptase inhibitor, plays an important role in anti-HIV regimens worldwide as one of the recommended antiretroviral drugs. However, due to its potential to cause DHRs, specifically named abacavir hypersensitivity reactions (AHRs), abacavir's safety profile has been questioned especially for use in children [1, 2]. A relationship between AHRs and certain alleles of human leukocyte antigen (HLA) has been reported. After administration of abacavir, AHRs occur in approximately 5 to 8% individuals carrying an HLA-B∗57:01 allele, which is a higher rate than the observed in people carrying other alleles [3–5].

Although many efforts have been made to investigate the mechanism by which AHRs occur, a complete explanation has not yet been obtained. According to previous studies, three distinct models have been reported: the hapten/prohapten model, the pharmacological interaction

(p-i) model, and the altered repertoire model [6, 7]. Recent studies revealed that abacavir forms noncovalent bonds with HLA-B∗57:01. This binding may change the repertoire of the HLA-B∗57:01-binding peptides and trigger "foreign antigen recognition" by T-cells [8–10]; these findings supported the third model. However, none of the current three models can explain the fact that about 40 percent of AHRs derived from T-cell clones react within less than 15 minutes of abacavir treatment [11, 12]. All three current models suggest that a much longer reaction time should be necessary.

More recently, a hypothesis referred to as the altered peptide-HLA (pHLA) model has been proposed to explain this phenotype; a partial detachment between the HLA molecule and self-peptide(s) may exist [13]. This hypothesis implies that the drug binds not only to the HLA molecule in the endoplasmic reticulum (ER) of the antigen-presenting cell but also to pHLA complexes on the cell surface. The latter event could be a subsequent result of the dissociation between the peptide and the HLA, creating a pocket where the drug enters (Figure 1). The immediate activation of TCCs can be

TABLE 1: Self-peptides used for this study.

Peptides	Protein name (human)
LSSPVTKSF (LF9) (PDB ID: 3VH8)	Ig kappa chain C region
IAVKVNHSY (IY9)	E3 SUMO-protein ligase PIAS4
VAKVCQYTF (VF9)	NADH dehydrogenase [ubiquinone] 1 alpha subcomplex subunit 11
VTYKNVPNW (VW9)	GTF-binding nuclear protein Ran

Protein name represents the proteins bound to HLA before processing into the self-peptides [8]. LF9 is the peptide derived from the crystal structure and obtained from the Protein Data Bank (PDB) [14].

well explained by this hypothesis, because, instead of passing through the ER, a direct conformational change triggered by interaction of abacavir with pHLA could shorten the reaction time.

In order to clarify this hypothesis, we performed molecular dynamics (MD) simulations using the structure of the pHLA complex. One of the simulation results implied that certain self-peptides are partially dissociated from HLA-B∗57:01, enabling accommodation of abacavir and thereby stabilizing the peptide-binding cleft. Our findings provide novel insights into abacavir-induced immediate activation of TCCs.

2. Materials and Methods

2.1. Modeling of pHLA Complexes. The models of three self-peptides, which were shown to bind to HLA-B∗57:01 before and after abacavir treatment [8], were constructed using the LSSPVTKSF (LF9) peptide (Protein Data Bank (PDB) ID: 3VH8) as a template [14] (Table 1). Subsequently, the self-peptides were docked with the HLA-B∗57:01 (PDB ID: 3VH8) to model pHLA complexes *in situ*. During this docking procedure, the ASEDock program [15] was used; flexibility of the ligand atoms was allowed and the backbone atoms of the receptors were tethered. Following the docking scores (U_dock), the top-scoring pose of each docking was collected. A series of these models were performed using MOE 2013.08 software [16].

2.2. MD Simulations. MD simulations were performed using the GROMACS 5.0.4 software package 1 and the OPLS-AA force field [17]. The four structures of pHLA (including the crystal structure (PDB ID: 3VH8)) were soaked using the TIP3P water model. A dodecahedral box was selected with a minimum distance of 1.4 nm between the edges of the protein and the box, and each of the systems was neutralized by adding counter ions at physiological concentrations (0.15 M). The energy of each system was minimized by using the steepest descent algorithm for 100 ps. The ν-rescale and Parrinello-Rahman methods were used to control temperature and pressure, respectively. The LINCS algorithm was used to constrain all bond lengths. The particle mesh Ewald (PME) method was used to compute long-range electrostatics. Finally, 500 ns MD simulations of all four complexes were performed at 310 K

using the TSUBAME 2.5 supercomputer at Tokyo Institute of Technology [18].

3. Results

3.1. The Root Mean Square Deviation (RMSD) Values for Self-Peptides Complexed with HLA-B∗57:01 during MD Simulations. Conformational changes of the four investigated self-peptides bound to HLA-B∗57:01 were calculated by RMSD during the period of the MD simulations. For these peptides, VF9 and IY9 peptides showed larger conformational changes after 100 ns with peptide RMSD values of about 2 to 3 Å (Figure 2(a)). More detailed conformational changes of the four peptides were analyzed by calculating the RMSD per residue over a 500 ns simulation period (Figure 2(b)). For VF9 and IY9 peptides, the C-terminal residues (residues 7–9), which are located in the abacavir binding site, showed larger conformational changes with RMSD values of about 2 to 3 Å.

3.2. The Distance between the Specific Residues of Self-Peptides and Those of HLA-B∗57:01. In normal states, self-peptides bind to the peptide-binding groove of HLA-B∗57:01 and there is no enough space for a drug to bind. According to the novel hypothesis, some self-peptides dissociate from the HLA, enabling accommodation of certain drugs. To confirm the partial detachment between the HLA molecule and self-peptides, distances between the specific residues of self-peptides and those of HLA-B∗57:01 which are implicated in abacavir binding were calculated during the MD simulation. The residues examined were (1) P7- (peptide residue 7-) Asp114, (2) P7-Ser116, and (3) P9-Ser116 (Figure 3(a)). For these pHLA complexes, only the IY9 peptide-HLA-B∗57:01 complex resulted in larger distances compared with the initial distances (Figure 3(b)). The distances increased gradually after 100 ns and showed peak values around 200 ns (15.7 Å, 13.3 Å, and 18.1 Å, resp.), compared with their initial distances (4.0 Å, 6.8 Å, and 4.4 Å, resp.). Interestingly, the distance of P7-Ser116 after 200 ns (4.7 Å at 500 ns) and that of P9-Ser116 after 400 ns decreased (8.3 Å at 500 ns). For the VF9 peptide-HLA-B∗57:01 complex, while the distances of P9-Ser116 became greater after 100 ns, the others stayed constant during the MD simulation. These results imply that the IY9 peptide is likely to dissociate from HLA.

3.3. The Distance between HLA-B∗57:01 α_1 and α_2 Helices Complexed with the IY9 Peptide Increased during MD Simulation. To further confirm the partial detachment between self-peptides and HLA-B∗57:01, we visualized the structures of IY9-HLA-B∗57:01 complexes at 0, 200, and 400 ns (Figure 4(a)). These snapshots also revealed that the IY9 peptide was dissociated from the HLA-B∗57:01. Surprisingly, at 200 ns and 400 ns, the distance between the HLA-B∗57:01 α_1 and α_2 helices, which enable the peptides to be accommodated and presented, became larger. To confirm the more detailed characteristics, the five representative distances between α_1 and α_2 helices of the HLA-B∗57:01, (1) Y59-R170, (2) N66-L163, (3) S70-E155, (4) Y74-A150, and (5) I80-K146, were calculated (Figure 4(b)). As expected, the

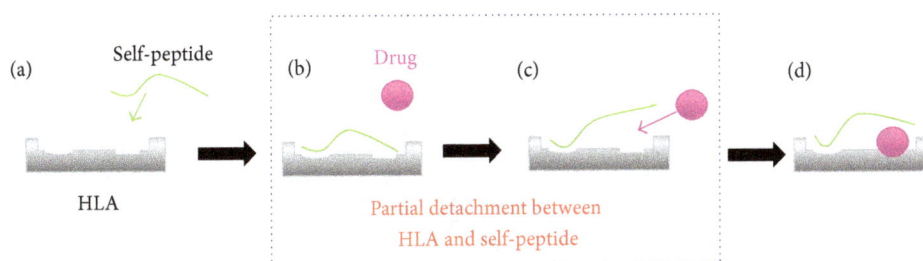

FIGURE 1: Schematic representation of the altered-pHLA model. First, self-peptides bind to HLA molecules in an HLA allele-dependent manner, forming the peptide-HLA complexes (a). Second, some peptide-HLA complexes undergo the partial detachments (b), enabling the accommodation of certain drugs into the space (c). Finally, peptide-drug-HLA complexes adopt stable conformations, leading to recognition by T-cells (d).

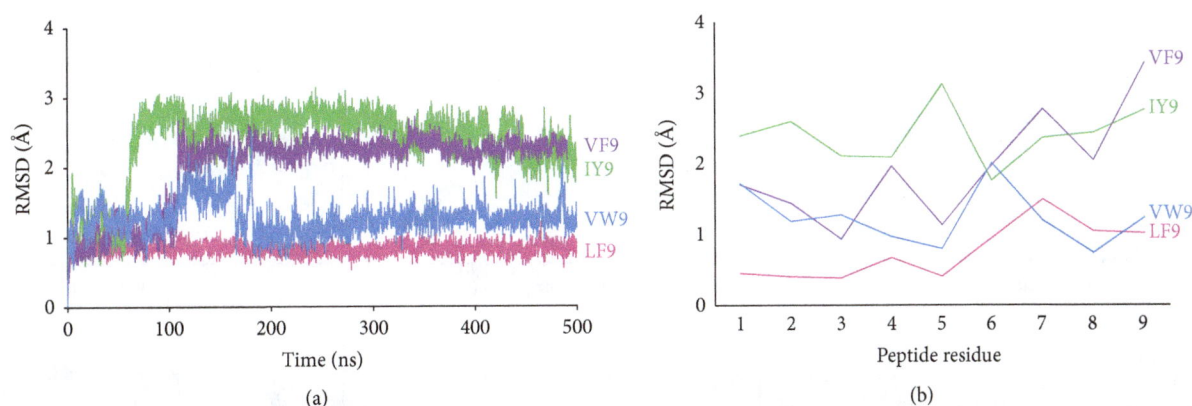

FIGURE 2: The RMSD values for the self-peptides. (a) RMSD values were calculated for Cα atoms of the peptide during the MD simulations. (b) The RMSD values were calculated per residue for the Cα atoms and averaged over 500 ns. Peptides VF9, IY9, VW9, and LF9 are shown in purple, green, blue, and magenta, respectively.

distances between (4) Y74-A150 and (5) I80-K146, which are both located near the abacavir binding site, became larger in comparison with their initial distances (17.1 Å (0 ns) and 19.2 Å (500 ns) for Y74-A150 and 12.7 Å (0 ns) and 17.5 Å (500 ns) for I80-K146) (Figure 4(c)). Together, these results suggested that increasing the distance between not only HLA and self-peptides but also HLA α_1 and α_2 helices is necessary for accommodation of abacavir in the peptide-binding cleft.

4. Discussion

Although DHRs are important problems that need to be resolved for both healthcare and pharmaceutical manufacturing, the mechanisms by which DHRs develop remain unclear. In this study, we performed MD simulations to validate a recently hypothesized mechanism (the altered-pHLA model) by which one of the most well-known DHRs, AHR, results in immediate activation of TCCs. For late hypersensitivity reactions of abacavir, Illing and her coworkers showed that abacavir binds specifically to HLA-B∗57:01, other than HLA-B∗57:03 or HLA-B∗58:01, using antigen-presenting cells [10]. However, to our knowledge, it is difficult to create in vitro assays to visualize a partial detachment of bounded peptide. Therefore, we carried out MD simulations in the current study. As it is well known, MD simulations are numerical

representations of Newton's equations of motion [19]. This technique enables us to simulate the dynamics of peptides bound to HLAs, which is difficult to accomplish in in vitro or in vivo experiments. Increasing simulation times are being used for MD simulation studies [20, 21], and at least 10 ns to 400 ns MD simulation lengths are needed to monitor the dynamics of pHLA [22].

We performed 500 ns MD simulations before and after abacavir binding for the four pHLA complexes whose peptides were known to bind to HLA-B∗57:01. The calculated dynamics of these peptides with the RMSD values imply that certain peptides dissociated from the HLA. However, a previous study using other pHLA complexes showed that the peptide residues dissociated from the HLA-B∗27 with the RMSD values of up to 10.0 Å during 400 ns MD simulations [23]. Considering these results, our simulation results show much lower RMSD values (about 2 to 3 Å). Therefore, to confirm sufficient partial detachment between HLA and self-peptides for the drug to be accommodated, we measured the distances between the peptide and HLA residues near the abacavir binding site during MD simulations. For the IY9 peptide-HLA-B∗57:01 complex, the distances became larger up to 200 ns and then decreased gradually. The distances at 200 ns (15.7 Å (p7-Asp114), 13.3 Å (p7-Ser116), and 18.1 Å (p7-Ser116)) are large enough for the drug to be accommodated,

(a)

(b)

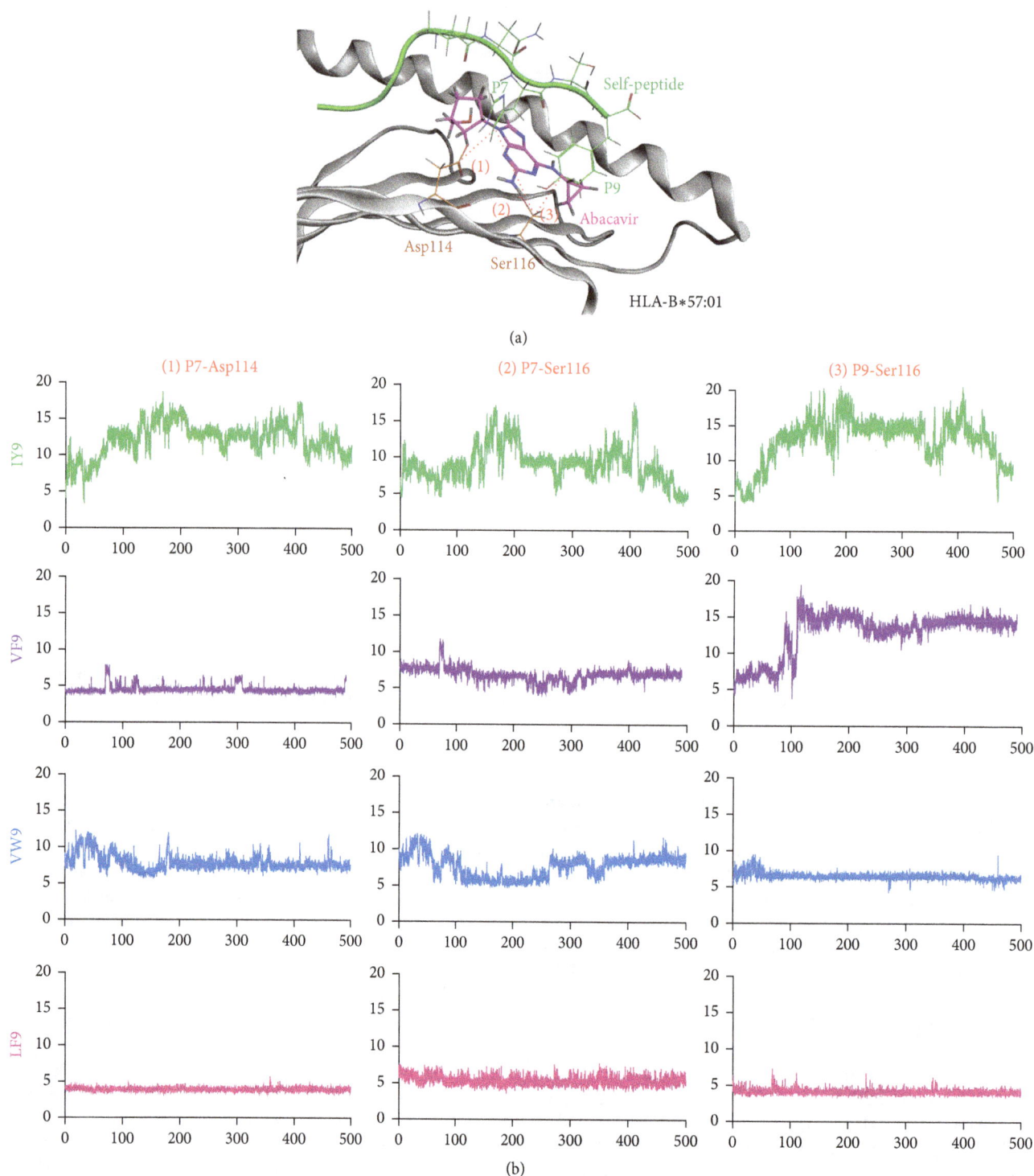

FIGURE 3: The distances between self-peptides and HLA-B*57:01. (a) Measurements of the distances between the HLA molecule and self-peptides. The distances between the specific residues of self-peptides and those of HLA-B*57:01 were measured during the MD simulations: (1) P7-Asp114, (2) P7-Ser116, and (3) P9-Ser116. HLA-B*57:01 is shown in gray, and Asp114 and Ser 116, the HLA residues implicated in abacavir binding, are shown in orange. The self-peptide (IY9 peptide is shown here) and abacavir are shown in green and magenta, respectively. (b) The distance between self-peptides and HLA-B*57:01. Horizontal and vertical axes of each graph represent time (ns) and RMSD values (Å), respectively. Color representation is the same as in (a).

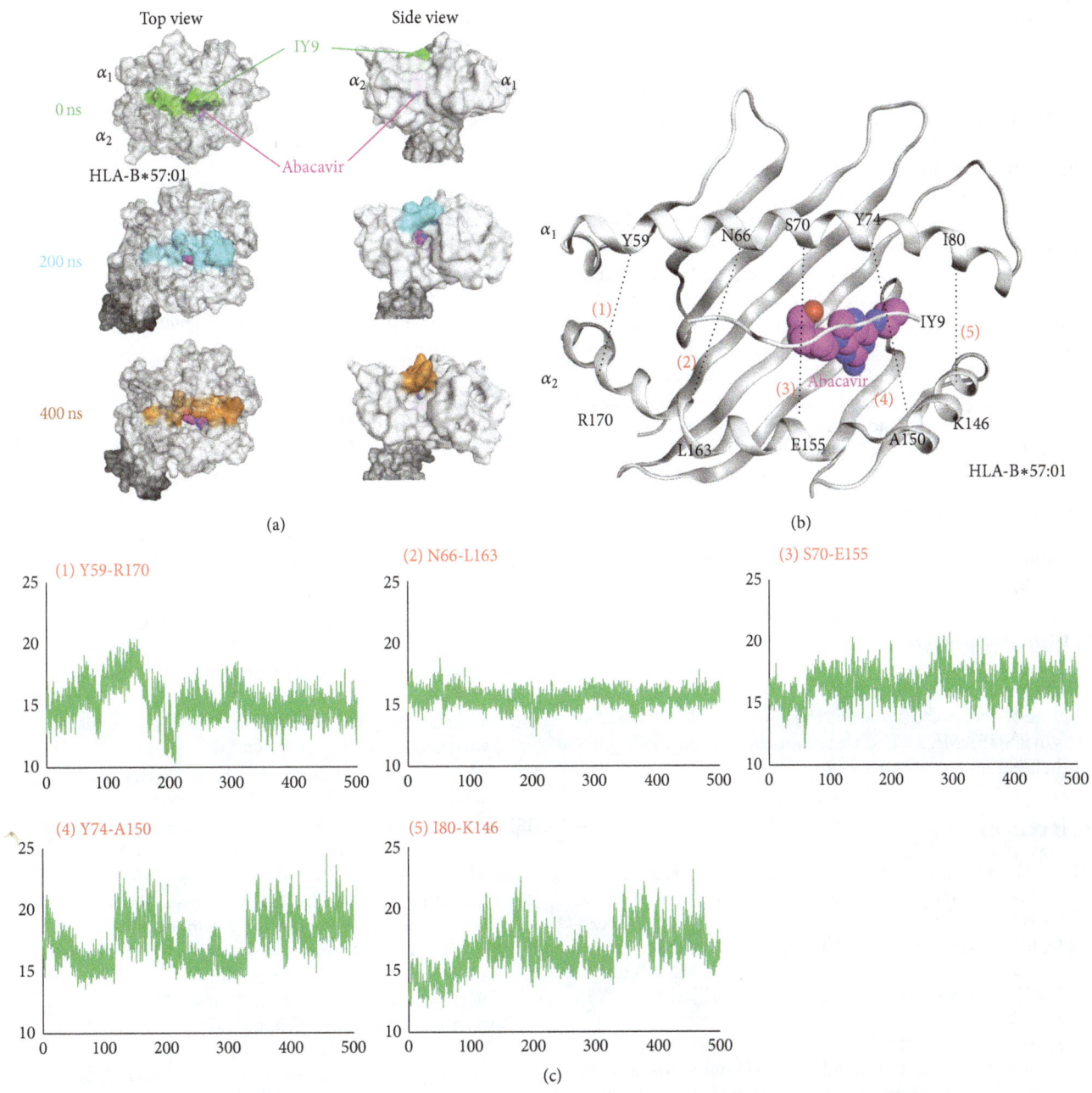

FIGURE 4: The distance between HLA-B*57:01 α_1 and α_2 helices complexed with IY9 peptide became larger during MD simulation. (a) Top view (left) and side view (right) of IY9-HLA-B*57:01 structures at 0, 200, and 400 ns. Abacavir was superposed with the structures of IY9-HLA-B*57:01 complexes during the MD simulation. The IY9 peptide at 0, 200, and 400 ns is shown in green, cyan, and orange, respectively. HLA-B*57:01 and the abacavir binding site are shown in gray and magenta, respectively. (b) Measurements of the distance between α_1 and α_2 helices of HLA-B*57:01. IY9 peptide and HLA-B*57:01 are shown in gray, and a superposed abacavir is shown in magenta. (c) The distance between α_1 and α_2 helices in the IY9-HLA-B*57:01 complex. Horizontal and vertical axes of each graph represent time (ns) and RMSD values (Å), respectively.

because the minimum distances calculated from the crystal structures of abacavir-peptide-HLA complexes (PDB ID: 3UPR) are 7.6 Å, 9.3 Å, and 7.2 Å, respectively. After 200 ns, the distances decreased over time, especially for p7-Ser116 and p9-Ser116, suggesting that the peptide directs the attachment to the HLA.

The snapshots obtained from MD simulations of the IY9 peptide-HLA-B*57:01 complex showed an enlarged distance not only between HLA and self-peptides but also between the α_1 and α_2 helices of HLA. The distances between HLA α_1 and α_2 helices, in particular those between residues Y74-A150 and I80-K146, became larger after 100 ns. However, the closure of these α_1 and α_2 helices was not confirmed during the period of our MD simulations. Performing MD simulations with a much longer timescale could be necessary for elucidating the complete mechanisms of the altered-pHLA model.

5. Conclusions

In this study, we performed MD simulations to elucidate the altered-pHLA model, which is a relatively new hypothesis to explain drug-induced immediate activation of TCCs, and concluded that one of our MD simulation results does indeed support this hypothesis. To our knowledge, this study is the first to test this hypothesis and support its validity. However, the results obtained from this study could not explain the detailed mechanisms by which only the IY9 peptide dissociates from HLA-B*57:01. Future studies will be required to elucidate the detailed characteristics, such as the peptide specificity and the mechanisms by which this peptide dissociates from the HLA. Our findings might also be applied to other DHRs, such as flucloxacillin- and allopurinol-induced DHRs [24]. Such long-term MD simulations could contribute to the identification of DHRs and various other mechanisms about pHLA.

Competing Interests

The authors declare that there is no conflict of interests regarding the publication of this paper.

Acknowledgments

The authors are grateful to TSUBAME group at the Tokyo Institute of Technology who were very helpful for the calculations in TSUBAME 2.5 and we are indebted to our colleagues for their valuable assistance.

References

[1] V. Musiime and A. J. Prendergast, "Can abacavir be used safely in children without HLA testing?" *The Lancet HIV*, vol. 3, no. 2, pp. e58–e59, 2016.

[2] J. Chakravarty, S. Sharma, A. Johri, A. Chourasia, and S. Sundar, "Clinical abacavir hypersensitivity reaction among children in India," *The Indian Journal of Pediatrics*, vol. 83, no. 8, pp. 855–858, 2016.

[3] S. Mallal, D. Nolan, C. Witt et al., "Association between presence of HLA-B*5701, HLA-DR7, and HLA-DQ3 and hypersensitivity to HIV-1 reverse-transcriptase inhibitor abacavir," *The Lancet*, vol. 359, no. 9308, pp. 727–732, 2002.

[4] S. Hetherington, A. R. Hughes, M. Mosteller et al., "Genetic variations in HLA-B region and hypersensitivity reactions to abacavir," *The Lancet*, vol. 359, no. 9312, pp. 1121–1122, 2002.

[5] S. Mallal, E. Phillips, G. Carosi et al., "HLA-B*5701 screening for hypersensitivity to abacavir," *The New England Journal of Medicine*, vol. 358, no. 6, pp. 568–579, 2008.

[6] R. Pavlos, S. Mallal, D. Ostrov et al., "T Cell-mediated hypersensitivity reactions to drugs," *Annual Review of Medicine*, vol. 66, pp. 439–454, 2015.

[7] K. D. White, W.-H. Chung, S.-I. Hung, S. Mallal, and E. J. Phillips, "Evolving models of the immunopathogenesis of T cell-mediated drug allergy: the role of host, pathogens, and drug response," *Journal of Allergy and Clinical Immunology*, vol. 136, no. 2, pp. 219–234, 2015.

[8] M. A. Norcross, S. Luo, L. Lu et al., "Abacavir induces loading of novel self-peptides into HLA-B*57: 01: an autoimmune model for HLA-associated drug hypersensitivity," *AIDS*, vol. 26, no. 11, pp. F21–F29, 2012.

[9] D. A. Ostrov, B. J. Grant, Y. A. Pompeu et al., "Drug hypersensitivity caused by alteration of the MHC-presented self-peptide repertoire," *Proceedings of the National Academy of Sciences of the United States of America*, vol. 109, no. 25, pp. 9959–9964, 2012.

[10] P. T. Illing, J. P. Vivian, N. L. Dudek et al., "Immune self-reactivity triggered by drug-modified HLA-peptide repertoire," *Nature*, vol. 486, no. 7404, pp. 554–558, 2012.

[11] J. Adam, K. K. Eriksson, B. Schnyder, S. Fontana, W. J. Pichler, and D. Yerly, "Avidity determines T-cell reactivity in abacavir hypersensitivity," *European Journal of Immunology*, vol. 42, no. 7, pp. 1706–1716, 2012.

[12] C. C. Bell, L. Faulkner, K. Martinsson et al., "T-cells from HLA-B*57:01+ human subjects are activated with abacavir through two independent pathways and induce cell death by multiple mechanisms," *Chemical Research in Toxicology*, vol. 26, no. 5, pp. 759–766, 2013.

[13] J. Yun, M. J. Marcaida, K. K. Eriksson et al., "Oxypurinol directly and immediately activates the drug-specific T cells via the preferential use of HLA-B*58:01," *Journal of Immunology*, vol. 192, no. 7, pp. 2984–2993, 2014.

[14] Protein Data Bank (PDB), http://pdb.org.

[15] J. Goto, R. Kataoka, H. Muta, and N. Hirayama, "ASEDock-docking based on alpha spheres and excluded volumes," *Journal of Chemical Information and Modeling*, vol. 48, no. 3, pp. 583–590, 2008.

[16] Molecular Operatiing Environment (MOE), Chemical Computing Group, Montreal, Canada, 2013.

[17] M. J. Abraham, D. van der, E. Lindahl, and B. Hess, "GROMACS User manual version 5.0.6," 2015, http://www.gromacs.org/.

[18] S. Matsuoka, T. Endo, N. Maruyama, H. Sato, and S. Takizawa, "The total picture of TSUBAME 2.0," *TSUBAME e-Science Journal, GSIC, Tokyo Institute of Technology*, vol. 1, pp. 2–4, 2010.

[19] R. O. Dror, R. M. Dirks, J. P. Grossman, H. Xu, and D. E. Shaw, "Biomolecular simulation: a computational microscope for molecular biology," *Annual Review of Biophysics*, vol. 41, no. 1, pp. 429–452, 2012.

[20] I. Kass, A. M. Buckle, and N. A. Borg, "Understanding the structural dynamics of TCR-pMHC interactions," *Trends in Immunology*, vol. 35, no. 12, pp. 604–612, 2014.

[21] B. Knapp, S. Demharter, R. Esmaielbeiki, and C. M. Deane, "Current status and future challenges in T-cell receptor/peptide/MHC molecular dynamics simulations," *Briefings in Bioinformatics*, vol. 16, no. 6, pp. 1035–1044, 2015.

[22] U. Omasitsa, B. Knappa, M. Neumannb et al., "Analysis of key parameters for molecular dynamics of pMHC molecules," *Molecular Simulation*, vol. 34, no. 8, pp. 781–793, 2008.

[23] D. Narzi, C. M. Becker, M. T. Fiorillo, B. Uchanska-Ziegler, A. Ziegler, and R. A. Böckmann, "Dynamical characterization of two differentially disease associated MHC class I proteins in complex with viral and self-peptides," *Journal of Molecular Biology*, vol. 415, no. 2, pp. 429–442, 2012.

[24] W. J. Pichler, "Consequences of drug binding to immune receptors: immune stimulation following pharmacological interaction with immune receptors (T-cell receptor for antigen or human leukocyte antigen) with altered peptide-human leukocyte antigen or peptide," *Dermatologica Sinica*, vol. 31, no. 4, pp. 181–190, 2013.

19

Porcine Pancreatic Lipase Inhibitory Agent Isolated from Medicinal Herb and Inhibition Kinetics of Extracts from *Eleusine indica* (L.) Gaertner

Siew Ling Ong, Siau Hui Mah, and How Yee Lai

School of Biosciences, Taylor's University, No. 1 Jalan Taylor's, 47500 Subang Jaya, Malaysia

Correspondence should be addressed to How Yee Lai; howyee.lai@taylors.edu.my

Academic Editor: Athar Ata

Eleusine indica (Linnaeus) Gaertner is a traditional herb known to be depurative, febrifuge, and diuretic and has been reported with the highest inhibitory activity against porcine pancreatic lipase (PPL) among thirty two plants screened in an earlier study. This study aims to isolate and identify the active components that may possess high potential as an antiobesity agent. Of the screened solvent fractions of *E. indica*, hexane fraction showed the highest inhibitory activity of 27.01 ± 5.68% at 100 μg/mL. Bioactivity-guided isolation afforded three compounds from the hexane fraction of *E. indica*, namely, β-sitosterol, stigmasterol, and lutein. The structures of these compounds were elucidated using spectral techniques. Lutein showed an outstanding inhibitory activity against PPL (55.98 ± 1.04%), with activity 60% higher than that of the reference drug Orlistat. The other compounds isolated and identified were β-sitosterol (2.99 ± 0.80%) and stigmasterol (2.68 ± 0.38%). The enzyme kinetics of *E. indica* crude methanolic extract on PPL showed mixed inhibition mechanism.

1. Introduction

Obesity is often defined as the excess accumulation of body fat resulting from a higher energy intake than energy expenditure [1]. In 2008, 10% of men and 14% of women in the world were obese, compared with 5% of men and 8% of women in 1980 [2]. Rates of both overweight and obesity are projected to increase in almost all countries, with 1.5 billion people overweight in 2015 [2]. Pancreatic lipase inhibition is one of the most widely studied mechanisms for antiobesity treatment, based on the principle that dietary fat will not be directly absorbed by the intestine unless the fat has been subjected to the action of pancreatic lipase [3, 4].

Phytochemicals or bioactive compound/extract identified from traditional medicinal plants had provided an exciting platform and opportunity for the development of safe and effective therapeutic drugs for the treatment of many metabolic diseases [5]. A review by Newman and Cragg (2007) [6] on the origin of drugs launched in the past 25 years showed about half of the compounds that were successful in clinical trials were derived from natural origin. Despite multiple research conducted in recent decades, the potential

of antiobesity therapeutic drug of natural product origin is still largely unexplored. Previous screening study on thirty two plants reported strongest porcine pancreatic lipase (PPL) activity in *E. indica* [7] and this has led to further investigation on this herb for potential antiobesity agent.

E. indica (Linnaeus) Gaertner (Poaceae) is an annual grass native in the tropics and subtropical regions [8, 9]. It is commonly widespread as weed in rice field and is known to be resistant to many herbicides (such as dinitroaniline) [10]. This plant is commonly known as goosegrass, wiregrass, "rumput sambari," or "rumput sambau" in Malaysia [11]. Its root is traditionally known to be depurative, febrifuge, diuretic, and laxative and thus is commonly used for treating hypertension, influenza, oliguria, and urine retention [8]. The decoctions of the boiled whole plant are consumed for antihelminthic and febrifuge treatment [12]. The seed of *E. indica* is sometimes used as famine food and in the treatment for liver complaints [13].

Several pharmacological properties on *E. indica* have been reported including hepatoprotective effect [13], antiplasmodial and antidiabetic [14], antioxidant and antimicrobial activity [8], anti-inflammatory [15], and cytotoxic effect towards several cancer cell lines [8, 16]. To date, only one study reported the isolation of secondary metabolites from *E. indica* where hexadecanoic acid and [[(2-aminoethoxy) hydroxyphosphinyloxy]methyl]-1,2–ethanediylester were isolated [17]. Hence, this paper is the first report on the kinetics of PPL enzyme inhibition by *E. indica* and the bioactivity-guided isolation of a potent PPL inhibitory compound (lutein) from *E. indica*.

2. Materials and Methods

2.1. Plant Materials, Extraction, and Preparation of Crude Extracts. The whole plants of *E. indica* (L.) Gaertn. were collected from Persatuan Pengkaji Herba Tradisional Negeri Sembilan (Pantai, Negeri Sembilan, coordinates: $2°46'13''$N, $101°59'40''$E). This plant was authenticated by Dr. Fadzureena Jamaludin from Forest Research Institute Malaysia (FRIM); the voucher specimen 003/15 (collection date: 11 February 2015) is kept at the School of Biosciences, Taylor's University (Lakeside Campus).

The whole plant of *E. indica* was cleaned from residual soil, freeze-dried, and pulverised. Analytical grade methanol was added and the extracts were then filtered and pooled, and the solvent was evaporated off.

2.2. Subextraction of the Main Extract. The crude extract of *E. indica* was suspended in distilled water (1 : 10, w/v) and sequentially extracted with solvents in increasing polarity (hexane, chloroform, ethyl acetate, and butanol), three times each (1 : 1, v/v), to obtain the respective solvent fractions. Each fraction was then assayed for porcine pancreatic lipase inhibition activity.

2.3. Porcine Pancreatic Lipase (PPL) Inhibition Assay. Porcine pancreatic lipase (PPL) inhibitory assay was performed as described by Bustanji et al. (2011) [18] with minor modification. The enzyme solutions was prepared immediately before use, by suspending crude porcine pancreatic lipase powder type II (Sigma, EC 3.1.1.3) in Tris-HCl buffer (50 mM Tris, 150 mM NaCl, 1 mM EDTA, 10 mM MOPS, pH 7.6) to give a concentration of 5 mg/mL (200 units/mL). The solution was then centrifuged at 1,500 rpm for 10 minutes and the clear supernatant was recovered. The plant extract (100 μg/mL) was preincubated with 200 μL of PPL solution for 5 minutes at 37°C, before the addition of 5 μL PNPB substrate solution (10 mM in acetonitrile). The total reaction volume was made to 1 mL using the Tris-HCl buffer before measuring the absorbance at 410 nm against blank using denatured enzyme. The denatured enzyme was prepared by boiling the enzyme solution for 5 minutes. Orlistat was used as a reference drug. The extract was dissolved in DMSO at a final concentration not exceeding 1% (v/v) which will not affect enzyme activity.

The activity of the negative control was checked with and without the inhibitor. The inhibitory activity (*I*%) was calculated according to the formula below [18]:

$$I\% = \left(1 - \frac{B - b}{A - a}\right) \times 100, \tag{1}$$

where A is the activity of the enzyme without inhibitor, a is the negative control without the inhibitor, B is the activity of the enzyme with inhibitor, and b is the negative control with inhibitor.

2.4. Kinetic Study. The inhibition mode of *E. indica* methanolic crude extract on porcine pancreatic lipase (PPL) was assayed with increasing concentrations (20, 40, 60, and 80 μM) of synthetic substrate, *p*-nitrophenyl butyrate (PNPB), in the presence and absence of two different concentrations of the extracts (100 and 200 μg/mL). The mode of inhibition was determined by Lineweaver-Burk plot of the data.

2.5. Chromatography and Spectral Instrumentation

2.5.1. Thin Layer Chromatography (TLC). The TLC was performed on the TLC Silica Gel 60 coated with fluorescent indicator F_{254} Aluminium sheets (Merck). Samples were spotted and viewed under UV lamp at 254 nm and 365 nm.

2.5.2. High Performance Liquid Chromatography (HPLC). The fingerprinting of the extracts was done on Shimadzu Prominence Series coupled with photodiode array (PDA) detector SPD-M20A using either reversed-phase or normal phase settings:

(i) Reversed-phase, Chromolith HighResolution RP-18 endcapped 100–4.6 mm (Merck): the mobile phase used was solvent A, acetonitrile and solvent B, water with a standard flow rate of 1.0 mL/min, and injection volume of 20 μL of 10 mg/mL extract; the gradient of the mobile phase was as follows: 0% to 50% A (0–45 min).

(ii) Normal phase, Phenomenex Luna Silica column (250 × 4.6 mm, 100 Å, 5 μm): the mobile phase used consists of solvent A, hexane and solvent B, 2-propanol with a flow rate of 1.0 mL/min, and injection volume of 20 μL of 10 mg/mL extract; the gradient program was as follows: 100% A (0–5 min), 100% to 0% A (5–25 min).

2.5.3. Infrared Spectroscopy (FT-IR). The IR spectra were measured by Perkin Elmer Spectrum 100 using potassium bromide pellet method.

2.5.4. Gas Chromatography–Mass Spectrometry Using Electron Impact Ionisation (GC-EI-MS). Mass spectra were recorded with EIMS using a Direct Injection Probe on a Shidmadzu GC-MS QP 5050A Spectrometer. GC-MS was performed to identify the purity and molecular weight of compounds.

2.5.5. UV-Visible Spectra. The UV-Vis spectra were recorded on a Thermo Scientific Genesys 10 UV Scanning Spectrophotometer.

2.5.6. Melting Point. Melting points were recorded using a melting point probe Electrothermal IA 9000 Series.

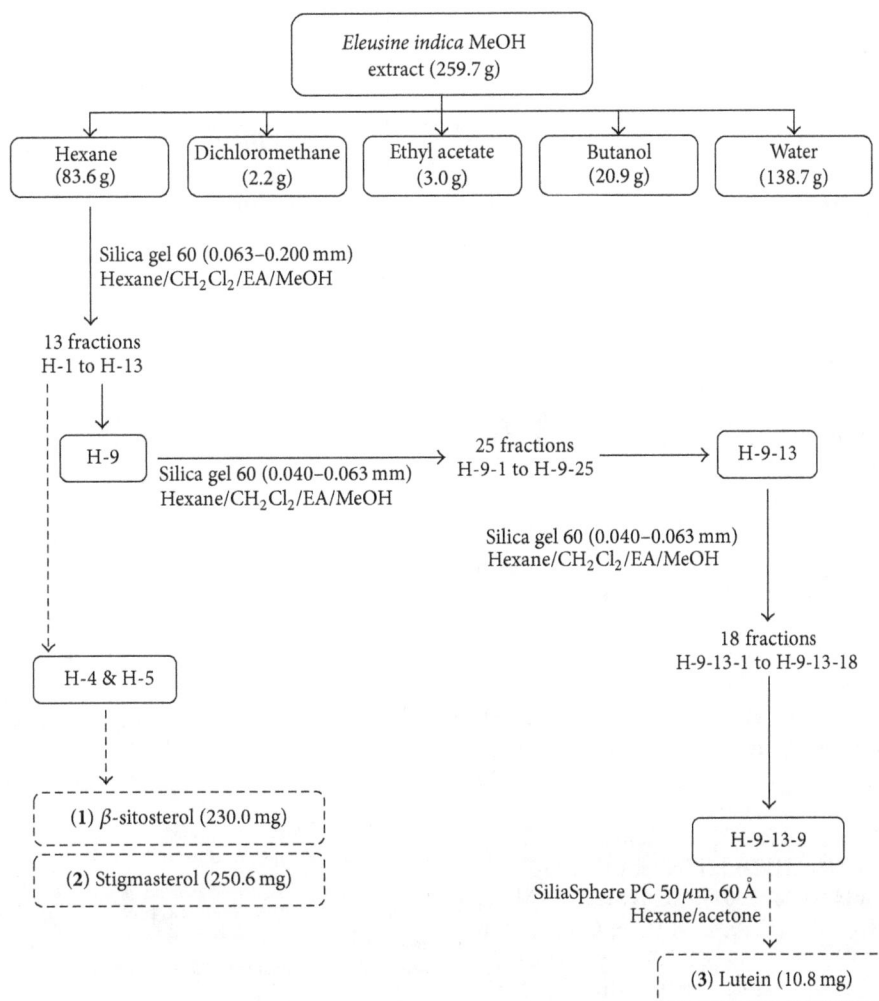

FIGURE 1: Schematic flow of the bioactivity-guided isolation on *E. indica* extract.

2.5.7. Nuclear Magnetic Resonance (NMR). The spectra were obtained from JEOL ECX500 FT NMR Spectrometer system. Deuterated chloroform (CDCl$_3$) was used as the solvent to dissolve the test samples. Tetramethylsilane (TMS) was used as internal standard for both ^{1}H (500 MHz) and ^{13}C (125 MHz). The chemical shifts from the spectra were recorded in ppm and coupling constants were given in Hertz (Hz).

2.6. Bioactivity-Guided Extraction and Isolation. The active fraction was subjected to gravitational column chromatography packed with suitable packing materials; the schematic flow is as shown in Figure 1. The weight of the selected packing materials introduced into the column was at least ten times the weight of the sample extract. Sample was separated using the solvent system as stated in Figure 1.

The isolated pure compounds were then characterised and elucidated employing several spectral methods as stated in Section 2.5.

β-sitosterol (**1**) White crystal; m.p. 134.5–137.6°C; UV (Hexane) λ_{max} nm (log ε): 210 (817), 230 (54); IR υ_{max} cm^{-1}: 3431, 2937, 1468, 1382, 1056; EIMS *m/z* (rel. int.): 414 [M$^+$], 329 (20), 145 (25), 107 (30), 105 (27), 91 (20), 93 (21), 95 (28), 81 (28), 69 (27), 57 (51), 55 (36), 43 (100), 41 (32); ^{1}H NMR (500 MHz, CDCl$_3$): δ 5.29 (m, 1H, H-3), 3.46 (m, 1H, H-6); ^{13}C NMR (125 MHz, CDCl$_3$): δ 140.7 (C-5), 121.8 (C-6), 79.1 (C-3 & C-13), 55.4 (C-14 & C-17), 50.6 (C-9), 48.7 (C-24), 42.1 (C-4), 39.5 (C-12), 39.0 (C-1), 38.4 (C-10), 37.2 (C-20), 33.4 (C-22), 32.7 (C-2), 31.2 (C-7 & C-8), 29.8 (C-25), 27.5 (C-16), 26.8 (C-23), 26.3 (C-15), 25.6 (C-28), 21.5 (C-11), 19.6 (C-26), 18.4 (C-19 & C-27), 17.8 (C-21), 15.5 (C-29), 14.9 (C-18).

Stigmasterol (**2**) White crystal; m.p. 168.0–170.0°C; UV (Hexane) λ_{max} nm (log ε): 210 (839), 230 (147); IR υ_{max} cm^{-1}: 3426, 2936, 1645, 1465, 1384, 1052 and 959; EIMS *m/z* (rel. int.): 412 [M$^+$] (61), 255 (52), 159 (56), 145 (61), 95 (58), 81 (78), 69 (65), 55 (100); ^{1}H-NMR (500 MHz, CDCl$_3$): δ 5.34 (d, 1H, J = 4.6 Hz, H-6), 5.16 (m, 1H, H-22), 5.03 (m, 1H, H-23), 3.53 (m, 1H, H-3), 1.00 (s, 3H, H-19), 0.916 (d, 1H, J = 5.75 Hz, H-21), 0.829 (m, 9H, H-26, H-27, H-29), 0.685 (s, 3H, H-18); ^{13}C NMR (125 MHz, CDCl$_3$): δ 140.8 (C-5), 138.4 (C-20), 129.4 (C-21), 121.8 (C-6), 71.9 (C-3), 56.9 (C-14), 56.2 (C-17), 51.3 (C-22), 50.2 (C-9), 42.4 (C-4), 42.3 (C-13), 39.9 (C-12), 39.8 (C-18), 37.4 (C-1), 36.6 (C-10), 32.0 (C-2), 31.7 (C-7), 29.2 (C-8), 29.0 (C-16), 28.3 (C-25), 25.5 (C-23), 24.4 (C-15),

TABLE 1: Kinetic analyses of PPL inhibition by methanolic crude extract of *E. indica*.

| | Velocity of enzyme activity in different concentration of substrate [S] (μM) | | | | V_{max} (μM min^{-1}) | K_m (μM) |
	20	40	60	80		
Control	0.035 ± 0.003	0.026 ± 0.005	0.022 ± 0.005	0.019 ± 0.003	65.79	26.36
100 μg/mL of methanolic *E. indica*	0.043 ± 0.003	0.029 ± 0.001	0.024 ± 0.002	0.023 ± 0.004	63.29	33.70
200 μg/mL of methanolic *E. indica*	0.047 ± 0.005	0.031 ± 0.001	0.029 ± 0.004	0.024 ± 0.003	57.14	34.11

Values are expressed as mean $\pm$ SD.

21.2 (C-11), 19.9 (C-27), 19.5 (C-26), 19.1 (C-19), 18.9 (C-28), 12.3 (C-29), 12.1 (C-24).

Lutein (**3**) orange crystal; m.p. 173.8–174.9°C; UV (Acetone) λ_{max} nm (log ε): 266, 426 (shoulder), 448 (628), 476 (564); IR v_{max} cm^{-1}: 3427, 2926, 1718, 1465, 1376, 1261; EIMS *m/z* (rel. int.): 568 [M$^+$], 145 (49), 119 (96), 105 (100), 93 (54), 91 (70); ^{1}H NMR (500 MHz, CDCl$_3$): δ 6.57 (m, 4H, H-11, H-15, H-11′, H-12′), 6.34 (d, 2H, J = 14.9 Hz, H-12), 6.23 (m, 2H, H-14, H-14′), 6.10 (m, 5H, H-8, H-10, H-7′, H-8′), 5.54 (s, 1H, H-4), 5.39 (dd, 1H, J = 10.4, 9.2 Hz, H-7), 4.24 (s, 1H, H-3), 3.98 (m, 1H, H-3′), 2.36 (m, 2H, H-6, H-4eq), 2.01 (dd, 1H, J = 10.3, 9.2 Hz, H-4ax′), 1.96 (s, 9H, H-20, H-19′, H-20′), 1.90 (s, 3H, H-19), 1.81 (dd, 1H, J = 5.7, 6.9 Hz, H-2eq), 1.73 (s, 3H, H-18′), 1.62 (s, 12H, H-18), 1.44 (t, 1H, J = 12.6, 11.5 Hz, H-2′), 1.34 (dd, 1H, J = 5.7, 6.9 Hz, H-2ax), 1.06 (s, 6H, H-16′, H-17′), 0.838 & 0.987 (s, 6H, H-16, H-17); ^{13}C NMR (125 MHz, CDCl$_3$): δ 138.6 (C-8′), 138.1 (C-8), 137.8 (C-5, C-12′), 137.6 (C-12, C-6′), 136.6 (C-13′), 136.5 (C-13), 135.8 (C-9′), 135.2 (C-9), 132.7 (C-14, C-14′), 131.4 (C-10′), 130.9 (C-10), 130.2 (C-15′), 130.1 (C-15), 128.8 (C-7), 126.2 (C-5′), 125.7 (C-7′), 125.0 (C-4), 124.9 (C-11′), 124.6 (C-11), 66.0 (C-3), 65.2 (C-3′), 55.1 (C-6), 48.5 (C-2′), 44.7 (C-2), 42.6 (C-4′), 37.2 (C-1′), 34.1 (C-1), 30.3 (C-17′), 29.6 (C-17), 28.8 (C-16′), 24.4 (C-16), 22.8 (C-18), 21.7 (C-18′), 13.2 (C-19), 12.9 (C-19′, C-20), 12.8 (C-20).

2.7. Statistical Analysis. All results were expressed as mean $\pm$ standard deviation. Significance of difference from the control was determined by Tukey's *post-hoc* test (one-way ANOVA) *p* value < 0.05 using SPSS software (version 16.0).

3. Results and Discussion

3.1. Kinetic Analysis. The inhibition mode of PPL by *E. indica* methanolic extract at 100 μg/mL and 200 μg/mL was analysed by double-reciprocal Lineweaver-Burk plot as shown in Figure 2. Kinetic parameters calculated from the double reciprocal trend lines showed that both the maximal velocity of the PPL enzyme-substrate extract reaction (V_{max}) and the affinity (K_m) were affected by the extract concentration, hence indicating a mixed mode inhibition. The Michaelis-Menten parameters are tabulated in Table 1, where the Michaelis-Menten constant (K_m) of PPL with synthetic substrate PNPB was 26.36 μM and maximal velocity (V_{max}) was 65.79 μM min^{-1}. The mixed mode inhibition exhibited by PPL indicates that the formation of enzyme-substrate

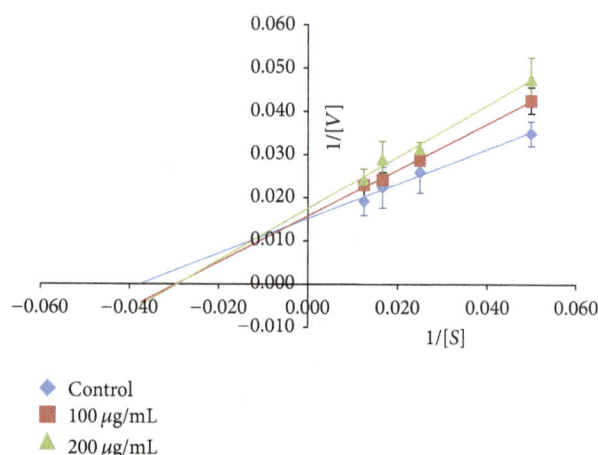

FIGURE 2: Lineweaver-Burk plot of *E. indica* methanolic extract against PPL at two different concentrations (100 and 200 μg/mL). Bar indicates the standard deviation.

complex was possible with the inhibitor binding at a distinct site from the active site resulting in reduction in the complex affinity, thus explaining the increase in K_m. Similar inhibition mode was observed in *Levisticum officinale* methanolic extract and regular cocoa extract against porcine pancreatic lipase [19, 20].

The methanolic crude extract of *E. indica* was then partitioned via liquid-liquid fractionation, to yield five (5) solvent extracts, that is, hexane, dichloromethane, ethyl acetate, butanol, and water. All solvent extracts were then assayed for their inhibitory activity against PPL. Table 2 shows that the hexane extract from *E. indica* possessed the highest PPL inhibitory activity, that is, 27.01 $\pm$ 5.68%. Although *E. indica* dichloromethane extract recorded a comparable value of 25.57 $\pm$ 3.26% PPL inhibitory activity, due to its low yield from the partition (1.18%), this extract was not further tested.

3.2. Fingerprinting of Solvent Extracts from E. indica. The HPLC chromatograms of all *E. indica* methanolic extract and solvent fractions are shown in Figure 3. Six major peaks were detected in elution profile of the crude methanolic extract of *E. indica* (Figure 3(a)). No peak was detected in hexane fraction (Figure 3(b)) due to the incompatibility of reverse phase column with the nature of the fraction, which was highly nonpolar. The hexane fraction was later

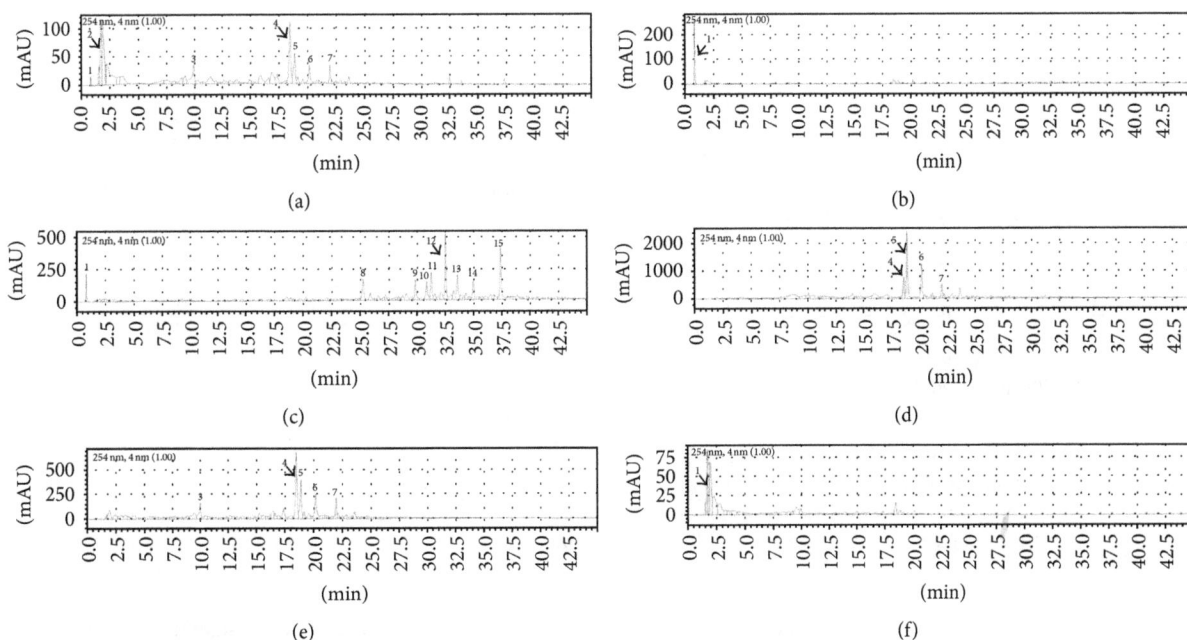

FIGURE 3: HPLC profiles of different fractions of *E. indica*: (a) crude methanolic extract; (b) hexane fraction; (c) dichloromethane fraction; (d) ethyl acetate fraction; (e) butanol fraction and; (f) aqueous fraction using Chromolith HighResolution RP-18 (Merck) HPLC column (reverse phase) at 254 nm using the gradient mobile phase 0% to 50% acetonitrile: 100% to 50% deionised water (0 to 45 minutes).

TABLE 2: Yield and PPL inhibitory activity of *E. indica* crude methanolic extract and solvent fractions.

	Yield (g/100 g crude extract)	PPL inhibition (%)
Crude methanolic extract	—	25.05 ± 3.58^c
Hexane fraction	34.16 ± 7.53	27.01 ± 5.68^c
Dichloromethane fraction	0.98 ± 0.47	25.57 ± 3.26^c
Ethyl acetate fraction	1.40 ± 0.47	10.38 ± 2.73^b
Butanol fraction	9.72 ± 2.36	5.23 ± 2.29^a
Aqueous fraction	52.78 ± 4.37	4.18 ± 1.91^a
Orlistat	—	34.49 ± 5.39^d

Values are expressed as mean $\pm$ SD, $n = 3$ values. The concentration of the tested extract against PPL was 100 μg/mL. Statistically significant effects were compared using one-way ANOVA (Tukey's *post-hoc* test), where different letters in superscripts indicated significance at $p < 0.05$.

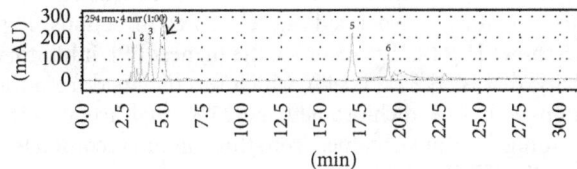

FIGURE 4: HPLC profiles of *E. indica* hexane fraction using Luna 5 μm Silica (Phenomenex) HPLC column (normal phase) at 254 nm using the gradient mobile phase 100% hexane for 5 minutes, followed by 100% to 0% of hexane: 0% to 100% 2-propanol (5 to 25 minutes).

optimised and run with Luna 5 μm Silica (Phenomenex), a normal phase column coupled with normal phase mobile phase, where six major peaks were detected as shown in Figure 4. A cluster of eight peaks were eluted in the second half end of the chromatogram in dichloromethane fraction (Figure 3(c)) due to its more nonpolar nature. Most of the peaks from this cluster (peak 8 to peak 15) were visible in the chromatogram of crude methanolic extract in Figure 3(a), but the concentration of these compound present in the crude extract was too low to be detected as the major peaks. Figures 3(d) and 3(e) which showed the elution profile of ethyl acetate and butanol extracts, respectively, recorded peak 4 to peak 7 which corresponded to the major peaks as detected in elution profile of crude methanolic extract where they represented

elution of semipolar compounds at the midrange of the chromatograms. The most polar compounds were eluted at the beginning of the spectrum (retention time less than 2.5 minutes) in the aqueous fraction (Figure 3(f)), which were also detected as one of the major peaks in the crude extract.

High PPL inhibitory activity was detected in hexane ($27.01 \pm 5.68\%$) and dichloromethane ($25.57 \pm 3.26\%$) fractions from *E. indica* (Table 2). Chromatogram of the hexane fraction (Figure 4) showed presence of six (6) major components (numbers 1 to 6) while chromatogram of the dichloromethane fraction (Figure 3(c)) showed eight major components (numbers 8 to 15). Attempts were made to identify the components by running with ten standards, namely, rutin, quercetin, neringenin, caffeic acid, chlorogenic acid, coumaric acid, gallic acid, esculin, kaempferol, and myricetin. However, none of the peaks' retention time matched those of the standards. As such, the components eluted from the hexane and dichloromethane fractions could not be identified from the chromatograms. Nevertheless, these chromatographic fingerprints obtained from the methanolic crude

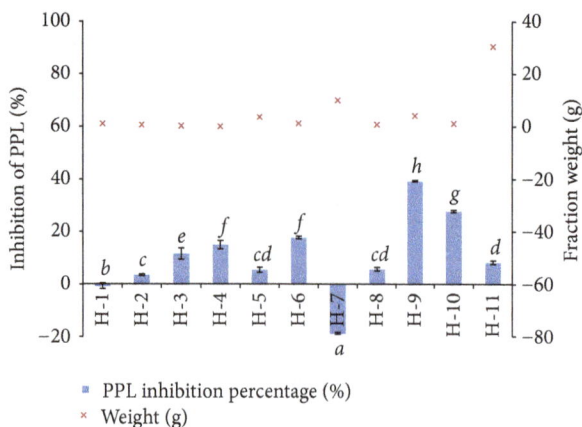

FIGURE 5: The fraction yield and PPL inhibitory activity of H-1 to H-11. Bar indicates the standard deviation. Statistically significant effects were compared using one-way ANOVA (Tukey's *post-hoc* test), where different letters indicated significance at $p < 0.05$.

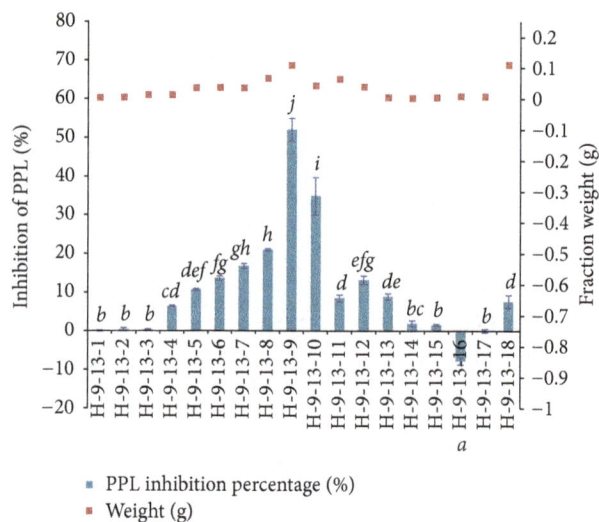

FIGURE 6: The fraction yield and PPL inhibitory activity of H-9-1 to H-9-25. Bar indicates the standard deviation. Statistically significant effects were compared using one-way ANOVA (Tukey's *post-hoc* test), where different letters indicated significance at $p < 0.05$.

and all solvent fractions may provide a simple guide for future identification and comparison of *E. indica* L. even if the geographical location and/or season of collection are different.

3.3. Bioactivity-Guided Extraction.

The hexane fraction of *E. indica* was further separated into eleven (11) fractions. Figure 5 shows H-9 (4.21 g) recorded the highest PPL inhibitory activity, that is, 39.35 ± 0.24%, which was obtained from the elution with 75% dichloromethane/25% ethyl acetate. The remaining fractions obtained from this column recorded less than 20% of PPL inhibitory activity.

Alongside with the separation of H-1 to H-11, two common sterols were isolated from the fractions H-4 and H-5, on elution with 90% dichloromethane/10% ethyl acetate. β-sitosterol (1) was isolated as a white flower-liked crystalline powder while stigmasterol (2) was in white needle-like crystals. The detailed physical properties of β-sitosterol and stigmasterol will be discussed in the later part of this paper. Both compounds were found to possess very low PPL inhibition activity, that is, 2.99 ± 0.80% (β-sitosterol) of inhibition at 100 µg/mL (242 µM) and 2.68 ± 0.38% (stigmasterol) of inhibition at 100 µg/mL (243 µM), respectively.

Fraction H-9 (4.21 g) was subjected to further separation due to its high PPL inhibitory activity and sufficient yield. Figure 6 shows the fraction yield and PPL inhibitory activity of twenty five (25) subfractions of H-9. Highest PPL inhibitory activity was captured in H-9-13 (32.15 ± 5.11%), followed by H-9-14 (29.26 ± 1.08%), where the yield was 0.32 g and 0.47 g, respectively. Subfractions of H-9-13, H-9-17, and H-9-21 recorded PPL inhibitory activity of more than 20% while other subfractions were either promoted or showed less than 20% PPL inhibition.

Both H-9-13 and H-9-14 were selected for further isolation due to their higher yield (323.6 mg and 465.3 mg, resp.). As both H-9-13 and H-9-14 showed comparable PPL inhibition as well as similar TLC spotting profile (data not shown), both subfractions were combined for further

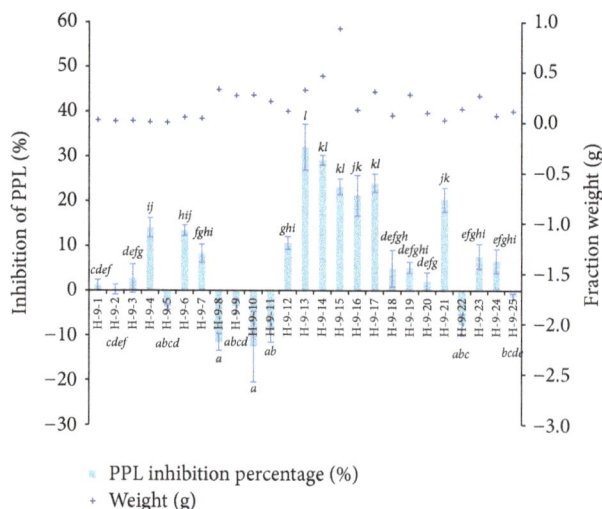

FIGURE 7: The fraction yield and PPL inhibitory activity of H-9-13-1 to H-9-13-18. Bar indicates the standard deviation. Statistically significant effects were compared using one-way ANOVA (Tukey's *post-hoc* test), where different letters indicated significance at $p < 0.05$.

isolation and the results of the PPL inhibitory activity of the resultant isolated subfractions are shown in Figure 7.

Highest PPL inhibitory activity was shown by H-9-13-9 (108.8 mg), that is, 52.08 ± 2.93%, which was about 18% higher than that recorded by Orlistat (34.49 ± 5.39%). Fraction H-9-13-10 recorded the second highest PPL inhibition, 34.96 ± 4.87%, which was similar to that of Orlistat.

The TLC profile from H-9-13-9 showed one prominent yellow spot where further isolation was then done, resulting in the isolation of lutein (3) (10.8 mg) from this fraction. This isolated pure compound (lutein) was subjected to few analysis including melting point analysis, UV, GC-MS (for the

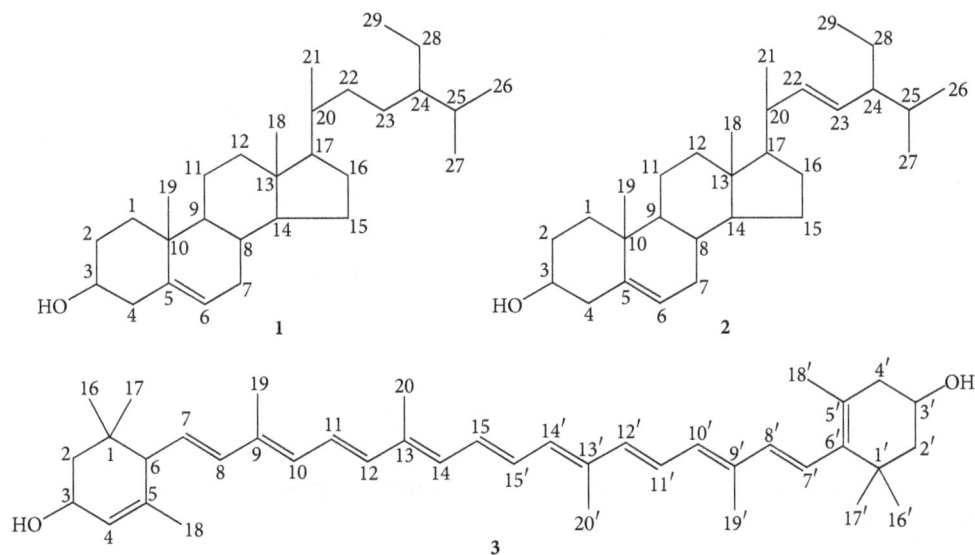

FIGURE 8: Chemical structures of β-sitosterol (1), stigmasterol (2), and lutein (3).

determination of molecular weight), FT-IR (determination of functional group), and NMR (structural elucidation). The characterised lutein was found to possess very strong PPL inhibitory activity, that is, 55.98 ± 1.04% at 100 μg/mL (176 μM), which was 21.5% higher than that recorded in Orlistat (34.49 ± 5.39%). To date, this is the first study to reveal the potential of lutein as a strong PPL inhibitory agent.

3.4. Isolation of Compounds from E. indica. The structures of the isolated compounds were shown in Figure 8. The white crystals of β-sitosterol (1) had melting point of 134.5–137.6°C [lit. 134-135°C [21]] and also showed IR absorptions at 3431 (O-H stretching), 2937 (aliphatic C-H stretching), 1468 (C-H$_2$ bending), 1382 (C-H$_3$ bend), and 1056 (=CH bend). EIMS has confirmed the molecular formula $C_{29}H_{50}O$ with the molecular ion peak at m/z 414. Similarly, stigmasterol (2) was isolated as white crystals with melting point of 168.0–170.0°C (lit 170°C [22]), and its mass spectral data suggested the molecular formula as $C_{29}H_{48}O$. The IR absorption of stigmasterol was similar to that of β-sitosterol with an additional absorption band at 1645 cm^{-1}indicative of an olefin group. Both β-sitosterol and stigmasterol recorded UV absorption maxima at 210 nm. Sterols normally absorb in the range of 190–210 nm, due to the transitions of π to ρ^* [23].

The ^{1}H NMR spectrum of β-sitosterol (1) had detected multiplet of signals at δ 3.21 of H-3 which belonged to the hydroxymethyl group at C-3, and another pair of multiplet resonated at δ 4.61 which is assigned to the olefinic proton at H-6. The ^{13}C NMR spectrum showed a total of 29 carbon signals were captured, which supported the molecular formula obtained in EIMS. These signals consist of a quaternary methine at C-5 (δ 145.3), an olefinic methine at C-6 (δ 121.8), as well as several methyl group at C-18, C-19, C-21, C-26, C-27, and C-29 (δ 14.9, 18.4, 17.8, 19.6, 18.4, and 15.5, resp.). And methylene group was located at δ 39.0 (C-1), δ 32.7 (C-2), δ 42.1 (C-4), δ 31.2 (C-7), δ 21.5 (C-11), δ 39.5 (C-12), δ 26.3 (C-15), δ 27.5 (C-16), δ 33.4 (C-22), δ 26.8 (C-23), and δ

25.6 (C-28). Both proton and carbon signals obtained were matched and in agreement with literature [24].

In the ^{1}H NMR spectrum of stigmasterol (2), there was presence of methyl singlets at δ 0.69 (H-18) and δ 1.00 (H-19); multiplets at δ 5.16 (H-22) and δ 5.03 (H-23) signified olefinic protons which were not found in β-sitosterol. Similarly, ^{13}C NMR had revealed 29 carbon peaks where olefinic carbons were identified at δ 140.8 (C-5), δ 121.8 (C-6), δ 51.3 (C-22), and δ 25.5 (C-23); methyl carbons were detected at δ 39.8 (C-18), δ 19.1 (C-19), δ 129.4 (C-21), δ 19.5 (C-26), δ 19.9 (C-27), and δ 12.3 (C-29); methylene carbons were detected at δ 37.4 (C-1), δ 32.0 (C-2), δ 42.4 (C-4), δ 31.7 (C-7), δ 21.2 (C-11), δ 39.9 (C-12), δ 24.4 (C-15), δ 29.0 (C-16), and δ 18.9 (C-28). Both spectra data were matched and in agreement with literature [25].

Lutein (3) was isolated as orange crystals with a melting point of 173.8–174.9°C and maxima wavelengths recorded at 426, 448, and 476 nm, which were in agreement with the data of the literature [26, 27]. Mass spectrum of lutein given the molecular ion at m/z 568, followed by fragments in m/z 550, is attributed to the loss of a hydroxy group. ^{1}H NMR spectra data revealed hydroxyl protons resonated at δ 4.24 (H-3) and δ 3.98 (H-3'); olefinic protons at δ 4.24 (H-3), δ 5.54 (H-4), δ 5.39 (H-7), δ 6.10 (H-8), δ 6.10 (H-10), δ 6.57 (H-11), δ 6.34 (H-12), δ 6.23 (H-14), δ 6.57 (H-15), δ 6.10 (H-7' and H-8'), δ 6.57 (H-11' and H-12'), and δ 6.23 (H-14'); allylic protons at δ 1.62 (H-18), δ 1.90 (H-19), δ 1.96 (H-20), δ 1.73 (H-18'), and δ 1.96 (H-19' and H-20'); methyl singlets at δ 0.838, δ 0.987 (H-16 and H-17), and δ 1.06 (H-16' and H-17'). The ^{13}C NMR spectra data revealed olefinic carbons resonated at δ 125.0 (C-4), δ 137.8 (C-5), δ 128.8 (C-7), δ 138.1 (C-8), δ 135.2 (C-8), δ 135.2 (C-9), δ 130.9 (C-10), δ 124.6 (C-11), δ 137.6 (C-12), δ 136.5 (C-13), δ 132.7 (C-14), δ 130.1 (C-15), δ 126.2 (C-5'), δ 137.6 (C-6'), δ 125.7 (C-7'), δ 138.6 (C-8'), δ 135.8 (C-9'), δ 131.4 (C-10'), δ 124.9 (C-11'), δ 137.8 (C-12'), δ 136.6 (C-13'), δ 132.7 (C-14'), and δ 130.2 (C-15'); hydroxyl attached carbon resonated at δ 66.0 (C-3) and δ 65.2 (C-3'); methyl carbons were detected at δ 24.4 (C-16), δ 29.6 (C-17), δ 22.8 (C-18), δ 13.2 (C-19), δ 12.8 (C-20), δ 28.8 (C-16$'$), δ 30.3 (C-17$'$), δ 21.7 (C-18$'$), and δ 12.9 (C-19$'$ & C-20$'$); and methylene carbons resonated at δ 44.7 (C-2), δ 48.5 (C-2$'$), and δ 42.6 (C-4$'$). Both ^{1}H and ^{13}C NMR values were in agreement with published values [26].

Common plant sterols like β-sitosterol and stigmasterol are important in cellular and developmental mechanisms in plants [28]. In therapeutic treatment via dietary options, food products supplemented with plant sterols helped in the reduction of plasma cholesterol and the risk of atherosclerosis [29]. However, the cholesterol lowering effect may not be attributed to the inhibition via pancreatic lipase since the PPL inhibition activity of both phytosterols obtained was less than 2%. Weak PPL inhibition activity of β-sitosterol and stigmasterol isolated from *Alpinia zerumbet* had also been reported by Chompoo et al. (2012) [30] with IC_{50} value of 99.99 $\pm$ 1.86 μg/mL and 125.05 $\pm$ 4.76 μg/mL, respectively, in comparison with the inhibition shown by curcumin (IC_{50} = 4.92 $\pm$ 0.21 μg/mL) and quercetin (IC_{50} = 18.60 $\pm$ 0.86 μg/mL) which were used as positive controls in their study. In our study, β-sitosterol and stigmasterol were recorded with weak PPL inhibitory activity of only 3.0 $\pm$ 0.8% and 2.7 $\pm$ 0.4% at 100 μg/mL, respectively, (i.e., 242 μM and 243 μM) in contrast with that obtained from Orlistat (34.5 $\pm$ 5.4% at 100 μg/mL), which were comparatively lower than that recorded in literature (i.e., 50% PPL inhibition at 100 μg/mL) [30]. This may be due to different experimental settings where concentrations of both subtrate and enzyme concentrations used were different in both studies.

Lutein, a member under the xanthophyll family, is the principal carotenoid in greens, leaves, and yellow flowers. The bioavailability of xanthophyll is highly dependent on the matrix due to its hydrophobicity of the long carbon skeletons, and thus dietary lipids are required to facilitate the dispersion of lutein, where similar matrix was adapted by pancreatic lipase [31]. Another study demonstrated xanthophyll ester hydrolysed by cholesteryl esterase, but not triacylglycerol lipase (pancreatic lipase), and thus ruled out the possibility of xanthophyll as a competitive substrate [32, 33]. To date, the mechanism and the inhibitory effect of xanthophyll on pancreatic lipase are still largely unknown, based on the literature findings that may lead to postulation that lutein may be a noncompetitive inhibitor by binding on the allosteric site of pancreatic lipase. Further study is thus required to fully understand the kinetic interactions between lutein and pancreatic lipase.

4. Conclusions

Bioactivity-guided isolation on hexane extract of *E. indica* has led to isolation and elucidation of potent PPL inhibitory agent lutein (3) with strong inhibitory activity of 55.98 $\pm$ 1.04%, alongside with the isolation of two other common sterols: (1) β-sitosterol and (2) stigmasterol. To date, this is the first report on the pancreatic lipase inhibitory activity of lutein.

Abbreviations

EI: *Eleusine indica*
PPL: Porcine pancreatic lipase
HPLC: High performance liquid chromatography
IR: Infrared
NMR: Nuclear magnetic resonance.

Competing Interests

The authors wish to confirm that there is no known conflict of interests associated with this publication and there has been no significant financial support for this work that could have influenced its outcome.

Acknowledgments

The authors wish to thank the Taylor's Research Grant Scheme TRGS/2/2011SOBS/012 and Postgraduate Research Scholarship Programme for financial supports.

References

[1] N. N. Finer, "Pharmacotherapy of obesity," *Best Practice & Research: Clinical Endocrinology & Metabolism*, vol. 16, no. 4, pp. 717–742, 2002.

[2] World Health Organization (WHO), *Obesity and Overweight*, 2015, http://www.who.int/mediacentre/factsheets/fs311/en/.

[3] R. B. Birari and K. K. Bhutani, "Pancreatic lipase inhibitors from natural sources: unexplored potential," *Drug Discovery Today*, vol. 12, no. 19-20, pp. 879–889, 2007.

[4] J. W. Yun, "Possible anti-obesity therapeutics from nature—a review," *Phytochemistry*, vol. 71, no. 14-15, pp. 1625–1641, 2010.

[5] R. Birari, V. Javia, and K. K. Bhutani, "Antiobesity and lipid lowering effects of *Murraya koenigii* (L.) spreng leaves extracts and mahanimbine on high fat diet induced obese rats," *Fitoterapia*, vol. 81, no. 8, pp. 1129–1133, 2010.

[6] D. J. Newman and G. M. Cragg, "Natural products as sources of new drugs over the last 25 years," *Journal of Natural Products*, vol. 70, no. 3, pp. 461–477, 2007.

[7] S.-L. Ong, S. Paneerchelvan, H.-Y. Lai, and N. K. Rao, "*In vitro* lipase inhibitory effect of thirty two selected plants in Malaysia," *Asian Journal of Pharmaceutical and Clinical Research*, vol. 7, no. 2, pp. 19–24, 2014.

[8] A. S. Al-Zubairi, A. B. Abdul, S. I. Abdelwahab, C. Y. Peng, S. Mohan, and M. M. Elhassan, "*Eleucine indica* possesses antioxidant, antibacterial and cytotoxic properties," *Evidence-Based Complementary and Alternative Medicine*, vol. 2011, Article ID 965370, 6 pages, 2011.

[9] M. H. Ricardus and T. S. Myrna, "Two new records from Lebanon: *Chamaesyce nutans* (Lag.) Small (Eiphorbiaceae) and *Eleusine indica* (L.) Gaertner (Poaceae)," *Turkish Journal of Botany*, vol. 31, pp. 341–343, 2007.

[10] A. I. Yemets, L. A. Klimkina, L. V. Tarassenko, and Y. B. Blume, "Efficient callus formation and plant regeneration of goosegrass [*Eleusine indica* (L.) Gaertn.]," *Plant Cell Reports*, vol. 21, no. 6, pp. 503–510, 2003.

[11] T. K. Lim, "Eleusine indica," in *Edible Medicinal and Non-Medicinal Plants*, pp. 228–236, Springer, Canberra, Australia, 2016.

[12] K. Julius, "A preliminary survey of traditional medicinal plants in the West Coast and Interior of Sabah," *Journal of Tropical Forest Science*, vol. 10, no. 2, pp. 271–274, 1997.

[13] M. Iqbal and C. Gnanaraj, "*Eleusine indica* L. possesses antioxidant activity and precludes carbon tetrachloride (CCl_4)-mediated oxidative hepatic damage in rats," *Environmental Health and Preventive Medicine*, vol. 17, no. 4, pp. 307–315, 2012.

[14] J. E. Okokon, C. S. Odomena, I. Effiong, J. Obot, and J. A. Udobang, "Antiplasmodial and antidiabetic activities of *Eleusine indica*," *International Journal of Drug Development and Research*, vol. 2, no. 3, pp. 493–500, 2010.

[15] G. O. De Melo, M. F. Muzitano, A. Legora-Machado et al., "C-glycosylflavones from the aerial parts of *Eleusine indica* inhibit LPS-induced mouse lung inflammation," *Planta Medica*, vol. 71, no. 4, pp. 362–363, 2005.

[16] P. Hansakul, C. Ngamkitidechakul, K. Ingkaninan, S. Sireeratawong, and W. Panunto, "Apoptotic induction activity of *Dactyloctenium aegyptium* (L.) P.B. and *Eleusine indica* (L.) Gaerth. Extracts on human lung and cervical cancer cell lines," *Songklanakarin Journal of Science and Technology*, vol. 31, no. 3, pp. 273–279, 2009.

[17] I. O. Alaekwe, V. I. E. Ajiwe, A. C. Ajiwe, and G. N. Aningo, "Phytochemical and anti-microbial screening of the aerial parts of *Eleusine indica*," *International Journal of Pure & Applied Bioscience*, vol. 3, no. 1, pp. 257–264, 2015.

[18] Y. Bustanji, M. Mohammad, M. Hudaib, K. Tawaha, and I. M. Al-Masri, "Screening of some medicinal plants for their pancreatic lipase inhibitory potential," *Jordan Journal of Pharmaceutical Sciences*, vol. 4, no. 2, pp. 81–88, 2011.

[19] A. Gholamhoseinian, B. Shahouzebi, and F. Sharifi-Far, "Inhibitory effect of some plant extracts on pancreatic lipase," *International Journal of Pharmacology*, vol. 6, no. 1, pp. 18–24, 2010.

[20] Y. Gu, W. J. Hurst, D. A. Stuart, and J. D. Lambert, "Inhibition of key digestive enzymes by cocoa extracts and procyanidins," *Journal of Agricultural and Food Chemistry*, vol. 59, no. 10, pp. 5305–5311, 2011.

[21] V. S. Chaturvedula and I. Prakash, "Isolation of Stigmasterol and β-Sitosterol from the dichloromethane extract of *Rubus suavissimus*," *International Current Pharmaceutical Journal*, vol. 1, no. 9, pp. 239–242, 2012.

[22] D. R. Lide, *CRC Handbook of Chemistry and Physics*, CRC Press, Taylor & Francis, Boca Raton, Fla, USA, 88th edition, 2007.

[23] P. Acuña-Johnson and A. C. Oehlschelager, "Identification of sterols and biologically significant steroids by ultraviolet and infrared spectroscopy," in *Analysis of Sterols and Other Biologically Significant Steroids*, pp. 267–284, Academic Press, San Diego, Calif, USA, 1989.

[24] F. Jamaluddin, S. Mohamed, and Md. Nordin Lajis, "Hypoglycaemic effect of *Parkia speciosa* seeds due to the synergistic action of β-sitosterol and stigmasterol," *Food Chemistry*, vol. 49, no. 4, pp. 339–345, 1994.

[25] D. Xie, L. Wang, H. Ye, and G. Li, "Isolation and production of artemisinin and stigmasterol in hairy root cultures of *Artemisia annua*," *Plant Cell, Tissue and Organ Culture*, vol. 63, no. 2, pp. 161–166, 2000.

[26] M. A. El-Raey, G. E. Ibrahim, and O. A. Eldahshan, "Lycopene and Lutein; a review for their chemistry and medicinal uses," *Journal of Pharmacognosy and Phytochemistry*, vol. 2, no. 1, pp. 245–254, 2013.

[27] A. Z. Mercadante, A. Steck, and H. Pfander, "Carotenoids from guava (*Psidium guajava* L.): isolation and structure elucidation," *Journal of Agricultural and Food Chemistry*, vol. 47, no. 1, pp. 145–151, 1999.

[28] Y. Sheng and X.-B. Chen, "Isolation and identification of an isomer of β-sitosterol by HPLC and GC-MS," *Health*, vol. 1, no. 3, pp. 203–206, 2009.

[29] L. Calpe-Berdiel, J. C. Escolà-Gil, and F. Blanco-Vaca, "New insights into the molecular actions of plant sterols and stanols in cholesterol metabolism," *Atherosclerosis*, vol. 203, no. 1, pp. 18–31, 2009.

[30] J. Chompoo, A. Upadhyay, S. Gima, M. Fukuta, and S. Tawata, "Antiatherogenic properties of acetone extract of *Alpinia zerumbet* seeds," *Molecules*, vol. 17, no. 6, pp. 6237–6248, 2012.

[31] E. Kotake-Nara and A. Nagao, "Absorption and metabolism of xanthophylls," *Marine Drugs*, vol. 9, no. 6, pp. 1024–1037, 2011.

[32] D. E. Breithaupt, A. Alpmann, and F. Carrière, "Xanthophyll esters are hydrolysed in the presence of recombinant human pancreatic lipase," *Food Chemistry*, vol. 103, no. 2, pp. 651–656, 2007.

[33] C. Chitchumroonchokchai and M. L. Failla, "Hydrolysis of zeaxanthin esters by carboxyl ester lipase during digestion facilitates micellarization and uptake of the xanthophyll by Caco-2 human intestinal cells," *The Journal of Nutrition*, vol. 136, no. 3, pp. 588–594, 2006.

20

Formulations of Amlodipine

Muhammad Ali Sheraz, Syed Furqan Ahsan, Marium Fatima Khan, Sofia Ahmed, and Iqbal Ahmad

Baqai Institute of Pharmaceutical Sciences, Baqai Medical University, 51 Deh Tor, Toll Plaza, Super Highway, Gadap Road, Karachi 74600, Pakistan

Correspondence should be addressed to Muhammad Ali Sheraz; ali_sheraz80@hotmail.com

Academic Editor: Francisco Javier Flores-Murrieta

Amlodipine (AD) is a calcium channel blocker that is mainly used in the treatment of hypertension and angina. However, latest findings have revealed that its efficacy is not only limited to the treatment of cardiovascular diseases as it has shown to possess antioxidant activity and plays an important role in apoptosis. Therefore, it is also employed in the treatment of cerebrovascular stroke, neurodegenerative diseases, leukemia, breast cancer, and so forth either alone or in combination with other drugs. AD is a photosensitive drug and requires protection from light. A number of workers have tried to formulate various conventional and nonconventional dosage forms of AD. This review highlights all the formulations that have been developed to achieve maximum stability with the desired therapeutic action for the delivery of AD such as fast dissolving tablets, floating tablets, layered tablets, single-pill combinations, capsules, oral and transdermal films, suspensions, emulsions, mucoadhesive microspheres, gels, transdermal patches, and liposomal formulations.

1. Introduction

Amlodipine (AD) belongs to the group of calcium channel blockers. The newer calcium channel blockers such as dihydropyridines, AD, felodipine, and nisoldipine have improved vascular selectivity and longer durations of action. They bind to target receptors in a slow and sustained pattern producing a smooth onset of action with a 24 h control of blood pressure. Once daily dosing of these longer acting calcium channel blockers improves patient compliance and is associated with minimum encounter of side effects. The calcium channel blockers are suitable for a wide range of hypertensive patients including the elderly, black, and those with concomitant diseases that preclude the use of other antihypertensives [1].

AD is commonly used in the treatment of heart diseases like angina and hypertension [2]. Efforts have been made to prepare various dosage forms of AD to improve its efficacy and stability. Therefore, a comprehensive review of various formulations of AD reported in the literature has been made which would be helpful for pharmaceutical scientists and formulators in identifying and developing the most suitable dosage form of AD.

2. Formulations of AD

Formulations of AD may contain its different salts such as besylate, mesylate, or maleate. These salts are considered interchangeably and the strength of the dosage form is determined in terms of the parent molecule, that is, AD [2]. Amlodipine besylate (ADB) is the most commonly used derivative of AD which is used for the preparation of its various dosage forms. The salts of AD are known to affect the physicochemical properties of the drug as the besylate salt is known to have better water solubility than AD alone. Some newer salts of AD such as adipate [3], camsylate [4], and nicotinate [5] were developed and compared with ADB for their pharmacokinetics. It was found that all newer salts were bioequivalent and showed similar pharmacokinetic characteristics to those of ADB. ADB and AD camsylate are known to exert similar neuroprotective effects on primary cultured cortical neuronal cells by reducing oxidative stress, enhancing survival signals, and inhibiting death signals [6]. Different types of formulations of AD have been reported by various workers which are presented as follows.

2.1. Tablets. AD is commercially available in tablet dosage form in once daily doses of 5 and 10 mg. It is usually given orally in the besylate form. A 6.9 mg of ADB is equivalent to 5 mg of AD. It is well absorbed after oral administration and has a bioavailability of around 60–65% [7]. A racemate and *S*-enantiomer of ADB (levamlodipine besylate) were prepared and compared with each other. It was found that the two compounds have different melting points, solubility, dissolution rate, crystal morphology, particle size distribution, and hygroscopicity. The melting point of *S*-enantiomer was lower as compared to the racemate form which was due to its better water solubility and intrinsic dissolution property [8]. Furthermore, it has been reported that the calcium channel blocking activity of AD is restricted to its *S*-enantiomer, that is, *S*-AD [9, 10], while the other form, that is, *R*-AD exhibits a 1000-fold lower activity [10, 11]. It is interesting to note that AD is therapeutically used as a racemic mixture and both *S*- and *R*-forms are available in 1:1 ratio in conventional formulations. Therefore, a tablet formulation containing only *S*-form was compared with the conventional tablets of AD. Both formulations were found to be bioequivalent and well tolerated and no difference was observed in terms of pharmacodynamic profiles and clinical effects. Both formulations were found to be well tolerated and no serious adverse effects were noted [10]. Similarly, a tablet formulation of *S*-enantiomer of ADB was prepared with compatible excipients. The formulation was optimized using full factorial design and was found within limits when compared to the commercial brands of ADB in terms of appearance, dissolution, and stability [8]. On the contrary, an in vitro study was performed to evaluate the ability of AD and its enantiomers (*S*- and *R*-) to release nitric oxide in isolated coronary microvessels and to regulate tissue oxygen consumption via nitric oxide release. It was found that AD and its *R*-form released nitric oxide in a concentration dependent manner and reduced oxygen consumption in canine cardiac tissues while no effect was observed by the *S*-form at any concentration in either case [11].

Since AD is a photosensitive drug, an attempt has been made to formulate tablets by liquisolid technique in order to provide photoprotection to the active drug. The tablets were prepared using propylene glycol as solvent in 1:1 ratio with AD, avicel PH102 as carrier, amorphous silicon (nanometer size), and titanium dioxide either alone or in combination as coating agents. These tablets were exposed to different radiations such as visible, UVA, and UVB for 8 h to determine the photoprotective effect of the coating material. The results indicated that liquisolid technique not only provided photoprotection but also improved the dissolution rate of AD. Therefore, this technique can be used as an alternative to conventional coating methods particularly in formulations containing photosensitive drugs [12].

2.1.1. Fast Dissolving/Orodispersible Tablets. In addition to the presently marketed AD tablets and capsules, the novel fast dissolving tablets (also known as orodispersible, fast melting, fast dispersing, rapid dissolve, rapid melt, and/or quick disintegrating tablet formulations) offer an option to the patients who have difficulty in swallowing (i.e., dysphagia). It is a convenient and modest method of administration without the need of water [13, 14] with good palatability [15, 16]. The dispersible tablets of ADB are comparatively bioequivalent to conventional tablets [17]. The main drawback of using orally disintegrating or crushed tablets of AD is their bitter taste [16, 18, 19] and, therefore, taste masking of such dosage forms is very important to increase palatability [15].

The fast dissolving oral ADB tablets were prepared by direct compression method using croscarmellose (Ac-Di-Sol), crospovidone (Kollidon CL), and sodium starch glycolate as superdisintegrants in varying concentrations of 2, 4, and 6%. Among the three disintegrants, croscarmellose in 6% concentration was found to be the most rapid by causing disintegration of the tablets within 11 s [20]. On the contrary, sodium starch glycolate and croscarmellose showed comparatively better results among the three disintegrants when used in the concentrations of 5–10% [21]. In another study, fast dissolving tablets of ADB were prepared by incorporating crospovidone and sodium starch glycolate either alone or in combination. The tablets prepared using a combination of both superdisintegrants were found to have most rapid disintegration and highest dissolution rate as compared to formulations containing a single superdisintegrants [22]. Therefore, it has been recommended to use a combination of superdisintegrants for the formulation of fast dissolving tablets of ADB [22, 23]. The solubility and dissolution of ADB was reported to increase when its solid dispersion was prepared with crospovidone by solvent evaporation method and then the mouth dissolving tablets were manufactured in 1:4 ratio [24]. The orodispersible tablets of AD are known to provide equivalent systemic effect to that of the conventional AD tablets or capsules when administered with or without water [25].

The dissolution of ADB was also enhanced when *Plantago ovata* mucilage (Ispaghol) was used as a natural superdisintegrant. The fast dissolving tablets were prepared by direct compression method and the concentration of the mucilage was found to be a key factor in affecting the rate of disintegration because a decrease in time with an increase in the concentration of the superdisintegrant has been noted [26]. Similarly, fenugreek seed mucilage and *Ocimum basilicum* (basil) gum were also employed as natural superdisintegrants in the formulation of fast dissolving tablets of ADB. The tablets were prepared by direct compression method using either of the superdisintegrants in varying concentrations (i.e., 2–10 mg). It was observed that the formulations containing the highest amount of the disintegrant showed the fastest disintegration due to rapid wetting, dispersion, and water-absorption ratio. Moreover, the tablets were also found stable for three months when stored at $25 \pm 20°C/60 \pm 5\%$ RH and $40 \pm 20°C/75 \pm 5\%$ RH [27].

2.1.2. Sustained Release Floating Tablets. Floating drug delivery systems or hydrodynamically balanced systems are those that have lower bulk density than the gastric fluids. Due to this property the tablet remains buoyant for prolonged period of time and thus releases the drug slowly at a desired rate. However, weight measurements and swelling properties are other two important parameters required for the buoyant capabilities of the tablets. Polymers play an important role in controlling the release of the drug in such systems. Sometimes an effervescent component is also added that liberates CO_2 when it comes in contact with the acidic gastric fluids. The liberated gas is entrapped in the gellified hydrocolloid and produces an upward motion causing floating of the tablet [28].

Pare et al. [29] formulated various floating effervescent tablets of ADB and studied their different physicochemical properties including the release of drug from its dosage form. The tablets were prepared by direct compression method using different hydrophilic (hydroxypropyl methylcellulose) and hydrophobic (Carbopol 934P) polymers and effervescing agents such as sodium bicarbonate and citric acid. The formulated tablets were compared with the commercial dosage forms and it was observed that their release was twice (i.e., 24 h) delayed to those of the marketed products (i.e., 12 h) [29].

2.1.3. Layered Tablets. Formulation of layered tablets has gained considerable popularity due to their certain advantages over conventional monolayer tablets. These advantages may include the use of two active drugs at the same time, formulation of two chemically incompatible substances in bilayer form, increased efficacy in case of combining two drugs with synergistic effect, use of two different release profile forms (quick and delayed release) of a single active drug, and better patient compliance due to decreased dosing burden [30, 31].

Layered tablets of ADB and atenolol were prepared as either monolayer (mixed matrix) or bilayer using similar excipients and processing technique. The bilayered tablet formulation was found to be more stable than the monolayered type. The packaging material also affected the stability of the formulations and it was observed that the stability of the tablets was increased when packed in aluminium strips compared to PVC blisters. In either case degradation in ADB was prominent whereas no decline in content was noted for atenolol [32]. In another study, an attempt was made to prepare bilayered effervescent floating tablets of ADB and hydrochlorothiazide by direct compression using various concentrations of polymers (various grades of hydroxypropyl methylcellulose such as K4M, K15M, K100M, and polyvinylpyrrolidone PVP K30). The tablets were formulated in a way to release ADB immediately in gas layer and hydrochlorothiazide with a sustained action. ADB was released more than 85% within 15 min while hydrochlorothiazide was released over a period of around 8 h [33]. Similarly, a bilayer combination of ADB with metoprolol succinate has also been reported with immediate and sustained release of each drug. The tablets were prepared by direct compression using sodium starch glycolate and pregelatinized starch as superdisintegrants and hydroxypropyl methylcellulose (K4M and K100) for sustained action. The tablets showed a first-order release of about 98% for ADB at 30 min and around 90% for metoprolol succinate in 20 h. The stability studies performed for blister packed tablets at 25°C/60% RH and 40°C/75% RH for three months were also found satisfactory [34].

2.1.4. Single-Pill (Fixed-Dose) Combinations. Film coated immediate release tablets of the combination of valsartan and AD were formulated and evaluated for their in vivo release profile and stability. The core tablets of the combination were prepared by dry granulation and the film coating was performed using Opadry aqueous coating dispersion. It was found that the release of each drug from the combination tablet meets the FDA guidelines for bioequivalence studies. The stability of the formulated tablets was evaluated according to the guideline of ICH. The film coated tablets were found stable both on long term (12 months) and accelerated stability studies [35]. Similarly, a study was performed to compare the pharmacokinetic profile of a combination of AD (5 mg) and benazepril (10 mg) in tablets and capsules. The results indicated both dosage forms containing the combination of actives to be bioequivalent and well tolerated [36].

A large number of pills for the treatment of a single or multiple diseases are a major source of noncompliance in patients. Therefore, a single-pill or fixed-dose combination therapy is often preferred to reduce the polypharmacy burden and improve patients' compliance [37, 38]. A number of workers have employed AD in combination with other drugs as a single-pill and used it clinically with reasonable success. Not much information regarding the formulations is available as the studies are more clinically oriented and the combinations have been discussed with respect to their clinical outcomes only in majority of the cases. The drugs most commonly employed in combination with AD (i.e., single drug + AD combination) include aliskiren [39–41], atorvastatin [42–52], azilsartan [53], benazepril [54, 55], fimasartan [56], indapamide [57, 58], irbesartan [59], olmesartan (olmesartan medoxomil) [39, 60–67], perindopril [68–72], telmisartan [73–77], and valsartan [70, 71, 78–97].

Some workers have tried triple combinations in a single pill and used it clinically, that is, two different drugs + AD. The drug combinations with AD include aliskiren and hydrochlorothiazide [98, 99], olmesartan and hydrochlorothiazide [67, 100–102], and valsartan and hydrochlorothiazide [88, 95, 101–103].

2.2. Capsules. Solid dispersion of drugs may provide fast dissolution but requires some time to initiate its release. For the drugs used in emergency conditions, like antihypertensive drugs, a lag time of almost zero is desirable. In order to reduce the lag time in drug release and enhance the dissolution, semisolid matrix-filled hard gelatin capsules of ADB were prepared by Tyagi et al. [104]. The solid dispersions of ADB were prepared through fusion method using varying concentrations of Poloxamer 407 and Plasdone S630. The solid dispersion that showed better dissolution profile was selected for the preparation of semisolid matrix. The optimized solid dispersion of ADB was mixed with Gelucire 44/14 and polyethylene glycol (PEG) 400 to make it semisolid and further mixed with PEG 6000 to suspend the particles in the matrix. The suspended particles were then transferred into hard gelatin capsules. Making semisolid matrix resulted in a threefold decrease in the lag time of ADB release as compared to its amorphous solid dispersions indicating that this approach can be used for the rapid therapeutic effect of the drug. The accelerated stability studies of these capsules revealed that the preparations were stable for at least three months when stored at $40 \pm 2°C$ and $75 \pm 5\%$ RH [104].

Asymmetric membrane capsules for simultaneous delivery of ADB and atenolol were formulated by dip coating (wet phase inversion) method using cellulose acetate as polymer in 10% concentration. Each active ingredient was mixed separately with the osmotic agents, that is, potassium chloride and citric acid monohydrate. Atenolol (50 mg) was filled manually in the body while ADB (5 mg) in the cap. Compartments in the capsules were formed by using paraffin wax plug. A layer of the polymer was applied over it to avoid any leakage from each compartment followed by outer sealing of the capsules with a solution (10% w/v cellulose acetate in a mixture of acetone and alcohol). The release data showed around 55% release of ADB at 12 h from capsules containing no osmotic agent while a 100% release was noted at 6 h for capsules containing 35 mg of citric acid and 20 mg of potassium chloride. In the latter case, the caps of the capsules were modified by increasing concentration of the polymer to 15%, which resulted in a sustained release of ADB (~95%) for 13 h indicating the role of the polymer in slowing down the disintegration of the capsules cap. A zero-order release was observed in the majority of cases. All capsules were found to be stable for three months when stored either in sealed or unsealed containers at $40 \pm 2.0°C/75 \pm 5\%$ RH [105].

2.3. Oral Films.
The in vitro disintegration studies for fast disintegrating films of ADB have been conducted by Shelke et al. [106] through the solvent casting technique. Sodium alginate was used as a film polymer and sodium starch glycolate as disintegrant in nine different concentrations. The study was carried out at pH 6.2 and it was observed that the sodium alginate film on the tablet started to disintegrate in 30 s and almost 75–80% of the drug was released after 6 min in all the formulations [106].

2.4. Suspensions.
In addition to many other formulations the extemporaneous suspensions of ADB (1 mg/mL) have also been prepared from the commercially available oral tablets. One of the suspensions was made by using methylcellulose (1%) in syrup and the other using a 1 : 1 mixture of commercially available extemporaneous syrup vehicles, Ora-Plus and Ora-Sweet. The suspensions were stored in plastic bottles at room (25°C) and refrigerated (5°C) temperatures and were analyzed for their physical and chemical stability for a period of three months. The results revealed that suspensions kept under refrigerator were more stable physically and chemically to those stored at room temperature. The assay results indicated that the suspensions stored in a refrigerator retained >90% of the drug for 91 days compared to only 56 days for the same concentration in the samples stored at room temperature. Moreover, a slight variation in pH was also observed in the suspensions containing methylcellulose and kept at room temperature. On the basis of these findings, it was suggested to use these suspensions as per body weight in pediatrics as well as in elderly patients who have difficulty in swallowing [107]. No significant difference in bioavailability has been reported between suspensions prepared from crushed tablets and oral tablets of AD when studied in healthy volunteers. However, the suspension was found to be very unpalatable [108].

A similar suspension formulation has also been used successfully by Rivero et al. [109] in the treatment of a 5 year old girl who developed hypertension due to a consequence of other complications. She was initially treated with nifedipine and captopril but due to poor prognosis was shifted to AD and enalapril, each in an oral dose of 2.5 mg/day that showed better therapeutic effect. The tablets for adults are available in a dose of 5 and 10 mg, therefore, the prescribed dose was administered in the form of a suspension in a similar dose of 1 mg/mL as reported by Nahata et al. [107] using a mixture of Ora-Plus and Ora-Sweet [109].

2.5. Nanoemulsions.
Targeted drug delivery system is gaining popularity day by day which has encouraged researchers towards the development of nanopreparations. Various oil-in-water nanoemulsions of AD were prepared by using different concentrations of oleic acid (oil phase), tween 20 (surfactant), Transcutol P (cosurfactant), and constructing pseudoternary phase diagrams. The transdermal effect of nanoemulsions on rat's skin was determined using Franz diffusion cell. The optimum concentration of excipients that showed highest rate of permeation in the formulation was 2% for oil, 20% for surfactant, and 10% for cosurfactant. The rate of permeation was found to be affected inversely with the excipient concentrations as the highest rate was achieved with the lowest oil and surfactants concentrations. The results showed a positive response in transdermal drug delivery and proved that the nanoemulsion is a potential vehicle for enhancing skin permeation of AD through transdermal preparations [110].

Similarly, oral nanoemulsions of ADB were prepared by spontaneous emulsification method with the purpose of obtaining increased bioavailability and targeted drug delivery to the site of action. Partition coefficient, droplet size, and in vitro release of drug were analyzed in nanoemulsions following construction of pseudoternary phase diagrams. The release of ADB from oral nanoemulsions was found to be much higher than those of the tablets available in the market. The oral administration of radiolabeled formulations (^{99m}Tc-labeled) in mice indicated about three times higher efficacy of nanoemulsions as compared to ADB suspensions. The higher bioavailability and biodistribution of ADB from nanoemulsions were due to better uptake of the drug in all organs, thus indicating the advantage of using nanoemulsions as carriers for the delivery of AD [111].

Another novel approach employed to enhance the bioavailability and photostability of AD was the preparation of redispersible dry emulsions by spray drying technique as oil-in-water emulsions. The redispersion of the dried emulsion in distilled water formed the emulsion but with a larger particle size which was 1.4-fold higher than the original emulsion (i.e., $0.24 \pm 0.30 \mu$ versus $0.17 \pm 0.02 \mu$). However, no further change in the droplet size of dry emulsions was observed during six months of storage at room temperature.

The dried emulsions showed a significant photoprotection of AD as only 6% of the drug was degraded in comparison to 70% in ethanolic solution and 23% as dry powder when exposed to UV irradiation for 12 h. Similarly, the in vitro release of dried emulsions (66%) was also found to be higher than that of the powder form (48%) at 60 min time interval with a 2.6–2.9-fold higher bioavailability as observed in rats after oral administration. All these results indicated that the dried emulsions of AD could be used as an effective alternative drug delivery system [112].

2.6. Mucoadhesive Microspheres for Nasal Delivery. Local or systemic delivery of drugs through nasal route has been used conventionally for the treatment of different local diseases. In the recent past, this route has gained considerable popularity because of its reliability for the delivery of drugs that are ineffective from oral route due to metabolism in the gastrointestinal tract [113, 114]. The recent developments and the factors affecting nasal drug delivery systems have been reviewed by Mainardes et al. [113] and Jadhav et al. [114]. Nasal delivery of AD as mucoadhesive microspheres is another field of interest for pharmaceutical scientists as some interesting progress has been made in this regard. AD loaded microspheres are known to provide highest photostability as compared to other dosage forms including ethanolic solutions, powder, tablets, liposomes, and cyclodextrin complexes [115].

A study has been performed in which mucoadhesive chitosan microspheres of ADB were prepared by simple emulsification cross-linking using glutaraldehyde as cross-linking agent. Various formulation parameters such as drug-polymer ratio (1:1, 1:2, 1:3, 1:4, and 1:5), stabilizing agent concentration (0.1, 0.2, and 0.3% w/v), and stirring rate (600 and 1200 rpm) were studied. It was observed that the in vitro mucoadhesive property and size of the microspheres increased from 28 μ to 52 μ with an increase in chitosan concentration which could be due to the amino groups available for binding with the sialic acid residues in mucus layer and cross-linking of the polymer. On the contrary, the release of ADB was slowed down with an increase in polymer concentration from about 85% to 76% after 8 h due to matrix formation. Increase in the stirring rate reduced the median particle size diameter of the microspheres from ~99 μ to 36 μ. The microspheres were found to be spherical with smooth surface without any aggregation and were, therefore, suggested as suitable for nasal administration [116].

Similarly, hydroxypropyl guar (HPG) microspheres containing ADB were formulated for nasal administration by water-in-oil emulsification solvent evaporation technique in order to investigate their suitability as nasal drug delivery system. The formulation variables which could affect the preparation of the microspheres including drug-polymer (0.5:3, 1:3, 1.5:3, and 2:3), polymer-drug (1:1, 2:1, 3:1, and 4:1), and emulsifier (0.2, 0.3, 0.4, and 0.5% w/v) concentrations, temperature (60, 70, 80, and 90°C), and agitation speed (1400, 1600, 1800, and 2000 rpm) were also studied. It was observed that an increase in emulsifier concentration, temperature, and agitation speed resulted in a decrease of particle size from about 132 μ to 19 μ. The microspheres were found to be spherical and free flowing and showed good

mucoadhesive and swelling properties. ADB was released from microspheres with a sustained action of over 8 h. The drug entrapment efficiency of the microspheres was found to be affected by drug and polymer concentrations. An increase in the HPG concentration resulted in higher ADB entrapment with an increase in the size of the microspheres. Similarly, an increase in the drug concentration also resulted in an increased particle size but the drug entrapment was found to decrease. The formulations were also found to be stable at room (25 ± 2°C/60 ± 5% RH), refrigeration (5 ± 3°C), and accelerated (40 ± 2°C/75 ± 5% RH) temperatures. No significant changes were observed at the end of 90 days indicating the suitability of ADB loaded microspheres for nasal administration [117].

2.7. Topical Formulations

2.7.1. Gels. Gel formulations containing dexamethasone (0.3%) and ADB (0.5%) have been formulated using carboxymethyl cellulose sodium as gelling agent, azone (laurocapram) as penetration enhancer, and propylene glycol as solvent and humectant. The gels were studied for drug penetration within flap tissues through excised rat skin. It was observed that the compound gel containing both drugs can penetrate into skin tissue which could significantly increase the survival of ischemic skin flap [118]. The gels of ADB have also been used for the treatment of feline hypertension (i.e., in cats). Gels were prepared in a commercially available vehicle, Lipoderm, which contains a proprietary liposomal component and has a smooth creamy texture and does not separate on refrigeration [119].

ADB loaded nanostructured lipid carrier gels or nanogels for intranasal delivery have been prepared by emulsion solvent diffusion and evaporation method followed by ultrasonication. Various properties of the nanogels including zeta potential, particle size, and entrapment efficiency were investigated. The gels were also characterized for drug content, pH, and in vitro and ex vivo drug diffusion. All these studies showed that the nanogels of ADB have good sustained action as compared to the pure drug solution and nanostructured lipid carrier dispersion and, therefore, can be used for intranasal delivery of ADB [120].

2.7.2. Transdermal Patches and Films. Drug-in-adhesive transdermal patches have been prepared using *S*-amlodipine (*S*-AD) free base (i.e., levamlodipine) and studied for in vitro and in vivo activity in rats after optimization of the formulation parameters. The *S*-AD (4%) loaded patches were prepared using appropriate amounts of pressure-sensitive adhesive. Penetration enhancers were added to acetic ether followed by agitation at room temperature and then applied to the surface of a fluoropolymer-treated polyester release liner (ScotchPak® 1022). The mixture was than subjected to drying, cutting, and covering with a polyester backing membrane (ScotchPak 9726) followed by storage in an aluminium-plastic membrane. The patches were applied transdermally to the rats and the plasma level of *S*-AD was measured at different time intervals. It was observed that the patches can maintain drug plasma level for up to 72 h without any first pass effect and hence can be used as an effective alternative dosage form in the treatment of hypertension [121].

In another study, an attempt was made to formulate various ADB (10%) loaded films by solvent evaporation technique using different polymers such as polycaprolactone, ethylcellulose, polylactic acid, and polyhydroxyethyl methacrylate. Polyethylene glycol 400 was used as a plasticizer in a 2% concentration in each formulation. The prepared films were evaluated for parameters such as weight variation, thickness, drug content, and in vitro permeation. All films showed good physicochemical performance. The in vitro release studies indicated sustained release of ADB from all films over a period of 24 h with the slowest rate in films prepared from polyhydroxyethyl methacrylate (i.e., 79%) [122].

2.8. Liposomal Formulations. Liposomes are spherical vesicles with at least a single lipid bilayer that are used to deliver a drug to a specific site or target in the body and to overcome any stability or toxicity related problems of the drug. Liposomes have gained tremendous popularity due to their ability of delivering both lipophilic and hydrophilic drugs [115]. AD is a lipophilic drug and is known to have better penetration ability into liposomal vesicles than other cardiovascular agents such as mexiletine and indapamide [123].

Since AD is sensitive to light, it requires protection to avoid degradation. To overcome this problem, a liposomal preparation of AD was prepared and evaluated for its photostability. It was observed that an inclusion complex between the liposome and drug was formed that resulted in a significant reduction in the photodegradation of AD which was higher than some other systems like solution and powder. The degradation time of 10% drug ($t_{0.1}$) was found to be about 220 min which was better than the ethanolic solutions ($t_{0.1}$ = ~10 min) and powder form of AD ($t_{0.1}$ = 111 min) [115].

AD possesses antioxidant properties and plays an important role in the apoptosis [124–129]. Due to this activity, targeted delivery of AD in liposomal preparations, either alone or in combination with other drugs, has been employed by various workers with significant success [124, 125, 129].

3. Conclusion

For an effective treatment, it is of utmost importance to deliver the drug in a suitable dosage form through an appropriate route. A dosage form must be designed in a way that not only provides stability to the formulation ingredients but also gives optimum therapeutic effect. Different formulations of AD have been developed and the majority of these have shown acceptable stability. However, further studies regarding their in vivo efficacy and more innovations in AD delivery systems would definitely help in the effective treatment of various diseases. Availability of different dosage forms of AD would also provide a choice to physicians and pharmacists to select the most appropriate delivery system based on the patient's condition.

Competing Interests

There is no conflict of interests regarding the publication of this paper.

References

[1] J. L. Palma-Gámiz, "High blood pressure and calcium antagonism," *Cardiology*, vol. 88, no. 1, pp. 39–46, 1997.

[2] *British National Formulary 61*, BMJ Group and RPS Publishing, London, UK, 2011.

[3] H.-Y. Lee, H.-J. Kang, B.-K. Koo et al., "Clinic blood pressure responses to two amlodipine salt formulations, adipate and besylate, in adult Korean patients with mild to moderate hypertension: a multicenter, randomized, double-blind, parallel-group, 8-week comparison," *Clinical Therapeutics*, vol. 27, no. 6, pp. 728–739, 2005.

[4] J.-Y. Park, K.-A. Kim, G.-S. Lee et al., "Randomized, open-label, two-period crossover comparison of the pharmacokinetic and pharmacodynamic properties of two amlodipine formulations in healthy adult male Korean subjects," *Clinical Therapeutics*, vol. 26, no. 5, pp. 715–723, 2004.

[5] J.-Y. Park, K.-A. Kim, P.-W. Park et al., "Comparative pharmacokinetic and pharmacodynamic characteristics of amlodipine besylate and amlodipine nicotinate in healthy subjects," *International Journal of Clinical Pharmacology and Therapeutics*, vol. 44, no. 12, pp. 641–647, 2006.

[6] Y. J. Lee, H.-H. Park, S.-H. Koh, N.-Y. Choi, and K.-Y. Lee, "Amlodipine besylate and amlodipine camsylate prevent cortical neuronal cell death induced by oxidative stress," *Journal of Neurochemistry*, vol. 119, no. 6, pp. 1262–1270, 2011.

[7] S. C. Sweetman, *Martindale: The Complete Drug Reference*, Royal Pharmaceutical Society, London, UK, 36th edition, 2009.

[8] Š. Hadžidedić, A. Uzunović, S. Šehić Jazić, and S. Kocova El-Arini, "The impact of chirality on the development of robust and stable tablet formulation of (S-) amlodipine besylate," *Pharmaceutical Development and Technology*, vol. 19, no. 8, pp. 930–941, 2014.

[9] S. Goldmann, J. Stoltefuss, and L. Born, "Determination of the absolute configuration of the active amlodipine enantiomer as (-)-S: a correction," *Journal of Medicinal Chemistry*, vol. 35, no. 18, pp. 3341–3344, 1992.

[10] J.-Y. Park, K.-A. Kim, P.-W. Park et al., "Pharmacokinetic and pharmacodynamic characteristics of a new S-amlodipine formulation in healthy Korean male subjects: a randomized, open-label, two-period, comparative, crossover study," *Clinical Therapeutics*, vol. 28, no. 11, pp. 1837–1847, 2006.

[11] X.-P. Zhang, E. L. Kit, S. Mital, S. Chahwala, and T. H. Hintze, "Paradoxical release of nitric oxide by an L-type calcium channel antagonist, the R+ enantiomer of amlodipine," *Journal of Cardiovascular Pharmacology*, vol. 39, no. 2, pp. 208–214, 2002.

[12] A. Khames, "Liquisolid technique: a promising alternative to conventional coating for improvement of drug photostability in solid dosage forms," *Expert Opinion on Drug Delivery*, vol. 10, no. 10, pp. 1335–1343, 2013.

[13] Y. Fu, S. Yang, S. H. Jeong, S. Kimura, and K. Park, "Orally fast disintegrating tablets: developments, technologies, taste-masking and clinical studies," *Critical Reviews in Therapeutic Drug Carrier Systems*, vol. 21, no. 6, pp. 433–475, 2004.

[14] V. Parkash, S. Maan, Deepika, S. Yadav, H. Hemlata, and V. Jogpal, "Fast disintegrating tablets: opportunity in drug delivery system," *Journal of Advanced Pharmaceutical Technology and Research*, vol. 2, no. 4, pp. 223–235, 2011.

[15] M. Fukui-Soubou, H. Terashima, K. Kawashima, O. Utsunomiya, and T. Terada, "Efficacy, safety, and palatability

of RACTAB® formulation amlodipine orally disintegrating tablets," *Drugs in R & D*, vol. 11, no. 4, pp. 327–336, 2011.

[16] T. Uchida, M. Yoshida, M. Hazekawa et al., "Evaluation of palatability of 10 commercial amlodipine orally disintegrating tablets by gustatory sensation testing, OD-mate as a new disintegration apparatus and the artificial taste sensor," *Journal of Pharmacy and Pharmacology*, vol. 65, no. 9, pp. 1312–1320, 2013.

[17] Y. Liu, J. Jia, G. Liu et al., "Pharmacokinetics and bioequivalence evaluation of two formulations of 10-mg amlodipine besylate: an open-label, single-dose, randomized, two-way crossover study in healthy chinese male volunteers," *Clinical Therapeutics*, vol. 31, no. 4, pp. 777–783, 2009.

[18] A. Ferrarini, A. A. Bianchetti, E. F. Fossali et al., "What can we do to make antihypertensive medications taste better for children?" *International Journal of Pharmaceutics*, vol. 457, no. 1, pp. 333–336, 2013.

[19] G. Milani, M. Ragazzi, G. D. Simonetti et al., "Superior palatability of crushed lercanidipine compared with amlodipine among children," *British Journal of Clinical Pharmacology*, vol. 69, no. 2, pp. 204–206, 2010.

[20] V. Bhardwaj, M. Bansal, and P. K. Sharma, "Formulation and evaluation of fast dissolving tablets of amlodipine besylate using different super disintegrants and camphor as sublimating agent," *American-Eurasian Journal of Scientific Research*, vol. 5, pp. 264–269, 2010.

[21] G. S. Krushnan, R. M. Britto, J. Perianayagam et al., "Formulation and evaluation of oro dispersible tablets of amlodipine besylate," *Indian Journal of Research in Pharmacy and Biotechnology*, vol. 1, pp. 472–477, 2013.

[22] B. S. Raj, I. S. R. Punitha, and S. Dube, "Formulation and characterization of fast disintegrating tablets of amlodipine using superdisintegrants," *Journal of Applied Pharmaceutical Science*, vol. 2, no. 8, pp. 118–123, 2012.

[23] P. S. Mohanachandran, P. R. Krishna Mohan, S. Fels, K. B. Bini, B. Beenu, and K. K. Shalina, "Formulation and evaluation of mouth dispersible tablets of amlodipine besylate," *International Journal of Applied Pharmaceutics*, vol. 2, no. 3, pp. 1–6, 2010.

[24] R. Dahima, A. Pachori, and S. Netam, "Formulation and evaluation of mouth dissolving tablet containing amlodipine besylate solid dispersion," *International Journal of ChemTech Research*, vol. 2, no. 1, pp. 706–715, 2010.

[25] V. Mascoli, U. Kuruganti, A. T. Bapuji, R. Wang, and B. Damle, "Pharmacokinetics of a novel orodispersible tablet of amlodipine in healthy subjects," *Journal of Bioequivalence and Bioavailability*, vol. 5, no. 2, pp. 76–79, 2013.

[26] G. Gokul Ghenge, S. D. Pande, A. Ahmad, L. Jejurkar, and T. Birari, "Development and characterisation of fast disintegrating tablet of amlodipine besylate using mucilage of plantago ovata as a natural superdisintegrant," *International Journal of PharmTech Research*, vol. 3, no. 2, pp. 938–945, 2011.

[27] S. Sukhavasi and V. S. Kishore, "Formulation and evaluation of fast dissolving tablets of amlodipine besylate by using Fenugreek seed mucilage and *Ocimum basilicum* gum," *International Current Pharmaceutical Journal*, vol. 1, no. 9, pp. 243–249, 2012.

[28] B. N. Singh and K. H. Kim, "Floating drug delivery systems: an approach to oral controlled drug delivery via gastric retention," *Journal of Controlled Release*, vol. 63, no. 3, pp. 235–259, 2000.

[29] A. Pare, S. K. Yadav, and U. K. Patil, "Formulation and evaluation of effervescent floating tablet of amlodipine besylate," *Research Journal of Pharmacy and Technology*, vol. 1, pp. 526–530, 2008.

[30] A. Abebe, I. Akseli, O. Sprockel, N. Kottala, and A. M. Cuitiño, "Review of bilayer tablet technology," *International Journal of Pharmaceutics*, vol. 461, no. 1-2, pp. 549–558, 2014.

[31] I. Akseli, A. Abebe, O. Sprockel, and A. M. Cuitiño, "Mechanistic characterization of bilayer tablet formulations," *Powder Technology*, vol. 236, pp. 30–36, 2013.

[32] S. Aryal and N. Škalko-Basnet, "Stability of amlodipine besylate and atenolol in multi-component tablets of mono-layer and bilayer types," *Acta Pharmaceutica*, vol. 58, no. 3, pp. 299–308, 2008.

[33] G. Hariharan, M. Sudhakar, and R. Vinay, "Development and optimization of bilayer hydrodyanamically balanced system of Amlodipine Besylate immediate release and Hydrochlorothiazide controlled release," *Asian Journal of Pharmaceutical and Clinical Research*, vol. 6, no. 3, pp. 243–246, 2013.

[34] S. Jayaprakash, S. M. Halith, K. Pillai, P. Balasubramaniyam, U. M. Firthouse, and M. Boopathi, "Formulation and evaluation of bilayer tablets of amlodipine besilate and metprolol succinate," *Der Pharmacia Lettre*, vol. 3, no. 4, pp. 143–154, 2011.

[35] A. N. Zaid, S. Natur, A. Qaddomi et al., "Formulation and bioequivalence of two valsartan/amlodipine immediate release tablets after a single oral administration," *Pakistan Journal of Pharmaceutical Sciences*, vol. 27, no. 4, pp. 755–762, 2014.

[36] K.-L. Chien, C.-L. Chao, and T.-C. Su, "Bioavailability study of fixed-dose tablet versus capsule formulation of amlodipine plus benazepril: a randomized, single-dose, two-sequence, two-period, open-label, crossover study in healthy volunteers," *Current Therapeutic Research—Clinical and Experimental*, vol. 66, no. 2, pp. 69–79, 2005.

[37] B. Farrell, V. French Merkley, and N. Ingar, "Reducing pill burden and helping with medication awareness to improve adherence," *Canadian Pharmacists Journal*, vol. 146, no. 5, pp. 262–269, 2013.

[38] A. Hagendorff, S. Freytag, A. Müller, and S. Klebs, "Pill burden in hypertensive patients treated with single-pill combination therapy—an observational study," *Advances in Therapy*, vol. 30, no. 4, pp. 406–419, 2013.

[39] C. Axthelm, C. Sieder, F. Meister, and E. Kaiser, "Efficacy and tolerability of the single-pill combination of aliskiren 300 mg/amlodipine 10 mg in hypertensive patients not controlled by olmesartan 40 mg/amlodipine 10 mg," *Current Medical Research and Opinion*, vol. 28, no. 1, pp. 69–78, 2012.

[40] N. Glorioso, M. Thomas, C. Troffa et al., "Antihypertensive efficacy and tolerability of aliskiren/amlodipine single- Pill combinations in patients with an inadequate response to aliskiren monotherapy," *Current Vascular Pharmacology*, vol. 10, no. 6, pp. 748–755, 2012.

[41] D. Pfeiffer, N. Rennie, C. C. Papst, and J. Zhang, "Efficacy and tolerability of aliskiren/amlodipine single-pill combinations in patients who did not respond fully to amlodipine monotherapy," *Current Vascular Pharmacology*, vol. 10, no. 6, pp. 773–780, 2012.

[42] K. Azushima, K. Uneda, K. Tamura et al., "Effects of single pill-based combination therapy of amlodipine and atorvastatin on within-visit blood pressure variability and parameters of renal and vascular function in hypertensive patients with chronic kidney disease," *BioMed Research International*, vol. 2014, Article ID 437087, 7 pages, 2014.

[43] S. Bashir, M. U. Sherwani, I. Shabbir, and A. Batool, "Efficacy of fix dose combination (atorvastatin and amlodipine) in treatment of uncontrolled hypertension and dyslipidemia," *Journal of Ayub Medical College Abbottabad*, vol. 23, no. 3, pp. 97–100, 2011.

[44] A. Delgado-Montero and J. L. Zamorano, "Atorvastatin calcium plus amlodipine for the treatment of hypertension," *Expert Opinion on Pharmacotherapy*, vol. 13, no. 18, pp. 2673–2685, 2012.

[45] J. Fedacko, D. Pella, P. Jarcuska et al., "Slovak trial on cardiovascular risk reduction following national guidelines with CaDUET (the STRONG DUET study)," *Advances in Therapy*, vol. 30, no. 1, pp. 60–70, 2013.

[46] M. A. Hussein, R. H. Chapman, J. S. Benner et al., "Does a single-pill antihypertensivelipid-lowering regimen improve adherence in us managed care enrolees? A non-randomized, observational, retrospective study," *American Journal of Cardiovascular Drugs*, vol. 10, no. 3, pp. 193–202, 2010.

[47] J. Hradec, J. Zamorano, and S. Sutradhar, "Post hoc analysis of the cluster randomized usual care versus caduet investigation assessing long-term risk (CRUCIAL) trial," *Current Medical Research and Opinion*, vol. 29, no. 6, pp. 589–596, 2013.

[48] J.-H. Kim, J. Zamorano, S. Erdine et al., "Reduction in cardiovascular risk using proactive multifactorial intervention versus usual care in younger (<65 years) and older (≥65 years) patients in the CRUCIAL trial," *Current Medical Research and Opinion*, vol. 29, no. 5, pp. 453–463, 2013.

[49] J. M. Neutel, W. H. Bestermann, E. M. Dyess et al., "The use of a single-pill calcium channel blocker/statin combination in the management of hypertension and dyslipidemia: a randomized, placebo-controlled, multicenter study," *Journal of Clinical Hypertension*, vol. 11, no. 1, pp. 22–30, 2009.

[50] J. Park, Y. Lee, S. Ko, and B. Cha, "Cost-effectiveness analysis of low density lipoprotein cholesterol-lowering therapy in hypertensive patients with type 2 diabetes in Korea: single-pill regimen (amlodipine/atorvastatin) versus double-pill regimen (amlodipine+atorvastatin)," *Epidemiology and Health*, vol. 37, Article ID e2015010, 2015.

[51] L. A. Simons, M. Ortiz, and G. Calcino, "Persistence with a single pill versus two pills of amlodipine and atorvastatin: the Australian experience, 2006–2010," *Medical Journal of Australia*, vol. 195, no. 3, pp. 134–137, 2011.

[52] M. Tanaka, R. Nishimura, T. Nishimura et al., "Effect of single tablet of fixed-dose amlodipine and atorvastatin on blood pressure/lipid control, oxidative stress, and medication adherence in type 2 diabetic patients," *Diabetology and Metabolic Syndrome*, vol. 6, no. 1, article 56, 2014.

[53] H. Rakugi, E. Nakata, E. Sasaki, and T. Kagawa, "Evaluation of the efficacy and tolerability of fixed-dose combination therapy of azilsartan and amlodipine besylate in Japanese patients with grade I to II essential hypertension," *Clinical Therapeutics*, vol. 36, no. 5, pp. 711–721, 2014.

[54] N. Reichek, R. B. Devereux, R. A. Rocha et al., "Magnetic resonance imaging left ventricular mass reduction with fixed-dose angiotensin-converting enzyme inhibitor-based regimens in patients with high-risk hypertension," *Hypertension*, vol. 54, no. 4, pp. 731–737, 2009.

[55] P. H. Skoglund, P. Svensson, J. Asp et al., "Amlodipine + benazepril is superior to hydrochlorothiazide + benazepril irrespective of baseline pulse pressure: subanalysis of the ACCOMPLISH Trial," *Journal of Clinical Hypertension*, vol. 17, no. 2, pp. 141–146, 2015.

[56] H.-Y. Lee, Y.-J. Kim, T. Ahn et al., "A randomized, multicenter, double-blind, placebo-controlled, 3 × 3 factorial design, phase II study to evaluate the efficacy and safety of the combination of fimasartan/amlodipine in patients with essential hypertension," *Clinical Therapeutics*, vol. 37, no. 11, pp. 2581–2596, 2015.

[57] U. Jadhav, J. Hiremath, D. J. Namjoshi et al., "Blood pressure control with a single-pill combination of indapamide sustained-release and amlodipine in patients with hypertension: the EFFICIENT study," *PLoS ONE*, vol. 9, no. 4, Article ID e92955, 2014.

[58] P. Kawalec, P. Holko, E. Stawowczyk, Ł. Borowiec, and K. J. Filipiak, "Economic evaluation of single-pill combination of indapamide and amlodipine in the treatment of arterial hypertension in the Polish setting," *Kardiologia Polska*, vol. 73, no. 9, pp. 768–780, 2015.

[59] K. P. Garnock-Jones, "Irbesartan/Amlodipine: a review of its use in adult patients with essential hypertension not adequately controlled with monotherapy," *American Journal of Cardiovascular Drugs*, vol. 13, no. 2, pp. 141–150, 2013.

[60] L. D. Esposti, S. Saragoni, S. Buda, and E. D. Esposti, "Drug adherence to olmesartan/amlodipine fixed combination in an Italian clinical practice setting," *ClinicoEconomics and Outcomes Research*, vol. 6, no. 1, pp. 209–216, 2014.

[61] G. Derosa, A. F. G. Cicero, A. Carbone et al., "Evaluation of safety and efficacy of a fixed olmesartan/amlodipine combination therapy compared to single monotherapies," *Expert Opinion on Drug Safety*, vol. 12, no. 5, pp. 621–629, 2013.

[62] G. Derosa, A. F. G. Cicero, A. Carbone et al., "RETRACTED: variation of some inflammatory markers in hypertensive patients after 1 year of olmesartan/amlodipine single-pill combination compared with olmesartan or amlodipine monotherapies," *Journal of American Society of Hypertension*, vol. 7, no. 1, pp. 32–39, 2013.

[63] G. Derosa, A. F. G. Cicero, A. Carbone et al., "Effects of an olmesartan/amlodipine fixed dose on blood pressure control, some adipocytokines and interleukins levels compared with olmesartan or amlodipine monotherapies," *Journal of Clinical Pharmacy and Therapeutics*, vol. 38, no. 1, pp. 48–55, 2013.

[64] G. Derosa, A. F. G. Cicero, A. Carbone et al., "Olmesartan/amlodipine combination versus olmesartan or amlodipine monotherapies on blood pressure and insulin resistance in a sample of hypertensive patients," *Clinical and Experimental Hypertension*, vol. 35, no. 5, pp. 301–307, 2013.

[65] G. Derosa, A. F. G. Cicero, A. Carbone et al., "Results from a 12 months, randomized, clinical trial comparing an olmesartan/amlodipine single pill combination to olmesartan and amlodipine monotherapies on blood pressure and inflammation," *European Journal of Pharmaceutical Sciences*, vol. 51, no. 1, pp. 26–33, 2014.

[66] G. Derosa, A. F. G. Cicero, A. Carbone et al., "Different aspects of sartan + calcium antagonist association compared to the single therapy on inflammation and metabolic parameters in hypertensive patients," *Inflammation*, vol. 37, no. 1, pp. 154–162, 2014.

[67] M. R. Weir, W. A. Hsueh, S. D. Nesbitt et al., "A titrate-to-goal study of switching patients uncontrolled on antihypertensive monotherapy to fixed-dose combinations of amlodipine and olmesartan medoxomil ± hydrochlorothiazide," *Journal of Clinical Hypertension*, vol. 13, no. 6, pp. 404–412, 2011.

[68] E. Angeloni, A. Vitaterna, P. Lombardo, M. Pirelli, and S. Refice, "Single-pill combination therapy in the initial treatment of marked hypertension: a propensity-matched analysis," *Clinical and Experimental Hypertension*, vol. 37, no. 5, pp. 404–410, 2015.

[69] W. J. Elliott, "Rationale for a single-pill combination of perindopril arginine and amlodipine besylate," *Journal of the American Society of Hypertension*, vol. 9, no. 4, pp. 257–265, 2015.

[70] P. Kizilirmak and Z. Ongen, "Comparison of single-pill strategies first line in hypertension: perindopril/amlodipine versus valsartan/amlodipine," *Journal of Hypertension*, vol. 33, no. 5, pp. 1114–1116, 2015.

[71] G. Mancia, R. Asmar, C. Amodeo et al., "Comparison of single-pill strategies first line in hypertension: perindopril/amlodipine versus valsartan/amlodipine," *Journal of Hypertension*, vol. 33, no. 2, pp. 401–411, 2015.

[72] A. J. Scheen and J. M. Krzesinski, "Fixed combination perindopril-amlodipine (Coveram) in the treatment of hypertension and coronary heart disease," *Revue Médicale de Liège*, vol. 64, no. 4, pp. 223–227, 2009.

[73] S. S. Billecke and P. A. Marcovitz, "Long-term safety and efficacy of telmisartan/amlodipine single pill combination in the treatment of hypertension," *Vascular Health and Risk Management*, vol. 9, no. 1, pp. 95–104, 2013.

[74] J. M. Neutel, G. Mancia, H. R. Black et al., "Single-pill combination of telmisartan/amlodipine in patients with severe hypertension: results from the TEAMSTA severe HTN study," *The Journal of Clinical Hypertension*, vol. 14, no. 4, pp. 206–215, 2012.

[75] A. M. Sharma, G. Bakris, J. M. Neutel et al., "Single-pill combination of telmisartan/Amlodipine versus amlodipine monotherapy in diabetic hypertensive patients: an 8-week randomized, parallel-group, double-blind trial," *Clinical Therapeutics*, vol. 34, no. 3, pp. 537–551, 2012.

[76] D. Zhu, P. Gao, W. Holtbruegge, and C. Huang, "A randomized, double-blind study to evaluate the efficacy and safety of a single-pill combination of telmisartan 80 mg/amlodipine 5 mg versus amlodipine 5 mg in hypertensive Asian patients," *Journal of International Medical Research*, vol. 42, no. 1, pp. 52–66, 2014.

[77] D. Zhu, P. Gao, N. Yagi, and H. Schumacher, "Efficacy and tolerability of telmisartan plus amlodipine in Asian patients not adequately controlled on either monotherapy or on low-dose combination therapy," *International Journal of Hypertension*, vol. 2014, Article ID 475480, 11 pages, 2014.

[78] O. Baser, L. M. Andrews, L. Wang, and L. Xie, "Comparison of real-world adherence, healthcare resource utilization and costs for newly initiated valsartan/amlodipine single-pill combination versus angiotensin receptor blocker/calcium channel blocker free-combination therapy," *Journal of Medical Economics*, vol. 14, no. 5, pp. 576–583, 2011.

[79] N. Braun, H.-J. Ulmer, A. Ansari, R. Handrock, and S. Klebs, "Efficacy and safety of the single pill combination of amlodipine 10 mg plus valsartan 160 mg in hypertensive patients not controlled by amlodipine 10 mg plus olmesartan 20 mg in free combination," *Current Medical Research and Opinion*, vol. 25, no. 2, pp. 421–430, 2009.

[80] R. Düsing, "Amlodipine/valsartan single pill combination therapy in Chinese patients not controlled on previous monotherapy," *Journal of Thoracic Disease*, vol. 7, no. 4, pp. 562–563, 2015.

[81] S. Eckert, S. B. Freytag, A. Müller, and S. H. G. Klebs, "Meta-analysis of three observational studies of amlodipine/valsartan in hypertensive patients with additional risk factors," *Blood Pressure*, vol. 22, no. 1, pp. 11–21, 2013.

[82] B. Ge, W. Peng, Y. Zhang, Y. Wen, C. Liu, and X. Guo, "Effectiveness of valsartan/amlodipine single-pill combination in hypertensive patients with excess body weight: subanalysis of China status II," *Journal of Cardiovascular Pharmacology*, vol. 66, no. 5, pp. 497–503, 2015.

[83] J. Huang, N.-L. Sun, Y.-M. Hao et al., "Efficacy and tolerability of a single-pill combination of amlodipine/valsartan in Asian

hypertensive patients not adequately controlled with valsartan monotherapy," *Clinical and Experimental Hypertension*, vol. 33, no. 3, pp. 179–186, 2011.

[84] D. Hu, L. Liu, and W. Li, "Efficacy and safety of valsartan/amlodipine single-pill combination in 11,422 Chinese patients with hypertension: an observational study," *Advances in Therapy*, vol. 31, no. 7, pp. 762–775, 2014.

[85] Y. Karpov, N. Dongre, A. Vigdorchik, and K. Sastravaha, "Amlodipine/valsartan single-pill combination: a prospective, observational evaluation of the real-life safety and effectiveness in the routine treatment of hypertension," *Advances in Therapy*, vol. 29, no. 2, pp. 134–147, 2012.

[86] Y.-N. Ke, J. Huang, and J.-R. Zhu, "Efficacy and safety of the single pill combination of valsartan 80 mg plus amlodipine 5 mg in mild to moderate essential hypertensive patients without adequate blood pressure control by monotherapy," *Zhonghua Xin Xue Guan Bing Za Zhi*, vol. 37, no. 9, pp. 794–799, 2009.

[87] Y. Ke, D. Zhu, H. Hong et al., "Efficacy and safety of a single-pill combination of amlodipine/valsartan in Asian hypertensive patients inadequately controlled with amlodipine monotherapy," *Current Medical Research and Opinion*, vol. 26, no. 7, pp. 1705–1713, 2010.

[88] W. Khan, N. Moin, S. Iktidar et al., "Real-life effectiveness, safety, and tolerability of amlodipine/valsartan or amlodipine/valsartan/hydrochlorothiazide single-pill combination in patients with hypertension from Pakistan," *Therapeutic Advances in Cardiovascular Disease*, vol. 8, no. 2, pp. 45–55, 2014.

[89] P. Kizilirmak, M. Berktas, M. R. Yalcin et al., "Efficacy and safety of valsartan and amlodipine single-pill combination in hypertensive patients (PEAK study)," *Türk Kardiyoloji Derneği Arşivi: Türk Kardiyoloji Derneğinin Yayın Organıdır*, vol. 41, pp. 406–417, 2013.

[90] P. Kızılırmak, I. Ar, and B. Ilerigelen, "Efficacy and safety of valsartan/amlodipine single-pill combination in patients with essential hypertension (PEAK LOW)," *Türk Kardiyoloji Derneği arşivi: Türk Kardiyoloji Derneğinin yayın organıdır*, vol. 42, no. 4, pp. 339–348, 2014.

[91] R. Lins, A. Aerts, N. Coen et al., "Effectiveness of amlodipine-valsartan single-pill combinations: hierarchical modeling of blood pressure and total cardiovascular disease risk outcomes (The Excellent Study)," *Annals of Pharmacotherapy*, vol. 45, no. 6, pp. 727–739, 2011.

[92] M. A. Malesker and D. E. Hilleman, "Comparison of amlodipine/valsartan fixed-dose combination therapy and conventional therapy," *Managed Care*, vol. 19, pp. 36–42, 2010.

[93] K. Motozato, S.-I. Miura, Y. Shiga et al., "Efficacy and safety of two single-pill fixed-dose combinations of angiotensin II receptor blockers/calcium channel blockers in hypertensive patients (EXAMINER study)," *Clinical and Experimental Hypertension*, vol. 38, no. 1, pp. 45–50, 2016.

[94] A. N. Odili, B. Ezeala-Adikaibe, M. B. Ndiaye et al., "Progress report on the first sub-Saharan Africa trial of newer versus older antihypertensive drugs in native black patients," *Trials*, 2012, article 59.

[95] J. Sison, S. H. Assaad-Khalil, R. Najem et al., "Real-world clinical experience of amlodipine/valsartan and amlodipine/valsartan/hydrochlorothiazide in hypertension: the EXCITE study," *Current Medical Research and Opinion*, vol. 30, no. 10, pp. 1937–1945, 2014.

[96] J.-G. Wang, W.-F. Zeng, Y.-S. He et al., "Valsartan/amlodipine compared to nifedipine GITS in patients with hypertension

inadequately controlled by monotherapy," *Advances in Therapy*, vol. 30, no. 8, pp. 771–783, 2013.

[97] D. Zhu, K. Yang, N. Sun et al., "Amlodipine/valsartan 5/160 mg versus valsartan 160 mg in Chinese hypertensives," *International Journal of Cardiology*, vol. 167, no. 5, pp. 2024–2030, 2013.

[98] Y. Huan and R. Townsend, "The single pill triple combination of aliskiren, amlodipine, and hydrochlorothiazide in the treatment of hypertension," *Expert Opinion on Pharmacotherapy*, vol. 13, no. 16, pp. 2409–2415, 2012.

[99] M. B. Hovater and E. A. Jaimes, "Optimizing combination therapy in the management of hypertension: the role of the aliskiren, amlodipine, and hydrochlorothiazide fixed combination," *Integrated Blood Pressure Control*, vol. 6, pp. 59–67, 2013.

[100] P. A. Sarafidis, "Patient Cases: 1. A patient with apparent compliance," *High Blood Pressure and Cardiovascular Prevention*, vol. 22, pp. 15–18, 2015.

[101] P. Stafylas, A. Mavrodi, G. Kourlaba, and N. Maniadakis, "8C.06: cost-effectiveness of two single-pill triple antihypertensive therapies based on the ambulatory blood pressure measurements," *Journal of Hypertension*, vol. 33, article e111, 2015.

[102] L. Xie, F. Frech-Tamas, E. Marrett, and O. Baser, "A medication adherence and persistence comparison of hypertensive patients treated with single-, double- and triple-pill combination therapy," *Current Medical Research and Opinion*, vol. 30, no. 12, pp. 2415–2422, 2014.

[103] P. Stafylas, G. Kourlaba, M. Hatzikou, D. Georgiopoulos, P. Sarafidis, and N. Maniadakis, "Economic evaluation of a single-pill triple antihypertensive therapy with valsartan, amlodipine, and hydrochlorothiazide against its dual components," *Cost Effectiveness and Resource Allocation*, vol. 13, no. 1, article 10, 2015.

[104] V. K. Tyagi, D. Singh, and K. Pathak, "Semisolid matrix-filled hard gelatin capsules for rapid dissolution of amlodipine besilate: development and assessment," *Journal of Advanced Pharmaceutical Technology and Research*, vol. 4, no. 1, pp. 42–49, 2013.

[105] S. Garg, K. Pathak, A. Philip, and D. Puri, "Osmotically regulated two-compartment asymmetric membrane capsules for simultaneous controlled release of anti-hypertensive drugs," *Scientia Pharmaceutica*, vol. 80, no. 1, pp. 229–250, 2012.

[106] P. V. Shelke, A. S. Dumbare, M. V. Gadhave et al., "Formulation and evaluation of rapidly disintegrating film of amlodipine besylate," *Journal of Drug Delivery and Therapeutics*, vol. 2, pp. 72–75, 2012.

[107] M. C. Nahata, R. S. Morosco, and T. F. Hipple, "Stability of amlodipine besylate in two liquid dosage forms," *Journal of the American Pharmaceutical Association*, vol. 39, no. 3, pp. 375–377, 1999.

[108] D. A. Lyszkiewicz, Z. Levichek, E. Kozer et al., "Bioavailability of a pediatric amlodipine suspension," *Pediatric Nephrology*, vol. 18, no. 7, pp. 675–678, 2003.

[109] N. L. Rivero, I. A. Santos, and A. P. Carreiro, "Amlodipine in pediatric patient with uncontrolled multifactorial hypertension. Formulation of amlodipine oral suspension," *European Review for Medical and Pharmacological Sciences*, vol. 16, no. 8, pp. 1117–1119, 2012.

[110] D. Kumar, M. Aqil, M. Rizwan, Y. Sultana, and M. Ali, "Investigation of a nanoemulsion as vehicle for transdermal delivery of amlodipine," *Pharmazie*, vol. 64, no. 2, pp. 80–85, 2009.

[111] G. Chhabra, K. Chuttani, A. K. Mishra, and K. Pathak, "Design and development of nanoemulsion drug delivery system of amlodipine besilate for improvement of oral bioavailability," *Drug Development and Industrial Pharmacy*, vol. 37, no. 8, pp. 907–916, 2011.

[112] D.-J. Jang, E. J. Jeong, H.-M. Lee, B.-C. Kim, S.-J. Lim, and C.-K. Kim, "Improvement of bioavailability and photostability of amlodipine using redispersible dry emulsion," *European Journal of Pharmaceutical Sciences*, vol. 28, no. 5, pp. 405–411, 2006.

[113] R. M. Mainardes, M. C. Urban, P. O. Cinto, M. V. Chaud, R. C. Evangelista, and M. P. D. Gremião, "Liposomes and micro/nanoparticles as colloidal carriers for nasal drug delivery," *Current Drug Delivery*, vol. 3, no. 3, pp. 275–285, 2006.

[114] K. R. Jadhav, M. N. Gambhire, I. M. Shaikh, V. J. Kadam, and S. S. Pisal, "Nasal drug delivery system-factors affecting and applications," *Current Drug Therapy*, vol. 2, no. 1, pp. 27–38, 2007.

[115] G. Ragno, E. Cione, A. Garofalo et al., "Design and monitoring of photostability systems for amlodipine dosage forms," *International Journal of Pharmaceutics*, vol. 265, no. 1-2, pp. 125–132, 2003.

[116] S. Patil and R. Murthy, "Preparation and in vitro evaluation of mucoadhesive chitosan microspheres of amlodipine besylate for nasal administration," *Indian Journal of Pharmaceutical Sciences*, vol. 68, no. 1, pp. 64–67, 2006.

[117] N. G. N. Swamy and Z. Abbas, "Preparation and in vitro characterization of mucoadhesive hydroxypropyl guar microspheres containing amlodipine besylate for nasal administration," *Indian Journal of Pharmaceutical Sciences*, vol. 73, no. 6, pp. 608–614, 2011.

[118] X. Wang, X. Zhang, Y. Qin, L. Zhong, K. Liu, and J. Zhang, "Percutaneous penetration ability of dexamethasone-amlodipine besylate compound gel and its effect on survival of ischemic random skin flap," *Zhongguo Xiu Fu Chong Jian Wai Ke Za Zhi*, vol. 24, no. 5, pp. 566–570, 2010.

[119] W. Mixon and S. R. Helms, "Transdermal amlodipine besylate in Lipoderm for the treatment of feline hypertension: a report of two cases," *International Journal of Pharmaceutical Compounding*, vol. 12, no. 5, pp. 392–397, 2008.

[120] M. S. Kamble, S. M. Dange, K. K. Bhalerao et al., "Development and evaluation of amlodipine besylate nanogel," *Journal of Bionanoscience*, vol. 9, no. 1, pp. 22–27, 2015.

[121] Y. Sun, L. Fang, M. Zhu et al., "A drug-in-adhesive transdermal patch for S-amlodipine free base: in vitro and in vivo characterization," *International Journal of Pharmaceutics*, vol. 382, no. 1-2, pp. 165–171, 2009.

[122] H. V. Patel, S. S. Patel, M. M. Raj et al., "Development and characterization of matrix-membrane controlled transdermal drug delivery system of amlodipine besylate," *Indo American Journal of Pharmaceutical Research*, vol. 4, pp. 5306–5314, 2014.

[123] M. G. Quaglia, F. Barbato, S. Fanali et al., "Direct determination by capillary electrophoresis of cardiovascular drugs, previously included in liposomes," *Journal of Pharmaceutical and Biomedical Analysis*, vol. 37, no. 1, pp. 73–79, 2005.

[124] X. Li, G.-R. Ruan, W.-L. Lu et al., "A novel stealth liposomal topotecan with amlodipine: apoptotic effect is associated with deletion of intracellular Ca^{2+} by amlodipine thus leading to an enhanced antitumor activity in leukemia," *Journal of Controlled Release*, vol. 112, no. 2, pp. 186–198, 2006.

[125] X. Li, W. L. Lu, G. W. Liang et al., "Effect of stealthy liposomal topotecan plus amlodipine on the multidrug-resistant

leukaemia cells in vitro and xenograft in mice," *European Journal of Clinical Investigation*, vol. 36, no. 6, pp. 409–418, 2006.

[126] R. P. Mason, I. T. Mak, M. W. Trumbore, and P. E. Mason, "Antioxidant properties of calcium antagonists related to membrane biophysical interactions," *American Journal of Cardiology*, vol. 84, no. 4, pp. 16–22, 1999.

[127] R. P. Mason, P. R. Leeds, R. F. Jacob et al., "Inhibition of excessive neuronal apoptosis by the calcium antagonist amlodipine and antioxidants in cerebellar granule cells," *Journal of Neurochemistry*, vol. 72, no. 4, pp. 1448–1456, 1999.

[128] R. P. Mason, M. W. Trumbore, and P. E. Mason, "Membrane biopphysical interactions of amlodipine result in antioxidant properties," *Drugs*, vol. 59, no. 2, pp. 9–16, 2000.

[129] Y. Zhang, R.-J. Li, X. Ying et al., "Targeting therapy with mitosomal daunorubicin plus amlodipine has the potential to circumvent intrinsic resistant breast cancer," *Molecular Pharmaceutics*, vol. 8, no. 1, pp. 162–175, 2011.

21

Pharmacological Investigation of the Wound Healing Activity of *Cestrum nocturnum* (L.) Ointment in Wistar Albino Rats

Hemant Kumar Nagar,[1] **Amit Kumar Srivastava,**[2] **Rajnish Srivastava,**[3] **Madan Lal Kurmi,**[1] **Harinarayan Singh Chandel,**[1] **and Mahendra Singh Ranawat**[4]

[1]*Department of Pharmacology, Truba Institute of Pharmacy, Karond Gandhi Nagar, Bhopal, Madhya Pradesh 462038, India*
[2]*Department of Pharmacology, Sapience Bioanalytical Research Lab, Bhopal, Madhya Pradesh 462021, India*
[3]*Faculty of Pharmacy, Moradabad Educational Trust Group of Institutions, Moradabad, Uttar Pradesh 244001, India*
[4]*Bhupal Nobles' College of Pharmacy, Udaipur, Rajasthan 313002, India*

Correspondence should be addressed to Hemant Kumar Nagar; hemant_nagar81@yahoo.co.in

Academic Editor: István Zupkó

Objectives. The present study was aimed at investigating the wound healing effect of ethanolic extract of *Cestrum nocturnum* (L.) leaves (EECN) using excision and incision wound model. *Methods.* Wistar albino rats were divided into five groups each consisting of six animals; group I (left untreated) considered as control, group II (ointment base treated) considered as negative control, group III treated with 5% (w/w) povidone iodine ointment (Intadine USP), which served as standard, group IV treated with EECN 2% (w/w) ointment, and group V treated with EECN 5% (w/w) ointment were considered as test groups. All the treatments were given once daily. The wound healing effect was assessed by percentage wound contraction, epithelialization period, and histoarchitecture studies in excision wound model while breaking strength and hydroxyproline content in the incision wound model. *Result.* Different concentration of EECN (2% and 5% w/w) ointment promoted the wound healing activity significantly in both the models studied. The high rate of wound contraction ($P < 0.001$), decrease in the period for epithelialization ($P < 0.01$), high skin breaking strength ($P < 0.001$), and elevated hydroxyproline content were observed in animal treated with EECN ointments when compared to the control and negative control group of animals. Histopathological studies of the EECN ointments treated groups also revealed the effectiveness in improved wound healing. *Conclusions.* Ethanolic extract of *Cestrum nocturnum* (EECN) leaves possesses a concentration dependent wound healing effect.

1. Introduction

Wound is defined as the disruption of the anatomic and cellular continuity of tissue caused by chemical, physical, thermal, microbial, or immunological injury to the tissue. Wound healing processes consist of integrated cellular and biochemical cascades leading to reestablishment of structural and functional integrity of the damaged tissue [1]. Various growth factors such as transforming growth factor beta (TGF-β), platelet activation factor (PAF), epidermal growth factor (EGF), and platelet-derived growth factors (PDGF) seem to be necessary for the initiation and promotion of wound healing [2].

Various treatment options (analgesics, antibiotics, and nonsteroidal anti-inflammatory drugs) are available for the wound management but majority of these therapies produce numerous unwanted side effects [3, 4]. In recent years, several studies have been carried out on herbal drugs to explicate their potential in wound management and these natural remedies proved their effectiveness as an alternative treatment to available synthetic drugs for the treatment of wound [5]. Many natural herbs have been pharmacologically reported possessing potent wound healing activity [6].

Solanaceae (*Cestrum nocturnum* (L.) family) is an evergreen woody shrub growing to 4 m in height. Leaves are dark green, oblong-ovate to oblong-lanceolate in shape with a pointed tip and 6–20 cm long with an entire margin. The nocturnal flowers are greenish white, having powerful sweet intoxicating fragrance [7]. Recent studies demonstrated the presence of important bioactive phytoconstituents in *Cestrum nocturnum* like alkaloids, flavonoids, glycosides, steroids, phenols, and essential oils [8]. It was also found to possess anti-inflammatory, antimicrobial, local anesthetic, and antioxidant properties that rationalized its more supportive and significant role as ideal wound healing drug [9–11].

Although need for scientific validation of herbal plants of ethnopharmacological relevance before these could be recommended for wound recovery as drugs is essential, therefore in the light of abovementioned facts about the plant, present study was designed to evaluate the wound healing potential of *Cestrum nocturnum* (L.) using excision and incision wound model in Wistar albino rats.

2. Materials and Methods

2.1. Plant Collection and Authentication. Fresh leaves of *Cestrum nocturnum* were collected in the month of February, locally from Govindpura, Bhopal, Madhya Pradesh, India. Plant material was identified and authenticated by Dr. Zia-Ul Hasan, Head of Department, Department of Botany, Safia Science College, Bhopal, and a specimen voucher (500/Bot/Safia/14), deposited in the Department of Pharmacology, Sapience Bioanalytical Research Lab, Bhopal, for future reference.

2.2. Extraction. The leaves of *Cestrum nocturnum* were shade-dried for 2 weeks, then pulverized to a coarse powder, and passed through sieve number 20 to maintain uniformity. Coarsely dried powder of the leaves was first defatted with petroleum ether (60–80°C) for 72 h to remove fatty materials and then extracted with ethanol (60–70°C) using soxhlet apparatus for 36 h; the extract was collected, filtered through Whatman filter paper, and concentrated in vacuum under reduced pressure and the dried extract was stored at 4°C for further study. The percentage yield of the extract was calculated.

2.3. Preliminary Phytochemical Screening. Ethanolic extract of *Cestrum nocturnum* leaves (EECN) was subjected to various phytochemical screening tests for the identification of the phytoconstituents present in *Cestrum nocturnum* leaves using standard procedures [12].

2.4. Determination of Total Polyphenolic and Total Flavonoid Contents. The total polyphenols content of the EECN was measured by UV spectrophotometrically according to the Folin-Ciocalteu method using gallic acid as a standard [13]. 0.1 mL of the extract solution was mixed with 0.5 mL of Folin-Ciocalteu reagent in a test tube and volume was made up to the 3 mL with distilled water. After 3 min of incubation, 2 mL of 20% sodium carbonate (Na_2CO_3) solution was added and mixed thoroughly. The resulting mixture was incubated for 5 min at 50°C and cooled at room temperature. Absorbance of the mixture was measured at 650 nm against the reagent blank. All measurements were carried out in triplicate. Content of phenolic compounds was expressed as mg of gallic acid equivalents (GAE)/g of dry extract using the linear equation

obtained from calibration curve of the standard gallic acid graph. The coefficient of determination (R^2) was 0.9971.

The total flavonoid content of the EECN was determined according to aluminum chloride method using quercetin as standard [14]. A volume of 0.5 mL of aluminum chloride ($AlCl_3$) ethanol solution (2%) was added to 0.5 mL of sample solution. Extract sample was evaluated at a final concentration of 0.1 mg/mL. After 1 h of incubation at room temperature, the absorbance was measured at 420 nm. All measurements were carried out in triplicate. The total flavonoid content was calculated as mg of quercetin equivalents (QE)/g of dry extract using the linear equation obtained from calibration curve of the standard quercetin graph. The coefficient of determination (R^2) was 0.9964.

2.5. Animals. Healthy Wistar albino rats weighing between 180 and 200 g were used for the present study. Animals were procured from the authorized animal house of Sapience Bioanalytical Research Lab, Bhopal, Madhya Pradesh. The animals were acclimatized to the standard laboratory conditions in cross ventilated animal house at 25 ± 2°C, relative humidity 44–56%, and light and dark cycle of 12 : 12 hours and fed with standard diet and water *ad libitum* during the study. The study protocol was approved by the Institutional Animal Ethics Committee (Approval Number 1413/PO/a/11/CPCSEA) as per Committee for the Purpose of Control and Supervision of Experiments on Animals guidelines, India.

2.6. Preparation of Formulation. Two types of ointment formulations, 2% and 5% (w/w), were prepared from the extract where 5 and 10 g of the extract were incorporated into 100 g of simple ointment base British Pharmacopoeia (BP), respectively [15]. Povidone iodine ointment (5% w/w) was used as a standard drug for comparing the wound healing potential of the extract.

2.7. Wound Healing Activities. For excision and incision wound model, animals were divided into five groups each consisting of six animals as follows: group I, left untreated and considered as control, group II, which served as negative control (ointment base treated), group III, which served as standard and was treated with 5% (w/w) povidone iodine ointment USP (Intadine), groups IV and V which were treated with 2% and 5% (w/w) ointments of extract, respectively. All the treatments were given once daily.

2.8. Excision Wound Model. Excision wound was created as per the method described [16]; five groups of animals each containing six rats were shaved on the dorsum portion using depilatory cream (Reckitt Benckiser, Inc., UK) and anesthetized using ketamine hydrochloride (50 mg/kg, i.p., body weight). An impression was made on shaved dorsal region and area of the wound to be created was marked. A full thickness excision wound with a circular area of 314 mm^2 was created along the marking using toothed forceps, a surgical blade, and pointed scissors. Rats were left undressed to the open environment. The simple ointment base, formulated extract ointment, and standard drug were applied once daily from the day of the operation until the complete healing. In this model, wound contraction and epithelialization period were evaluated. Wound contraction was measured as percent contraction every 4th day after wound formation. At the end of the study, all the rats were anesthetized and from the healed wounds, specimen samples of tissue were collected from each rat, leaving a 5 mm margin of normal skin around the edges of the healed wound. Specimen tissues were stored in 10% formalin solution and used for histopathological and biochemical studies.

2.9. Incision Wound Model. Incision wound was created according to the method already described [17]. The animals were grouped and treated the same as in the excision wound model. All rats were anesthetized using ketamine hydrochloride (50 mg/kg, i.p., body weight). Paravertebral incision of 6 cm length was made through the entire thickness of the shaved skin, on either side of the vertebral column of the rats with the help of a sharp scalpel. After complete hemostasis, the wound was stitched by means of interrupted sutures placed approximately 1 cm apart using black silk surgical thread (number 000) and a curved needle (number 11). After stitching, the wound was left undressed and animals were treated daily for 10 days. On the 10th day, all rats were anesthetized and sutures were removed and tensile strength of cured wound skin was measured using tensiometer.

2.10. Wound Healing Evaluation Parameters

2.10.1. Measurement of Wound Contraction and Epithelialization Period. In the excision wound model, wound area was measured by tracing the wound with the help of transparent sheet using millimeter based graph paper on days 0, 4, 8, 12, and 16 for all groups. Wound contraction was measured every 4th day until complete wound healing and represented as percentage of healing wound area [18]. Percentage of wound contraction was calculated taking the initial size of the wound as 100% using the following formula:

% wound contraction

$$= \frac{(\text{Intial wound area} - \text{Specific day wound area})}{\text{Intial wound area}} \quad (1)$$

$$\times 100.$$

Epithelialization period was calculated as the number of days required for falling off the dead tissue remnants of the wound without any residual raw wound [19].

2.11. Measurement of Tensile Strength. The tensile strength of a healing skin wound indicates the degree of wound healing. It represents how much the healed tissue resists to breaking under tension and may identify the quality of healing tissue. On the 10th day, all the animals were anesthetized by injecting ketamine hydrochloride (50 mg/kg, i.p., body weight), the sutures were removed, and the healed tissue was excised from all animals. Tensile strength of excised tissue was measured with the help of tensiometer [20].

2.12. Hydroxyproline Estimation. Excised wound tissues from all rats were analyzed for the estimation of hydroxyproline.

TABLE 1: Percentage yield, phytochemical screening, and quantitative phytochemical standardization of EECN.

Percentage yield	11.78% (w/w)
Phytochemical screening	
Alkaloids	+
Flavonoids	+
Tannins	+
Glycosides	+
Triterpenoids	+
Carbohydrates	+
Steroids	−
Saponins	−
Standardization of content of phytochemicals	
Total polyphenolic content[a]	238.64 ± 1.29
Total flavonoid content[b]	61.39 ± 0.57

For phytochemical screening: (+) presence of phytoconstituents and (−) absence of phytoconstituents; values of standardization of the content of the phytochemicals represent mean ± SD (n = 3). [a]Expressed as mg of gallic acid equivalents (GAE)/g of the dry extract. [b]Expressed as mg of quercetin equivalents (QE)/g of the dry extract.

Tissues were dried in a hot air oven at 60°C to constant weight and were hydrolyzed in 6 N HCl for 4 h at 130°C. The hydrolysates were then neutralized to pH 7.0 and were subjected to Chloramine-T oxidation for 20 min. After 5 min, the reaction was terminated by the addition of 0.4 M perchloric acid and developed color with Ehrlich reagent at 60°C. After thorough stirring the samples were analyzed at 557 nm in ultraviolet (Systronics-2203) spectrophotometer. The hydroxyproline content in the tissue samples was calculated using a standard curve of the pure L-hydroxyproline [21].

2.13. Histopathological Study. At the end of the study, all the animals were anesthetized using ketamine and specimens of wound tissue were collected and preserved in glass vials containing 10% formalin solution for histological examination. Sections of wound tissue specimens (about 5 μm thickness) were prepared by microtomy and stained with hematoxylin and eosin (H&E) dye for histological examination.

2.14. Statistical Analysis. The results are expressed as mean ± standard error of mean (SEM). The statistical significance was analyzed using one-way analysis of variance (ANOVA) followed by Tukey-Kramer Multiple Comparisons Test employing statistical software, GraphPad, InStat 3. Differences between groups were considered significant at $P < 0.05$ levels.

3. Results

3.1. Preliminary Phytochemical Screening. The percentage yield of EECN was found to be 11.78% w/w. The preliminary phytochemical investigation of the EECN revealed the presence of alkaloids, flavonoids, glycosides, tannins, triterpenoids, polyphenols, carbohydrates, and proteins (Table 1).

TABLE 2: Effect of EECN on % wound contraction and epithelialization period of wound in excision wound model.

Group	% wound contraction				Epithelialization period (days)
	4th day	8th day	12th day	16th day	
Group I (untreated)	4.39 ± 0.82	18.62 ± 0.69	42.62 ± 2.56	68.87 ± 0.91	19.16 ± 0.7
Group II (ointment base treated)	4.21 ± 0.19	19.48 ± 0.93	42.76 ± 1.36	71.2 ± 0.93	19.66 ± 0.66
Group III (standard)	14.55 ± 0.87 a***, b***	38.39 ± 0.46 a***, b***, c***	67.38 ± 2.01 a***, b***	94.3 ± 0.43 a***, b***	17.33 ± 0.4 a**, b**
Group IV (2% w/w, ointment)	13.83 ± 1.0 a***, b***	31.11 ± 0.83 a***, b***, c**	56.46 ± 0.79 a***, b***, c**	80.21 ± 0.27 a***, b***, c**	18.33 ± 0.22
Group V (5% w/w, ointment)	14.33 ± 0.94 a***, b***	34.82 ± 0.67 a***, b***	59.64 ± 1.18 a***, b***, c**	93.58 ± 0.76 a***, b***	17.66 ± 0.7 a**, b**

All values are represented as mean ± SEM, $n = 6$ animals in each group. Data were analyzed by one-way ANOVA, followed by Tukey-Kramer Multiple Comparisons Test. a: significant difference as compared to untreated group (group I); b: significant difference as compared to ointment base treated group (group II); c: significant difference as compared to standard group (group III), and $^{**}P < 0.01$, $^{***}P < 0.001$.

3.2. Determination of Total Polyphenolic and Total Flavonoid Contents. The phenolic and flavonoid contents of the EECN are represented in Table 1. The amount of phenolic contents was 238.64 ± 1.29 mg of gallic acid equivalents (GAE)/g of extract. The flavonoid content was 61.39 ± 0.57 mg of quercetin equivalents (QE)/g of extract.

3.3. Effect of EECN on Percentage Wound Contraction and Epithelialization Period. During the course of treatment the extract was found to show its preliminary effect from day 4 up to day 16 (Figure 1). The credentials found on day 16 anonymously favor the potential curative effect of the test drug (Table 2), which shows its maximum significant effect by increasing wound contraction with respect to control ($P < 0.001$) and ointment base treated ($P < 0.001$) and standard groups ($P < 0.01$) that proportionally confer healing process. As per rate of epithelialization concern the test drug was found to show its contributory role in the accelerating epithelialization rate and required lesser time to complete epithelialization process ($P < 0.01$) as compared to control and the ointment base treated group (Table 2).

3.4. Effect of EECN on Tissue Hydroxyproline Content. Increased hydroxyproline content ultimately responsible for increasing the collagen level confirmed the increased viability or microcirculation of collagen fibrils around the wound area. The hydroxyproline level was found to be significantly elevated ($P < 0.01$) in treated group animals in a concentration dependent manner in comparison to control and ointment base treated group (Table 3). The relative order for different groups in accordance to collagen stability or wound strength was at standard 5% povidone iodine > extract 5% > extract 2% > ointment base treated > control.

3.5. Effect of EECN on Tensile Strength of the Wound. An ideal wound healing agent must have the property of increasing the viability of collagen fibrils around the wound area that increases the tensile strength of the wound that was assessed by evaluating the tensile strength of the healed wound using tensiometer (Table 4). The EECN was found to possess significant concentration dependent action in increasing the tensile strength as compared to control and ointment base treated group ($P < 0.01$ and $P < 0.001$).

3.6. Histopathological Study. The histopathological studies of the tissue of the excision wound were performed on the 16th day and histopathological features of the tissue of all groups of animals are shown in Figures 2(a)–2(e). Section of group I (control) animals showed inflammatory cells, reduced collagen fibers, fibroblast cells, and blood vessels; there is also a presence of visible scar tissue (Figure 2(a)). Group II (ointment base treated) displayed the necrotic cells and less collagen fibers and blood vessels (Figure 2(b)). Group III (standard) showed complete tissue regeneration which was evident by increased fibroblast cell, collagen fibers, and blood vessels and reduced inflammatory cells (Figure 2(c)). Section of group IV (2% w/w ointment) showed less cellular necrosis along with increased collagen fibers and blood vessels (Figure 2(d)). However group V (5% w/w ointment) showed prominently increased fibroblast cells, blood vessels, and well organized collagen fibers as compared to the control (Figure 2(e)). Extract ointment treated and standard groups also showed the proliferation of epithelial tissue along with keratinization.

4. Discussion

Wound healing is an intricate process following damage to the skin and other soft tissues of the body. Wound healing involves the dynamic process of multiple biochemical consequences towards restoration of the damaged cellular structure to its regular and original state [22]. A classical cascade of wound healing involves three sequential and overlapping phases: inflammation, proliferation, and remodeling [23]. Topical application of prepared ointments (2% and 5% w/w) of EECN improved the wound healing in both excision and incision wound model in rats.

TABLE 3: Effect of EECN on tissue hydroxyproline content in excision wound model.

Group	Dry weight of tissues (mg)	Hydroxyproline content (μg/100 mg tissues)
Group I (untreated)	42.66 ± 1.13	27.50 ± 0.71
Group II (ointment base treated)	44.31 ± 0.8	28.13 ± 0.92
Group II (standard)	44.33 ± 2.0	34.50 ± 0.84 a[***], b[***]
Group III (2% w/w, ointment)	41.66 ± 1.22	31.83 ± 0.74 a[**], b[**]
Group IV (5% w/w, ointment)	39.0 ± 3.12	32.16 ± 0.65 a[**], b[**]

All values are represented as mean ± SEM, $n = 6$ animals in each group. Data were analyzed by one-way ANOVA, followed by Tukey-Kramer Multiple Comparisons Test. a: significant difference as compared to untreated group (group I); b: significant difference as compared to ointment base treated group (group II), and [**]$P < 0.01$, [***]$P < 0.001$.

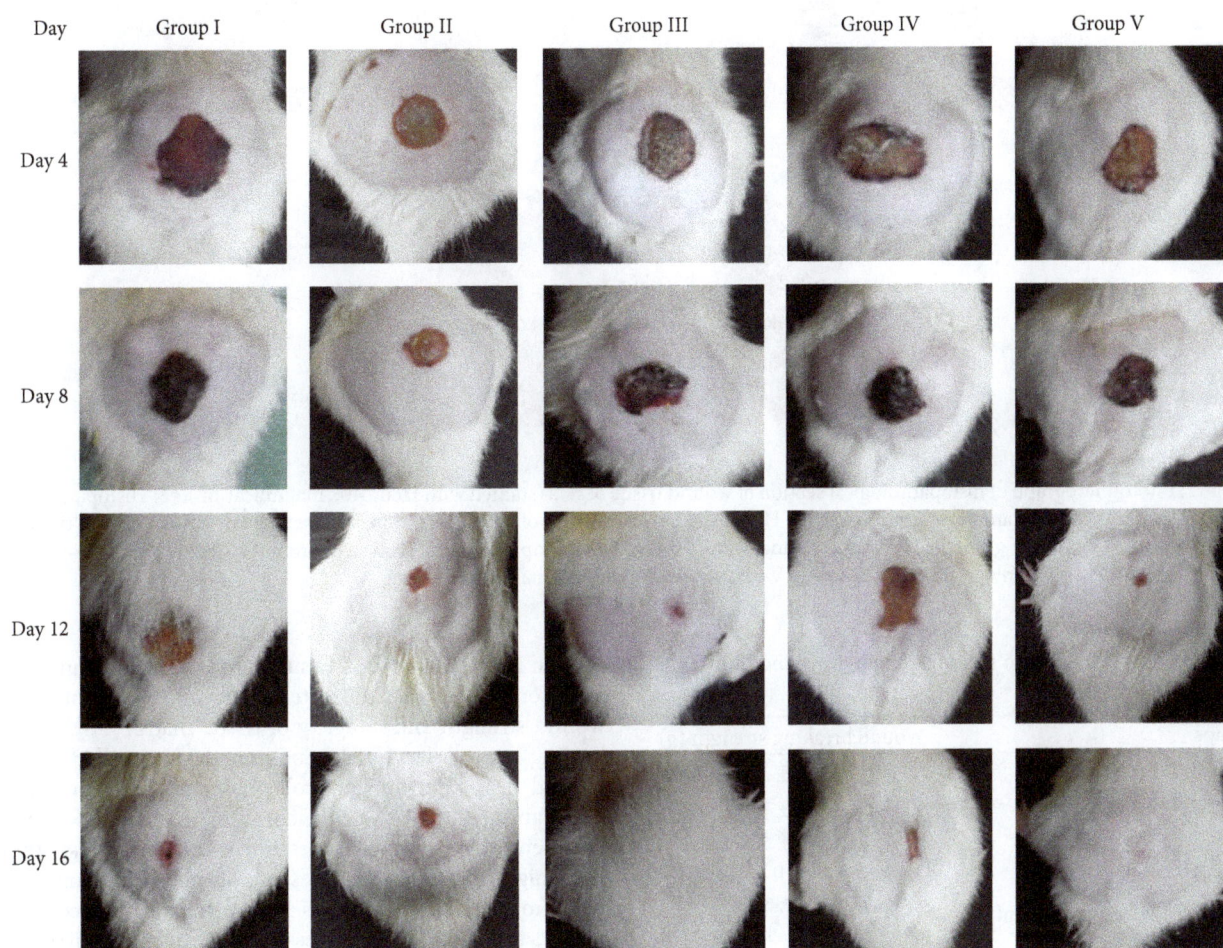

FIGURE 1: Photographs of wound repair at different time interval in excision wound model in rats.

The preliminary qualitative phytochemical screening of the EECN showed the presence of alkaloids flavonoids, terpenoids, glycosides, and tannins. Quantitative analysis of the EECN revealed rich amount of phenolic and flavonoidal content in the leaves of *Cestrum nocturnum*. Recent studies suggested the valuable role of flavonoids, triterpenoids, and tannins in promoting the wound healing by multiple mechanisms, for example, wound contraction, increased rate of epithelialization, and prevention of secondary bacterial infection that would have complicated and delayed wound healing [24, 25]. In the present study, wound healing potency of EECN may be attributed to its high phenolics and flavonoidal content owing to their astringent, anti-inflammatory, and antimicrobial activity. Povidone iodine as standard treatment is a well reported agent as antimicrobial and is used to prevent secondary wound infections. In contrast to that, the EECN

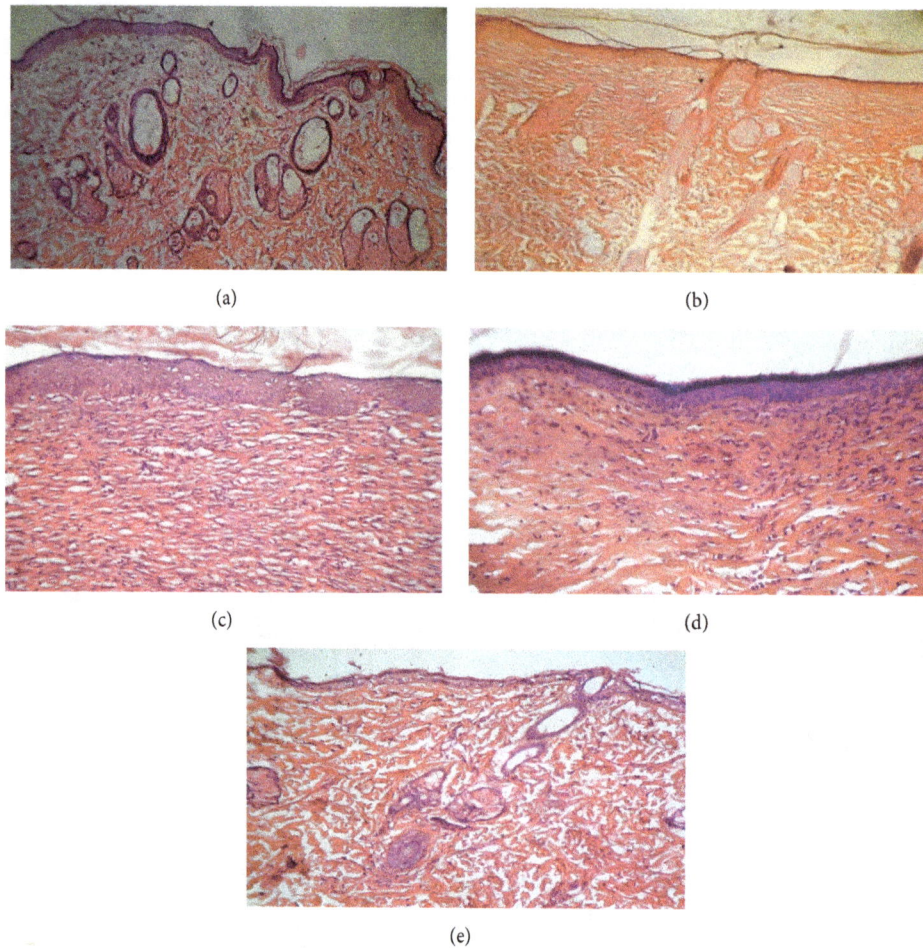

(a)

(b)

(c)

(d)

(e)

FIGURE 2: Photomicrograph of histopathological section of wound tissue of rats (stained with H&E, 40x magnification). (a) Histopathological section of group I (control) animal wound tissue. (b) Histopathological section of group II (ointment base treated) animal wound tissue. (c) Histopathological section of group III (standard) animal wound tissue. (d) Histopathological section of group IV (2% w/w ointment) animal wound tissue. (e) Histopathological section of group V (5% w/w ointment) animal wound tissue.

TABLE 4: Effect of EECN on tensile strength of wound in incision wound model.

Groups	Wound breaking strength (g)
Group I (untreated)	168.35 ± 3.53
Group II (ointment base treated)	172.95 ± 1.24
Group III (standard)	210.76 ± 6.65 a***, b**
Group IV (2% w/w, ointment)	191.35 ± 6.43 a**, b**, c*
Group V (5% w/w, ointment)	201.83 ± 4.98 a***, b***

All values are represented as mean $\pm$ SEM, $n = 6$ animals in each group. Data were analyzed by one-way ANOVA, followed by Tukey-Kramer Multiple Comparisons Test. a: significant difference as compared to untreated group (group I); b: significant difference as compared to ointment base treated group (group II); c: significant difference as compared to standard group (group III), and $^*P < 0.05$, $^{**}P < 0.01$, and $^{***}P < 0.001$.

extract ointment as already mentioned reveals rich phenolic and flavonoids presence that might have multiple mechanism in favor of wound healing. Collagen is a key extracellular protein in the granulation tissue of healing wound and is the vital component that ultimately plays an important role in wound strength and integrity of tissue matrix [26]. Wound healing process largely depends on the controlled synthesis and deposition of new collagens and their consequent maturation [27]. As wound contraction in EECN treated ointment shows better venerability of collagen synthesis that might be due to the presence of phenolic compounds [28], however the flavonoids might prevent the secondary wound infections as it possesses antiviral and antibacterial activities [29]. In the present study, we evaluate the level of hydroxyproline as a biochemical marker of collagen turnover. Significantly increased ($P < 0.001$) hydroxyproline levels in the granulation tissue of ointment of extract (2% and 5% w/w) treated rats indicate the elevated level of collagen content leading to swift wound healing and this venerable finding might be due to presence of flavonoid [30]. An increase in the tensile strength of the treated wounds was observed and this may be owing to the increased collagen level and stabilization of the collagen fibers [31]. Histopathological study of the ointments treated rat wound tissues also revealed the effectiveness of EECN in improved wound healing.

5. Conclusion

In conclusion, the results of the present study revealed that the ethanolic extract ointment of EECN contains the phytoconstituents that promote natural healing process and it could be effectively used as a wound healing agent. EECN ointment efficiently stimulates the wound strength and increases the rate of epithelialization, tensile strength, and collagen viability around the wound area. Further studies are in-process to isolate the active compound(s) responsible for wound healing and efforts shall be taken to develop the commercial preparation for wound healing.

Conflict of Interests

The authors declare that they have no conflict of interests.

Acknowledgment

The authors extend their thanks to Dr. Zia-Ul Hasan, Head of Department, Department of Botany, Safia Science College, Bhopal, Madhya Pradesh, India, for his kind help in the authentication of plant material.

References

[1] J. S. Boateng, K. H. Matthews, H. N. E. Stevens, and G. M. Eccleston, "Wound healing dressings and drug delivery systems: a review," *Journal of Pharmaceutical Sciences*, vol. 97, no. 8, pp. 2892–2923, 2008.

[2] N. B. Menke, K. R. Ward, T. M. Witten, D. G. Bonchev, and R. F. Diegelmann, "Impaired wound healing," *Clinics in Dermatology*, vol. 25, no. 1, pp. 19–25, 2007.

[3] R. R. Shenoy, A. T. Sudheendra, P. G. Nayak, P. Paul, N. G. Kutty, and C. M. Rao, "Normal and delayed wound healing is improved by sesamol, an active constituent of *Sesamum indicum* (L.) in albino rats," *Journal of Ethnopharmacology*, vol. 133, no. 2, pp. 608–612, 2011.

[4] M. N. Muscará, W. McKnight, S. Asfaha, and J. L. Wallace, "Wound collagen deposition in rats: effects of an NO-NSAID and a selective COX-2 inhibitor," *British Journal of Pharmacology*, vol. 129, no. 4, pp. 681–686, 2000.

[5] B. Kumar, M. Vijayakumar, R. Govindarajan, and P. Pushpangadan, "Ethnopharmacological approaches to wound healing-Exploring medicinal plants of India," *Journal of Ethnopharmacology*, vol. 114, no. 2, pp. 103–113, 2007.

[6] T. K. Biswas and B. Mukherjee, "Plant medicines of Indian origin for wound healing activity: a review," *The International Journal of Lower Extremity Wounds*, vol. 2, no. 1, pp. 25–39, 2003.

[7] A. Kamboj, S. Kumar, and V. Kumar, "Evaluation of antidiabetic activity of hydroalcoholic extract of cestrum nocturnum leaves in streptozotocin-induced diabetic rats," *Advances in Pharmacological Sciences*, vol. 2013, Article ID 150401, 4 pages, 2013.

[8] G. Bouchbaver, L. Jirovetz, and V. K. Koul, "Volatiles of the absolute of *Cestrum nocturnum* L.," *Journal of Essential Oil Research*, vol. 7, no. 1, pp. 5–9, 1995.

[9] A. Mazumder, A. Bhatt, V. A. Bonde, A. Shaikh, and R. Mazumder, "Evaluation of *Cestrum nocturnum* for its anti-inflammatory and analgesic potentiality," *Journal of Herbal Medicine and Toxicology*, vol. 4, no. 1, pp. 113–117, 2010.

[10] J. Zeng, X. H. Huang, and F. Lai, "Study of local anesthetic effect of *Cestrum nocturnum* water extract," *Gannan Yixueyuan Xuebao*, vol. 23, pp. 1–3, 2002.

[11] S. M. Al-Reza, A. Rahman, Y.-S. Cho, and S. C. Kang, "Chemical composition and antioxidant activity of essential oil and organic extracts of *Cestrum nocturnum* L.," *Journal of Essential Oil Bearing Plants*, vol. 13, no. 5, pp. 615–624, 2010.

[12] K. R. Khandelwal, *Practical Pharmacognosy Techniques and Experiments*, Nirali Prakashan, Pune, India, 22nd edition, 2005.

[13] S. Sadasivam and A. Manickam, *Biochemical Methods*, New Age International, New Delhi, India, 2nd edition, 1996.

[14] A. A. L. Ordoñez, J. D. Gomez, M. A. Vattuone, and M. I. Isla, "Antioxidant activities of *Sechium edule* (Jacq.) Swartz extracts," *Food Chemistry*, vol. 97, no. 3, pp. 452–458, 2006.

[15] A. Bhaskar and V. Nithya, "Evaluation of the wound-healing activity of *Hibiscus rosa* sinensis L (Malvaceae) in Wistar albino rats," *Indian Journal of Pharmacology*, vol. 44, no. 6, pp. 694–698, 2012.

[16] P. K. Mukherjee, R. Verpoorte, and B. Suresh, "Evaluation of in-vivo wound healing activity of *Hypericum patulum* (Family: Hypericaceae) leaf extract on different wound model in rats," *Journal of Ethnopharmacology*, vol. 70, no. 3, pp. 315–321, 2000.

[17] S. Hemalata, N. Subramanian, V. Ravichandran, and K. Chinnaswamy, "Wound healing activity of *Indigofera ennaphylla* Linn.," *Indian Journal of Pharmaceutical Sciences*, vol. 63, no. 4, pp. 331–333, 2001.

[18] F. Sadaf, R. Saleem, M. Ahmed, S. I. Ahmad, and Navaid-ul-Zafar, "Healing potential of cream containing extract of *Sphaeranthus indicus* on dermal wounds in Guinea pigs," *Journal of Ethnopharmacology*, vol. 107, no. 2, pp. 161–163, 2006.

[19] B. K. Manjunatha, S. M. Vidya, K. V. Rashmi, K. L. Mankani, H. J. Shilpa, and S. D. J. Singh, "Evaluation of wound-healing potency of *Vernonia arborea* Hk.," *Indian Journal of Pharmacology*, vol. 37, no. 4, pp. 223–226, 2005.

[20] H. Kuwano, K. Yano, S. Ohno et al., "Dipyridamole inhibits early wound healing in rat skin incisions," *Journal of Surgical Research*, vol. 56, no. 3, pp. 267–270, 1994.

[21] J. F. Woessner Jr., "The determination of hydroxyproline in tissue and protein samples containing small proportions of this imino acid," *Archives of Biochemistry and Biophysics*, vol. 93, no. 2, pp. 440–447, 1961.

[22] R. A. F. Clark, "Cutaneous tissue repair: basic biologic considerations. I.," *Journal of the American Academy of Dermatology*, vol. 13, no. 5, part 1, pp. 701–725, 1985.

[23] T. Kondo and Y. Ishida, "Molecular pathology of wound healing," *Forensic Science International*, vol. 203, no. 1–3, pp. 93–98, 2010.

[24] S. Lodhi and A. K. Singhai, "Wound healing effect of flavonoid rich fraction and luteolin isolated from *Martynia annua* Linn. on streptozotocin induced diabetic rats," *Asian Pacific Journal of Tropical Medicine*, vol. 6, no. 4, pp. 253–259, 2013.

[25] K. Li, Y. Diao, H. Zhang et al., "Tannin extracts from immature fruits of *Terminalia chebula* Fructus Retz. promote cutaneous wound healing in rats," *BMC Complementary and Alternative Medicine*, vol. 11, article 86, 2011.

[26] S. W. Hassan, M. G. Abubakar, R. A. Umar, A. S. Yakubu, H. M. Maishanu, and G. Ayeni, "Pharmacological and toxicological properties of leaf extracts of *Kingelia africana* (Bignoniaceae)," *Journal of Pharmacology and Toxicology*, vol. 6, no. 2, pp. 124–132, 2011.

[27] A. Puratchikody, C. Devi, and G. Nagalakshmi, "Wound healing activity of *Cyperus rotundus* Linn.," *Indian Journal of Pharmaceutical Sciences*, vol. 68, no. 1, pp. 97–101, 2006.

[28] I. Binic, V. Lazarevic, M. Ljubenovic, J. Mojsa, and D. Sokolovic, "Skin ageing: natural weapons and strategies," *Evidence-Based Complementary and Alternative Medicine*, vol. 2013, Article ID 827248, 10 pages, 2013.

[29] J. Yang, J. Guo, and J. Yuan, "In vitro antioxidant properties of rutin," *LWT—Food Science and Technology*, vol. 41, no. 6, pp. 1060–1066, 2008.

[30] S. Lodhi, A. P. Jain, V. K. Sharma, and A. K. Singhai, "Wound-healing effect of flavonoid-rich fraction from *Tephrosia purpurea* Linn. on streptozotocin-induced diabetic rats," *Journal of Herbs, Spices & Medicinal Plants*, vol. 19, no. 2, pp. 191–205, 2013.

[31] A. L. Udupa, D. R. Kulkarni, and S. L. Udupa, "Effect of *Tridax procumbens* extracts on wound healing," *International Journal of Pharmacognosy*, vol. 33, no. 1, pp. 37–40, 1995.

22

Self-Medication Pattern among Social Science University Students in Northwest Ethiopia

Dessalegn Asmelashe Gelayee

Department of Pharmacology, College of Medicine and Health Sciences, University of Gondar, Gondar, Ethiopia

Correspondence should be addressed to Dessalegn Asmelashe Gelayee; desefikir@gmail.com

Academic Editor: Giuseppina De Simone

Background. Inappropriate self-medication causes wastage of resources among others. *Method*. This survey study was conducted to determine self-medication pattern of 404 social science university students in Northwest Ethiopia, who were selected through stratified random sampling technique. Data were collected using self-administered questionnaire and analyzed with SPSS version 20 statistical software. Binary Logistic Regression analysis was employed with *P* value < 0.05 considered statistically significant. *Result*. At 95.3% response rate, mean age of 21.26 ± 1.76 years, and male/female ratio of 1.26, the prevalence of self-medication during the six month recall period was 32.7%. Headache (N = 87, 69.1%) was the primary complaint that prompted the practice and hence analgesics (N = 67, 53.2%) were the mostly used drugs followed by antimicrobials (N = 50, 39.7%). The top two reasons driving the practice were nonseverity of the illness (N = 41, 32.5%) and suggestions from friends (N = 33, 26.2%). Female sex (P = 0.042) and higher income (P = 0.044) were associated with the practice. *Conclusion*. Self-medication practice, involving the use of both nonprescription and prescription drugs such as antimicrobials, among the social science university students is high. Therefore health education interventions regarding the risks of inappropriate self-medication are essential.

1. Introduction

Illness or symptoms of an illness are a common human experience for which the actions taken vary depending on the perceptions and experiences of individuals and other factors. Self-care is the major form of care in illness, which is the oldest and most widely used behavior that affects the health of individuals [1]. Self-medication is the selection and use of medicines by individuals to treat self-recognized illnesses or symptoms. Recognition of the responsibility of individuals for their own health and the awareness that professional care for minor illness is often unnecessary have contributed to the concept of self-medication. A responsible self-medication involves the use of medicines which are approved and available without prescription and which are safe and effective when used as directed [2]. The practice however also involves the use of herbal medicines and prescription only drugs such as antibiotics [3, 4]. Acquiring medicines without a prescription, resubmitting old prescriptions to purchase medicines, sharing medicines with relatives or members of

one's social circle, or using leftover medicines stored at home is considered as self-medication practice [5].

This practice has been on the rise worldwide with huge variation in its prevalence among developing and developed nations due to inherent differences in cultural and socioeconomic factors and disparities in health care systems such as reimbursement policies and access to healthcare and drug dispensing policies [6]. Different factors at individual level such as age, sex, income, self-care orientation, education level in general and medical knowledge in particular, access to drugs, and exposure to advertisements also influence the practice [7, 8].

In economically deprived countries most episodes of illness are treated by self-medication [9] imposing much public and professional concern about the irrational use of drugs [10]. A lot has been done on improving access to essential drugs and rational drug use including self-medication practice has been a subject of interest. Medical care in Ethiopia is largely based on out of pocket expenditure of the patients and there are student clinics where the care is given to college students for free. In the nation, few studies have been carried on self-medication practice of the general public as well as among healthcare university students. However data on social science university students is unavailable. It is assumed that the pattern of self-medication may differ in these populations as their curriculum is devoid of medical training. Hence, to make tailored interventions, it is important to characterize the problem in such population. In addition, investigating self-medication among tertiary level students is important as they constitute a segment of the society that is highly educated and more inclined to information about health [4]. This study was therefore carried out to assess the pattern of self-medication among social science students of University of Gondar, Northwest Ethiopia.

2. Material and Methods

A cross-sectional study was conducted from February to June 2014 at University of Gondar, Northwest Ethiopia, which at the time had five campuses. One of them, Maraki Campus, was selected for the study because of convenience for data collection. There were a total of 5685 social science students during the study. The sample size was determined using a formula of $n = z^2 P (1 - P)/w^2$ and 5% contingency with the following assumptions: a P value of 0.05, $z = 1.96$ and CI = 95%, and $w = 0.05$. Thus 404 respondents were chosen with a stratified random sampling technique based on seniority and sex. The inclusion criterion was enrollment in one of the social science programs in the campus during the study period. Ethical approval was obtained from the Department of Pharmacology, College of Medicine and Health Science, University of Gondar, and then data was collected using a pretested self-administered questionnaire with both open and closed ended questions. The instrument was adapted from previous similar studies [5–7] and had items regarding sociodemography as well as pattern of self-medication. Finally, the collected data were checked for completeness and entered to SPSS version 20 statistical software for further analysis using Binary Logistic Regression with P value < 0.05 taken as statistically significant.

3. Results

Among the four hundred and four participants, 385 completed the questionnaire making a 95.3% response rate. Most of the respondents were males (55.8%), third-year students (33.8%), and with an average monthly middle income of 200–500 Eth birr (64.7%). The mean age ± SD of the respondents was 21.26 ± 1.76 years (Table 1).

As shown in Table 2, one hundred and twenty-six (32.7%) respondents practiced self-medication within the 6-month recall period preceding this study. The majority of them (40.5%) did the practice more than twice and 22.2% respondents described that their self-medication practice extended for a period of one week up to a month. Analgesics were the most commonly used drugs ($N = 67$, 53.2%) followed by antimicrobials ($N = 50$, 39.7%), antacids (10.3%), and vitamins (8.7%).

TABLE 1: Sociodemography of respondents.

Sociodemographic characteristics	Frequency	Percent (%)
Sex		
Male	215	55.8
Female	170	44.2
Year of study		
First year	116	30.1
Second year	113	29.4
Third year	130	33.8
Fourth year	12	3.1
Fifth year	14	3.6
Monthly income		
Less than 200 Eth birr	80	20.8
200–500 Eth birr	249	64.7
Greater than 500 Eth birr	56	14.5

1USD = 19.95 Eth birr.

TABLE 2: Prevalence, frequency, and duration of self-medication practice.

Variable	Response	
	Number of students	(%)
Did SM in the past 6 months ($N = 385$)		
Yes	126	32.7
No	259	67.3
Frequency of SM in the past 6 months ($N = 126$)		
Once	42	33.3
Twice	33	26.2
More than twice	51	40.5
Duration of SM ($N = 126$)		
For <1 week	87	69.1
For 1 week-1 month	28	22.2
For >1 month	11	8.7

Note: SM = self-medication.

The main medical conditions that prompted self-medication were headache ($N = 87$, 69.1%), common cold ($N = 20$, 15.9%), fever ($N = 20$, 15.9%), and abdominal discomfort ($N = 19$, 15.1%) (Figure 1). Mildness of the disease (32.5%), suggestions of friends (26.2%), and inexpensiveness of the practice (25.4%) were the top three driving reasons (Table 3).

In the present study, the practice of self-medication was significantly associated with female sex (AOR = 1.658, CI [1.020–2.696], $P = 0.042$) and higher income (AOR = 2.153 CI [1.020–4.545], $P = 0.044$) (Table 4).

4. Discussion

The study population in this cross-sectional study was social science students of University of Gondar, Northwest Ethiopia. They were young people of similar age group

TABLE 3: Reasons for practicing self-medication ($N = 126$).

Reasons	Frequency	(%)
Mildness of the problem	41	32.5
Friends' suggestion	33	26.2
Self-medication is cheaper	32	25.4
Previous experience	25	19.8
Do not trust health professionals	20	15.9
Obtaining drugs easily	20	15.9
Being embarrassed to tell about disease	10	7.9
Long waiting time	9	7.1
Long distance from health facility	4	3.2
Can afford cost of drugs	3	2.4

Note: it is multiple response question.

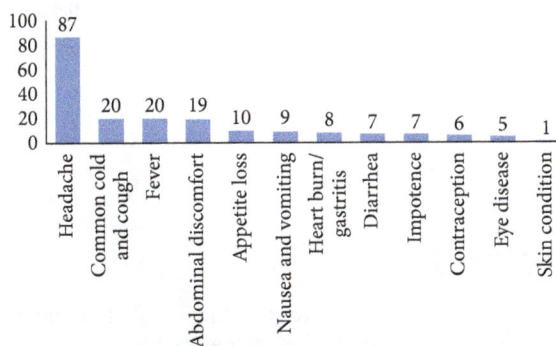

FIGURE 1: Medical conditions for which self-medication was practiced ($N = 126$). Note: it is multiple response questions.

and academic backgrounds. The 32.7% prevalence of self-medication practice found in the present study is relatively higher than the 27.2% prevalence among the general public in and around the study area reported in a previous study [11]. The difference might be due to increased academic status of the respondents in this study as the positive impact of literacy on self-medication practice is documented in previous studies and the ratio of literate people who are practicing self-medication is high as compared to those of illiterate people [12]. However, the prevalence in the present study is relatively lower than 38.5% [13], 43.24% [14], and 45.89% [15] prevalence reports in studies carried out in Ethiopia. The medical training background of the respondents in the latter three studies may explain the difference because such training was shown to influence self-medication by students in other studies [16]. On the other hand the prevalence of self-medication practice in this study varies inconsistently with studies done abroad among university students: 19% in Portugal [17], 59% in United Arab Emirates [18], 75.7% in India [19], 86.4% in Brazil [20], and 92.3% in Slovenia [7]. The difference might arise due to variation in the socioeconomic factors and sociodemographic characteristics as well as the methodologies used to assess self-medication practice.

While appropriate and responsible self-medication practice is good in that it can save time and readily relieve acute health problems and may save life in such serious conditions and may be economical too for the individual as

well as the health care system [2, 21], it can however also bring several harms when practiced inappropriately. With wrong self-medication practice resources are wasted, drug resistance of pathogens is increased, adverse drug reactions happen, drug dependency develops, and the health suffering increases [21, 22]. In relation to this, irrational use of drugs is a huge global concern with half of the medicines worldwide being prescribed, dispensed, or sold irrationally and 50% of patients failing to adhere to the prescribers' advice and not taking them correctly [23]. In the face of such challenges, more frequent and extended self-medication practice among a population of individuals without medical background may be inappropriate. In the present study, the respondents were engaged in more frequent (more than twice for 40.5% respondents) and more extended self-medication practice (for longer than a week by 31% of respondents who did self-medication). Such pattern of self-medication in the 6-month recall period may be associated with too many problems described above and it needs appropriate interventions.

Several previous studies have shown that headache, fever, gastrointestinal disease, and respiratory tract infection are some of the common medical conditions that prompted self-medication [14, 19, 24, 25]. Similarly in this study headache was the top first condition that prompted self-medication and hence analgesics were the mostly used drugs. Another study showed that headache is highly prevalent (as high as 87.7%) among university students [26].

In the present study, headache was followed by common cold and cough and fever as well as abdominal discomforts which is very similar to previous studies [13, 15, 17, 20, 24, 27].

Antimicrobials were the second mostly used drugs (39.68%) during self-medication and this should be considered an alarming problem as misuse of these drugs is a threat to development of drug resistance. Inappropriate use of antimicrobials is known to be common in the developing countries where there is increased access to such drugs without a prescription [28]. Paralleling this, a high prevalence of self-medication with antibiotics among college students is reported in Ghana (70%) [4] and Iran (53%) [29]. In the current study using antimicrobials for self-medication is however higher (more than twice) than that reported by Abay and Amelo [13] among healthcare university students in the same area few years back. The difference may arise from decreased awareness of drug resistance in the social science students of this study and accordingly they might be more likely to be engaged in indiscriminate use of antimicrobials for self-medication practice.

The nonseverity of the health problem, previous experience, and friends' suggestion as well as inexpensiveness were identified to be the reasons for practicing self-medication in this study. It is consistent with previous studies conducted among university students as well as the general public [4, 5, 13, 14, 18, 25, 27, 30]. However such reasons may sometimes be unacceptable as treatment on the bases of previous experience may result in misdiagnosis and wrong choice of drugs since diseases may share similar symptoms. Therefore incorrect treatment of even mild problems may prolong the suffering or may worsen the problem and this is likely because the respondents are social science students and lack medical

TABLE 4: Determinants of self-medication practice.

Variable	Number of students who did self-medication		Crude Odds ratio	Adjusted odds ratio	P value
	Yes	No			
Sex					
Male	64	151	1	1	
Female	62	108	1.354	1.658 [1.020–2.696]	**0.042*****
Monthly income (Eth. birr)					
<200	27	53	1	1	
200–500	67	182	0.723	0.661 [0.371–1.176]	0.159
>500	32	24	2.617	2.153 [1.020–4.545]	**0.044*****
Year of study					
First year	38	78	1	1	
Second year	29	84	0.709	0.782 [0.427–1.432]	0.426
Third year	45	85	1.087	1.154 [0.633–2.105]	0.640
Fourth year	7	5	2.874	2.977 [0.818–10.841]	0.098
Fifth year	7	7	2.053	1.819 [0.546–6.058]	0.330

background which enhances disease diagnosis. In line with this, previous study in Ethiopia reported that 55.4% of those who practiced self-medication admitted deterioration of their condition following self-medication [31]. The present study however identified reasons for self-medication which are not commonly reported so far such as lack of trust on the healthcare professionals as well as easy access to drugs. The unregulated drug dispensing practice which is a feature of developing countries may be associated with the latter reason.

In this study, sex (being female) encouraged self-medication practice ($P = 0.042$) and is in agreement with previous studies [6, 14]. It may be due to higher medication sharing practice among females compared to males which encourages self-medication practice. This however needs to be further studied. High monthly income (>500 Eth Birr) was also shown to encourage self-medication practice ($P = 0.044$) which may be related to high purchasing power as reported in previous studies [32]. However seniority in educational level did not significantly influence self-medication practice ($P > 0.05$) unlike that of Osemene and Lamikanra [6], Klemenc-Ketis et al. [7], Abay and Amelo [13], and Gutema et al. [14]. Lack of medical training for the respondents in this study may explain the difference as seniority did not add any medical knowledge in contrary to respondents in the other studies.

5. Conclusion

There is high prevalence of self-medication practice among the social science university students including the use of antimicrobials. This is significantly influenced by sex and income of the respondents. Therefore health education intervention regarding the risks of inappropriate self-medication is essential.

Competing Interests

The author declares that there is no conflict of interests regarding the publication of this paper.

References

[1] J. H. Kilwein, "The pharmacist and public health," in *Pharmacy Practice, Social and Behavioural Aspects*, A. I. Wertheimer and M. C. Smith, Eds., p. 389, Williams and Wilkins Publishing, Philadelphia, Pa, USA, 3rd edition, 1989.

[2] World Health Organization, *Guidelines for the Regulatory Assessment of Medicinal Products for Use in Self-Medication*, WHO/EDM/QSM/00.1, World Health Organization, 2000.

[3] L. Y. Goh, A. I. Vitry, S. J. Semple, A. Esterman, and M. A. Luszcz, "Self-medication with over-the-counter drugs and complementary medications in South Australia's elderly population," *BMC Complementary and Alternative Medicine*, vol. 9, article 42, 2009.

[4] E. S. Donkor, P. B. Tetteh-Quarcoo, P. Nartey, and I. O. Agyeman, "Self-medication practices with antibiotics among tertiary level students in Accra, Ghana: a cross-sectional study," *International Journal of Environmental Research and Public Health*, vol. 9, no. 10, pp. 3519–3529, 2012.

[5] S. N. Zafar, R. Syed, S. Waqar et al., "Self-medication amongst university students of Karachi: prevalence, knowledge and attitudes," *Journal of the Pakistan Medical Association*, vol. 58, no. 4, pp. 214–217, 2008.

[6] K. P. Osemene and A. Lamikanra, "A study of the prevalence of self-medication practice among university students in southwestern Nigeria," *Tropical Journal of Pharmaceutical Research*, vol. 11, no. 4, pp. 683–689, 2012.

[7] Z. Klemenc-Ketis, Z. Hladnik, and J. Kersnik, "Self-medication among healthcare and non-healthcare students at University of Ljubljana, Slovenia," *Medical Principles and Practice*, vol. 19, no. 5, pp. 395–401, 2010.

[8] D. Bennadi, "Self-medication: a current challenge," *Journal of Basic and Clinical Pharmacy*, vol. 5, no. 1, pp. 19–23, 2014.

[9] P. W. Geissler, K. Nokes, R. J. Prince, R. A. Odhiambo, J. Aagaard-Hansen, and J. H. Ouma, "Children and medicines: Self-treatment of common illnesses among Luo schoolchildren in western Kenya," *Social Science & Medicine*, vol. 50, no. 12, pp. 1771–1783, 2000.

[10] A. I. de Loyola Filho, M. F. Lima-Costa, and E. Uchôa, "Bambuí Project: a qualitative approach to self-medication," *Cadernos de Saude Publica*, vol. 20, no. 6, pp. 1661–1669, 2004.

[11] T. Abula and A. Worku, "Self-medication in three towns of North West Ethiopia," *Ethiopian Journal of Health Development*, vol. 15, no. 1, pp. 25–30, 2001.

[12] S. Jain, R. Malvi, and J. K. Purviya, "Concept of self-medication: a review," *International Journal of Pharmaceutical and Biological Archive*, vol. 2, pp. 831–836, 2011.

[13] S. M. Abay and W. Amelo, "Assessment of self-medication practices among medical, pharmacy, and health science students in Gondar University, Ethiopia," *Journal of Young Pharmacists*, vol. 2, no. 3, pp. 306–310, 2010.

[14] G. B. Gutema, D. A. Gadisa, Z. A. Kidanemariam et al., "Self-medication practices among health sciences students: the case of Mekelle University," *Journal of Applied Pharmaceutical Science*, vol. 1, no. 10, pp. 183–189, 2011.

[15] M. T. Angamo and N. T. Wabe, "Attitude and practice of self medication in Southwest Ethiopia," *International Journal of Pharmaceutical Sciences and Research*, vol. 3, no. 4, pp. 1005–1010, 2012.

[16] H. James, S. S. Handu, K. A. J. Al Khaja, and R. P. Sequeira, "Influence of medical training on self-medication by students," *International Journal of Clinical Pharmacology and Therapeutics*, vol. 46, no. 1, pp. 23–29, 2008.

[17] J. Cabrita, H. S. Ferreira, P. Iglésias et al., "Study of drug utilization among students at Lisbon University in Portugal," *Pharmacoepidemiology and Drug Safety*, vol. 11, no. 4, pp. 333–334, 2002.

[18] I. Sharif and S. Sharif, "Self-medication among social science students of the University of Sharjah, United Arab Emirates," *Archives of Pharmacy Practice*, vol. 5, no. 1, pp. 35–41, 2014.

[19] R. Parakh, N. Sharma, k. Kothari, R. Parakh, and P. Parakh, "Self -medication practice among engineering students in an engineering college in North India," *The Journal of Phytopharmacology*, vol. 2, no. 4, pp. 30–36, 2013.

[20] M. G. Corrêa Da Silva, M. C. F. Soares, and A. L. Muccillo-Baisch, "Self-medication in university students from the city of Rio Grande, Brazil," *BMC Public Health*, vol. 12, article 339, 2012.

[21] K. A. J. Al Khaja, S. S. Handu, H. James, S. Otoom, and R. P. Sequeira, "Evaluation of the knowledge, attitude and practice of self-medication among first-year medical students," *Medical Principles and Practice*, vol. 15, no. 4, pp. 270–275, 2006.

[22] H. Ullah, S. A. Khan, S. Ali et al., "Evaluation of self-medication amongst university students in Abbottabad, Pakistan; prevalence, attitude and causes," *Acta Poloniae Pharmaceutica*, vol. 70, no. 5, pp. 919–922, 2013.

[23] S. Kumar, W. Raja, J. Sunitha et al., "Household survey on rational use of medicines in India," *International Journal of Pharmacy and Therapeutics*, vol. 4, no. 1, pp. 59–69, 2013.

[24] L. Mohan, M. Pandey, and R. K. Verma, "Evaluation of self-medication among professional students in North India: proper statutory drug control must be implemented," *Asian Journal of Pharmaceutical and Clinical Research*, vol. 3, no. 1, pp. 60–64, 2010.

[25] T. Eticha, H. Araya, A. Alemayehu, G. Solomon, and D. Ali, "Prevalence and predictors of self-medication with antibiotics among Adi-haqi Campus students of Mekelle University, Ethiopia," *International Journal of Pharmaceutical Sciences and Research*, vol. 5, no. 10, pp. 678–684, 2014.

[26] A. S. Lima, R. C. de Araújo, M. R. D. A. Gomes et al., "Prevalence of headache and its interference in the activities of daily living in female adolescent students," *Revista Paulista de Pediatria*, vol. 32, no. 2, pp. 256–261, 2014.

[27] C. Omolase, O. Adeleke, A. Afolabi, and O. Ofolabi, "Self medication amongst general outpatients in a Nigerian community hospital," *Annals of Ibadan Postgraduate Medicine*, vol. 5, no. 2, pp. 64–67, 2011.

[28] A. A. Bin Abdulhak, M. A. Altannir, M. A. Almansor et al., "Non prescribed sale of antibiotics in Riyadh, Saudi Arabia: a cross sectional study," *BMC Public Health*, vol. 11, article 538, 2011.

[29] S. Sarahroodi and A. Arzi, "Self medication with antibiotics, is it a problem among Iranian college students in Tehran?" *Journal of Biological Sciences*, vol. 9, no. 8, pp. 829–832, 2009.

[30] S. Worku and A. G/Mariam, "Practice of self-medication in Jimma town," *Ethiopian Journal of Health Development*, vol. 17, no. 2, pp. 111–116, 2003.

[31] S. Suleman, A. Ketsela, and Z. Mekonnen, "Assessment of self-medication practices in Assendabo town, Jimma zone, southwestern Ethiopia," *Research in Social and Administrative Pharmacy*, vol. 5, no. 1, pp. 76–81, 2009.

[32] L. Yuefeng, R. Keqin, and R. Xiaowei, "Use of and factors associated with self-treatment in China," *BMC Public Health*, vol. 12, no. 1, article 995, 2012.

23

A Comparison of the Effects of Alpha and Medical-Grade Honey Ointments on Cutaneous Wound Healing in Rats

Shahram Paydar,[1,2] **Majid Akrami,**[2,3] **Amirreza Dehghanian,**[1,4]
Roshanak Alavi Moghadam,[1] **Mohsen Heidarpour,**[1] **Amir Bahari Khoob,**[1]
and Behnam Dalfardi[5,6]

[1]*Trauma Research Center, Shahid Rajaee (Emtiaz) Trauma Hospital, Shiraz University of Medical Sciences, Fars Province, Shiraz, Iran*
[2]*Department of General Surgery, Shiraz University of Medical Sciences, Fars Province, Shiraz, Iran*
[3]*Breast Diseases Research Center, Shiraz University of Medical Sciences, Fars Province, Shiraz, Iran*
[4]*Department of Pathology, School of Medicine, Shiraz University of Medical Sciences, Fars Province, Shiraz, Iran*
[5]*Student Research Committee, Shiraz University of Medical Sciences, Shiraz, Iran*
[6]*Department of Internal Medicine, Shiraz University of Medical Sciences, Shiraz, Iran*

Correspondence should be addressed to Behnam Dalfardi; dalfardibeh@gmail.com

Academic Editor: Giuseppina De Simone

Introduction. This study compared the healing efficacy and possible adverse effects of topical Alpha and medical-grade honey ointments on cutaneous wounds in rats. *Methods*. To conduct the study, 22 male Sprague-Dawley rats were randomly allocated into two equal groups: (1) rats with Alpha ointment applied to the wound surface area and (2) rats with medical-grade honey ointment applied to their wounds. The ointments were applied daily during the 21-day study period. Wound contraction was examined photographically with images taken on days 0, 7, and 21 after wounding. The healing process was histopathologically assessed using skin biopsies taken from the wound sites on days 7 and 21. *Results*. No statistically significant difference in mean wound surface area was observed between the two study groups. According to histopathological assessment, a significant reduction in the amount of collagen deposition (P value: 0.007) and neovascularisation (P value: 0.002) was seen in the Alpha-treated rats on day 21. No tissue necrosis occurred following the application of Alpha ointment. *Conclusion*. Daily topical usage of Alpha ointment on a skin wound can negatively affect the healing process by inhibiting neovascularization. Topical Alpha ointment can reduce the possibility of excessive scar formation by reducing collagen deposition.

1. Introduction

Wounds, especially chronic ones, are now a major health concern affecting a large number of patients and causing a considerable reduction in their health-related quality of life [1, 2]. For this reason, research on wound healing agents is currently an attractive and developing field in biomedical sciences [2, 3].

One group of drugs that has shown significant capabilities in the area of wound care and management is herbal medicines [3]. The use of plant materials has been a common medical practice since early times, especially in eastern countries; even now, various wound care products contain herbal ingredients [2, 3]. One such herbal medicine presently

available in Iran and claimed to improve wound healing is Alpha ointment [4, 5].

Alpha ointment contains the active ingredient Lawsone (available in natural henna (*Lawsonia inermis* Linn.)) and unsaturated fatty acids [4–6]. According to previous research, this composition has antioxidant and anti-inflammatory features [5, 6]. It has also been claimed that Alpha ointment is beneficial in improving wound healing [4]. As we see in our daily clinical practice, Alpha ointment is one of the prescriptions commonly used for the management of lower extremity chronic wounds, particularly diabetic ulcers. However, data regarding its efficacy in wound management is insufficient, and there are no strong and well-documented recommendations for its use. Based on these facts, the current

TABLE 1: The histopathological scoring system for evaluation of wound healing [8].

Parameter	Score			
	0	1	2	3
Acute and chronic inflammation	None	Scant	Moderate	Abundant
Amount of granulation tissue	None	Scant	Moderate	Abundant
Granulation tissue maturation	Immature	Mild maturation	Moderate maturation	Fully mature
Amount of collagen deposition	None	Scant	Moderate	Abundant
Reepithelialization	None	Partial	Complete but immature or thin	Complete and mature
Neovascularization	None	Up to five vessels per HPF*	6 to 10 vessels per HPF	More than 10 vessels per HPF

*HPF: microscopic high power field.

experimental study evaluated the ability of Alpha ointment to improve skin wound healing and compared it with the effects of medical-grade honey ointment, a product that received U.S. Food and Drug Administration (FDA) approval for use in conditions like leg ulcers, burns, diabetic foot ulcers, traumatic wounds, and so forth [7].

2. Materials and Methods

2.1. Ethical Approval. The study protocol was approved by the Animal Ethics Committee of Shiraz University of Medical Sciences, Shiraz, Iran. All procedures were performed under general anesthesia, and all efforts were made to minimize the animals' suffering.

2.2. Animals and Excisional Wound Model. In this study, we used a previously examined method [9]. A total of 22 healthy adult male Sprague-Dawley rats (mean weight: 350 g) were selected for this experimental study. The rats were kept in separate clean cages and had free access to equal amounts of standard food (Center of Comparative and Experimental Medicine, Shiraz University of Medical Sciences, Shiraz, Iran) and water. They were housed in temperature-controlled (22 ± 2°C) and humidity-controlled (55 ± 15%) rooms with 12-hour light/dark photoperiods and allowed to adapt to their environment for one week before experiments began.

The rats were randomly and equally allocated into two groups ($n = 11$): (1) rats for which Alpha ointment (Rejuderm, Iran) was applied to the wound surface area (Alpha-treated group) and (2) rats for which medical-grade honey ointment (Medihoney®, Comvita Ltd., New Zealand) was applied to the wounds (honey-treated group). During the 21-day study period, the ointments were applied to the wound surface areas at 24-hour intervals with disposable applicators in a manner that created a thin layer that fully covered the wound.

To generate the wounds, the rats were first anesthetized with an intramuscular injection of thiopental sodium (40 mg/kg; Biochemie, GmbH, Austria) and xylazine (10 mg/kg; Alfasan International, Woerden, Netherlands). Then, their back hair was shaved, and the wound site was disinfected using alcohol ethylic solution. Next, a full-thickness circular excisional skin wound (20 mm in diameter and 2 mm deep) was created on the back of each rat using scissors and forceps.

Throughout the study period, the rats' wounds were carefully examined every day for any possible complications, particularly any macroscopical manifestation of infection. Of note, rats were to be excluded from the experiment if death occurred.

2.3. Photographical Evaluation of Wound Healing. Wound contraction was assessed photographically with images taken using a digital camera (PowerShot G9 12.1 Megapixel Camera; Canon, Tokyo, Japan) on days 0, 7, and 21 after wounding. The camera was fixed at a distance of 10 cm from the wound surface (in a vertical view), and a fine-line ruler was held at wound level at the time of photography in order to calibrate the magnification of the photographs. Photos were analyzed using Adobe Photoshop CS program (Adobe Systems, San Jose, CA, USA) (analysis menu > record measurements command).

2.4. Histopathological Evaluation of Wound Healing. Semicircular full-thickness skin biopsies from wound sites in both groups were taken on days 7 (half of the wound site with a margin of 2 mm) and 21 (the remaining part with a 2 mm margin) after wounding. Animals were first anesthetized with inhaled *ether* on day 7 and then euthanized with *ether* on day 21.

After the biopsy, specimens were washed with sterile normal saline. Tissue samples were immediately fixed in buffered formaldehyde (10% formalin) and then sent for histopathological assessments (haematoxylin and eosin and Masson-trichrome staining and light microscopic evaluation).

The scoring system described by Abramov et al. for the histopathological evaluation of physiological parameters involved in the wound healing process was adapted for use in this study (Table 1) [8]. Abramov's scoring system examines the following criteria: amount of acute and chronic inflammatory infiltrates, amount of granulation tissue, maturation of granulation tissue, collagen deposition, neovascularization, and reepithelialization. All investigators who assessed tissue samples or analyzed images in this study were blinded to the agents given.

2.5. Statistical Analysis. The results are presented as mean ± standard deviation (SD). Statistical comparisons were made using the Mann–Whitney U test (SPSS Statistics software,

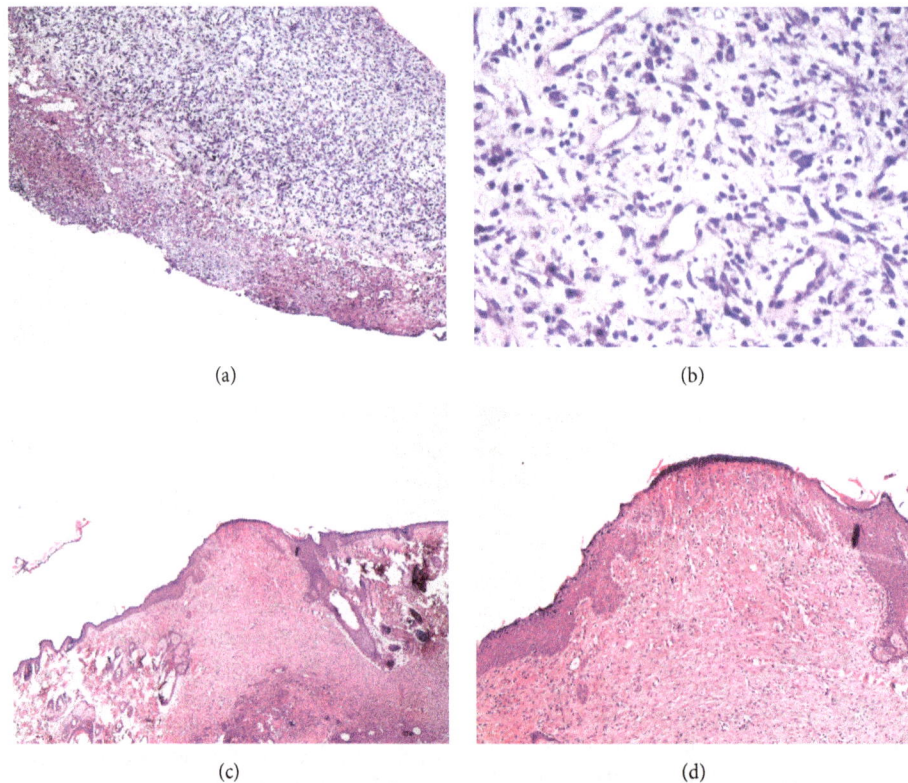

FIGURE 1: Histopathologic changes of ulcers in Alpha-treated group on day 7 showed ulceration, chronic inflammation, and granulation tissue formation: (a) ×400 and (b) ×400. Histopathologic changes in lesions of the same group on day 21 showed full reepithelialization and neovascularization: (c) ×40 and (d) ×100.

TABLE 2: Mean ± SD of wound surface area (mm^2) in Alpha- and honey-treated groups on different days after wounding.

Day	0	7	21
Alpha-treated	318.16 ± 13.22	46.54 ± 11.34	0.0 ± 0.00
Honey-treated	316.87 ± 13.67	50.83 ± 9.49	0.26 ± 0.49
P value	0.177	0.387	0.347

version 16; Chicago, Illinois, USA). A P value less than 0.05 was considered significant.

3. Results

3.1. Wound Contraction. The mean ± SD values of wound surface area were calculated for each group using images taken on days 0, 7, and 21 after wounding (Table 2). The results indicated no statistically significant difference between the two groups on the aforementioned study days. Of note, all rats survived the experiment, and their wounds showed no apparent signs of infection during the study period.

3.2. Histopathological Examinations. The results of the histopathological assessment (Figures 1 and 2) are summarized in Table 3. According to the findings, there was no statistically significant difference between the Alpha- and honey-treated groups regarding the factors of acute and chronic inflammation, amount and maturation of granulation tissue, and reepithelialization on days 7 and 21. However, significant differences in collagen deposition (P value: 0.007) and neovascularisation (P value: 0.002) between the two groups were observed on day 21. The histopathological examination of the skin biopsies revealed no tissue necrosis following the application of Alpha ointment.

4. Discussion

Finding new agents to accelerate wound healing and improve currently available products is the main concern for researchers in biomedical sciences [10]. Herbal medicines are a favourite agent used for this purpose [3]. One such agent, Alpha ointment containing Lawsone from henna and some other ingredients, has been produced in Iran in recent years [4–6]. Issues concerning herbal-derived wound care products are their efficacy and possible adverse dermatological effects associated with their use [11]. Because of these issues and the fact that documented evidence about Alpha ointment is insufficient, this study examined the effects of this product on the parameters involved in the skin healing process and compared it with the FDA-approved product medical-grade honey ointment [7].

Some previous studies defend the antibacterial properties of *Lawsonia inermis* and its efficacy in acceleration of wound repair [12–14]. The experiment of Shivananda Nayak et al.,

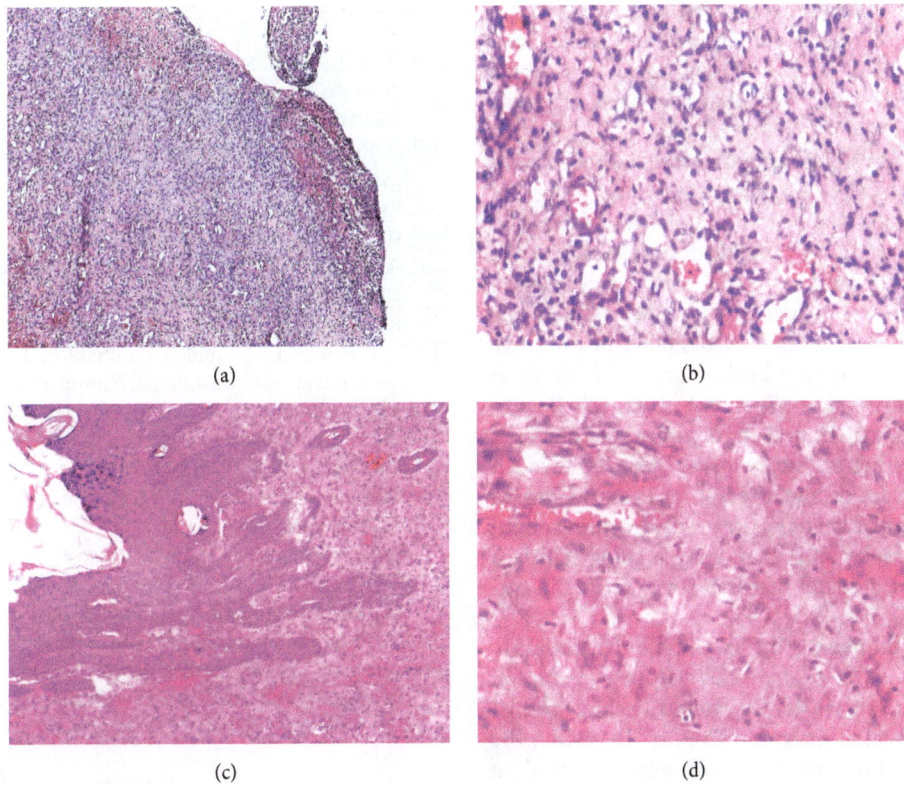

FIGURE 2: Histopathologic changes in the ulcers of honey-treated group on day 7 showed ulceration, chronic inflammation, and granulation tissue formation: (a) ×40 and (b) ×400. Histopathologic changes in the lesions of the same group on day 21 showed full reepithelialization, subepidermal fibrosis, and scar formation: (c) ×100 and (d) ×400.

TABLE 3: Mean ± SD values of histopathological scores of wound healing among different study groups.

Parameter	Groups					
	Day 7		P value	Day 21		P value
	Alpha-treated	Honey-treated		Alpha-treated	Honey-treated	
Acute and chronic inflammation	1.27 ± 0.46	1.90 ± 0.94	0.15	1.36 ± 0.67	1.81 ± 0.87	0.24
Amount of granulation tissue	2.54 ± 0.52	2.54 ± 0.52	1.00	0.81 ± 0.87	0.81 ± 0.75	0.89
Granulation tissue maturation	2.45 ± 0.52	2.63 ± 0.50	0.47	1.63 ± 1.36	2.09 ± 1.37	0.36
Amount of collagen deposition	1.72 ± 0.64	2.00 ± 0.44	0.33	0.90 ± 0.70	2.00 ± 0.89	0.007*
Reepithelialization	0.63 ± 1.02	0.54 ± 1.03	0.79	2.45 ± 0.93	2.72 ± 0.64	0.51
Neovascularization	3.00 ± 00	3.00 ± 00	1.00	2.18 ± 0.60	3.00 ± 0.00	0.002*

* indicates significant differences ($P < 0.05$).

who conducted an animal study to evaluate the impact of ethanol extract of *Lawsonia inermis* (the plant on which Alpha ointment is based), is an example for this case [12]. According to their results, this agent had the ability to increase the rate of wound contraction, decrease the period of epithelialization, and significantly increase the granulation tissue weight when compared with controls [12]. These authors' histological findings from the extract-treated group showed an increased amount of well-organized collagen bands (consequently the increased skin-breaking strength), increased number of fibroblasts, and reduced number of inflammatory cells compared with the controls [12].

However, few studies have directly assessed the efficacy of Alpha ointment for wound healing [4–6]. Ansari

et al., using their study criteria, compared the efficacy of topical Alpha ointment with that of topical hydrocortisone (1%) in healing radiation-induced dermatitis in cases of breast cancer [6]. After following up the patients for three weeks, the authors concluded that the topical application of Alpha ointment was more effective in healing radiation-induced dermatitis than topical hydrocortisone cream (1%) [6]. Hosseini et al. compared the impact of Alpha ointment with that of silver sulfadiazine on the healing process of standard third-degree and *Pseudomonas aeruginosa* infected burn wounds [4]. According to their results, Alpha ointment significantly decreased the rate of wound infection, positive cultures, and scar formation compared with the other groups [4]. The authors reported that another notable advantage of Alpha ointment compared with some other products used in burn wound care, like silver sulfadiazine, was its lower price [4]. Moreover, they noted that Alpha ointment had very few and acceptable adverse reactions [4].

In the current study, significant differences were observed between Alpha- and honey-treated groups regarding the two factors of collagen deposition and neovascularisation on day 21. In contrast to Shivananda Nayak et al.'s work, this study revealed significantly lesser collagen deposition in the Alpha-treated group than in the honey-treated one [12]. This phenomenon reduces the possibility of excessive scar formation after the wound healing process (similar to what was seen in Hosseini et al.'s work) [4, 15–17]. Due to the role of collagen matrix and its organization in tissue tensile strength, the other probable aspect of reduced collagen deposition is its impact on the strength of the final healed tissue [18, 19]. However, a prerequisite for commenting about the significance of this event is examining it using standard methods and devices, a matter that was not evaluated in this work.

Another important point is the angioinhibitory property of Alpha ointment. It is evident that neovascularization (neoangiogenesis) is critical during wound healing to provide tissues with essential materials [20, 21]. Therefore, the inhibition of such event could negatively affect the healing process. However, in spite of the angioinhibitory function of Alpha ointment, photographical examinations in the current study revealed no statistically significant difference between the two examined groups regarding wound contraction and wound surface areas on the specified days.

This study had some limitations that need to be mentioned. First of all, for each rat, biopsies were obtained from the same healing wound on days 7 and 21 (half of the wound area was biopsied in each day), and this restricted the interpretation of wound surface area on day 21. Another limitation of this work was the limited number of skin biopsies obtained from each rat. In fact, to better monitor the healing process and better recognize possible differences, additional biopsies should have been taken early after wounding (e.g., on day 4) and between days 7 and 21.

5. Conclusion

According to this histopathological study, daily topical usage of Alpha ointment on a skin wound in rats can negatively affect the healing process by inhibiting neovascularization. Furthermore, because of the reduced collagen deposition within the healing tissues, there is lesser possibility of excessive scar formation after the topical application of Alpha ointment. However, further human *in vivo* studies are recommended to examine the clinical importance of these findings.

Competing Interests

The authors declare that there are no competing interests regarding the publication of this paper.

References

[1] G. A. James, E. Swogger, R. Wolcott et al., "Biofilms in chronic wounds," *Wound Repair and Regeneration*, vol. 16, no. 1, pp. 37–44, 2008.

[2] B. Kumar, M. Vijayakumar, R. Govindarajan, and P. Pushpangadan, "Ethnopharmacological approaches to wound healing—exploring medicinal plants of India," *Journal of Ethnopharmacology*, vol. 114, no. 2, pp. 103–113, 2007.

[3] A. A. Dorai, "Wound care with traditional, complementary and alternative medicine," *Indian Journal of Plastic Surgery*, vol. 45, no. 2, pp. 418–424, 2012.

[4] S. V. Hosseini, N. Tanideh, J. Kohanteb, Z. Ghodrati, D. Mehrabani, and H. Yarmohammadi, "Comparison between Alpha and silver sulfadiazine ointments in treatment of *Pseudomonas* infections in 3rd degree burns," *International Journal of Surgery*, vol. 5, no. 1, pp. 23–26, 2007.

[5] M. Mohsenikia, H. Nuraei, F. Karimi et al., "Comparing effects of *Arnebia euchroma* and Alpha ointment on wound healing process," *Thrita*, vol. 4, no. 1, article e25781, 2014.

[6] M. Ansari, D. Farzin, A. Mosalaei, S. Omidvari, N. Ahmadloo, and M. Mohammadianpanah, "Efficacy of topical alpha ointment (containing natural henna) compared to topical hydrocortisone (1%) in the healing of radiation-induced dermatitis in patients with breast cancer: a randomized controlled clinical trial," *Iranian Journal of Medical Sciences*, vol. 38, pp. 293–300, 2013.

[7] D. S. Lee, S. Sinno, and A. Khachemoune, "Honey and wound healing: an overview," *American Journal of Clinical Dermatology*, vol. 12, no. 3, pp. 181–190, 2011.

[8] Y. Abramov, B. Golden, M. Sullivan et al., "Histologic characterization of vaginal vs. abdominal surgical wound healing in a rabbit model," *Wound Repair and Regeneration*, vol. 15, no. 1, pp. 80–86, 2007.

[9] H. Khoshmohabat, B. Dalfardi, A. Dehghanian, H. R. Rasouli, S. M. J. Mortazavi, and S. Paydar, "The effect of CoolClot hemostatic agent on skin wound healing in rats," *Journal of Surgical Research*, vol. 200, no. 2, pp. 732–737, 2016.

[10] T. Abdelrahman and H. Newton, "Wound dressings: principles and practice," *Surgery*, vol. 29, no. 10, pp. 491–495, 2011.

[11] E. Ernst, "Adverse effects of herbal drugs in dermatology," *British Journal of Dermatology*, vol. 143, no. 5, pp. 923–929, 2000.

[12] B. Shivananda Nayak, G. Isitor, E. M. Davis, and G. K. Pillai, "The evidence based wound healing activity of *Lawsonia inermis* Linn.," *Phytotherapy Research*, vol. 21, no. 9, pp. 827–831, 2007.

[13] F. Malekzadeh, "Antimicrobial activity of Lawsonia inermis L.," *Applied microbiology*, vol. 16, no. 4, pp. 663–664, 1968.

[14] H. S. Muhammad and S. Muhammad, "The use of Lawsonia inermis linn. (henna) in the management of burn wound infections," *African Journal of Biotechnology*, vol. 4, no. 9, pp. 934–937, 2005.

[15] G. Gabbiani, "The myofibroblast in wound healing and fibrocontractive diseases," *Journal of Pathology*, vol. 200, no. 4, pp. 500–503, 2003.

[16] B. J. Larson, M. T. Longaker, and H. P. Lorenz, "Scarless fetal wound healing: a basic science review," *Plastic and Reconstructive Surgery*, vol. 126, no. 4, pp. 1172–1180, 2010.

[17] S. Jahanabadi, M. Y. Karami, S. Paydar et al., "Albusite: a novel synthetic gel for promotion of skin wound healing in rats," *OnLine Journal of Biological Sciences*, vol. 15, no. 3, pp. 104–110, 2015.

[18] H. W. Hopf and M. D. Rollins, "Wounds: an overview of the role of oxygen," *Antioxidants and Redox Signaling*, vol. 9, no. 8, pp. 1183–1192, 2007.

[19] H. Derici, E. Kamer, H. R. Ünalp et al., "Effect of sildenafil on wound healing: an experimental study," *Langenbeck's Archives of Surgery*, vol. 395, no. 6, pp. 713–718, 2010.

[20] J. Jacobi, J. J. Jang, U. Sundram, H. Dayoub, L. F. Fajardo, and J. P. Cooke, "Nicotine accelerates angiogenesis and wound healing in genetically diabetic mice," *American Journal of Pathology*, vol. 161, no. 1, pp. 97–104, 2002.

[21] Z. Zhou, J. Wang, R. Cao et al., "Impaired angiogenesis, delayed wound healing and retarded tumor growth in perlecan heparan sulfate-deficient mice," *Cancer Research*, vol. 64, no. 14, pp. 4699–4702, 2004.

Permissions

List of Contributors

João Tavares Calixto-Júnior
Juazeiro do Norte College (FJN), Juazeiro do Norte, CE, Brazil

Selene Maia de Morais
Biotechnology Postgraduation Programme (RENORBIO), Laboratory of Natural Products, State University of Ceará, Itaperi Campus, Fortaleza, CE, Brazil

Aracélio Viana Colares
UNILEAO University Center, Juazeiro do Norte, CE, Brazil

Henrique Douglas Melo Coutinho
Department of Biological Chemistry, Regional University of Cariri, Crato, CE, Brazil

Pajaree Sakdiset
Faculty of Pharmaceutical Sciences, Josai University, 1-1 Keyakidai, Sakado, Saitama 350-0295, Japan
School of Pharmacy,Walailak University, 222 Thai Buri, Tha Sala, Nakhon SiThammarat 80160,Thailand

Yuki Kitao, Hiroaki Todo and Kenji Sugibayashi
Faculty of Pharmaceutical Sciences, Josai University, 1-1 Keyakidai, Sakado, Saitama 350-0295, Japan

Kanakapura Basavaiah and Nagib A. S. Qarah
Department of Chemistry, University of Mysore, Manasagangotri, Mysore 570 006, India

Sameer A. M. Abdulrahman
Department of Chemistry, Faculty of Education and Sciences Rada'a, Al-Baydha University, Al Bayda, Yemen

Shahram Paydar
Trauma Research Center, Shahid Rajaee (Emtiaz) Trauma Hospital, Shiraz University of Medical Sciences, Shiraz, Iran
Department of General Surgery, School of Medicine, Shiraz University of Medical Sciences, Shiraz, Iran

Ali Noorafshan and Seyedeh-Saeedeh Yahyavi
Histomorphometry and Stereology Research Centre, Shiraz University of Medical Sciences, Shiraz, Iran

Behnam Dalfardi
Student Research Committee, Shiraz University of Medical Sciences, Shiraz, Iran
Department of Internal Medicine, Shiraz University of Medical Sciences, Shiraz, Iran

Shahram Jahanabadi
International Branch, Shiraz University of Medical Sciences, Shiraz, Iran

Seyed Mohammad Javad Mortazavi
Medical Physics Department, School of Medicine, Shiraz University of Medical Sciences, Shiraz, Iran
Ionizing and Non-Ionizing Radiation Protection Research Center (INIRPRC), Shiraz University of Medical Sciences, Shiraz, Iran

Hadi Khoshmohabat
Trauma Research Center, Baqiyatallah University of Medical Sciences, Tehran, Iran

Archana Vyas, Heera Ram and Ashok Purohit
Department of Zoology, Jai Narain Vyas University, Jodhpur, Rajasthan 342001, India

Rameshwar Jatwa
Molecular Medicine and Toxicology Lab, School of Life Sciences, Devi Ahilya University, Indore, Madhya Pradesh 452001, India

Ashlesha P. Pandit, Vaibhav V. Pol and Vinit S. Kulkarni
Department of Pharmaceutics, JSPM's Rajarshi Shahu College of Pharmacy & Research, Pune-Mumbai Bypass Highway, Tathawade, Pune, Maharashtra 411033, India

Regina Au
BioMarketing Insight, Boston, MA, USA

Ebrahim Abbasi Oshaghi, Iraj Khodadadi and Heidar Tavilani
Department of Clinical Biochemistry, School of Medicine, Hamadan University of Medical Sciences, Hamadan, Iran

Fatemeh Mirzaei
Student Research Committee, Kermanshah University of Medical Sciences, Kermanshah, Iran

Mozafar Khazaei
Fertility and Infertility Research Center, Kermanshah University of Medical Sciences, Kermanshah, Iran

Mohammad Taghi Goodarzi
Department of Clinical Biochemistry, School of Medicine, Hamadan University of Medical Sciences, Hamadan, Iran
Research Center for Molecular Medicine, Hamadan University of Medical Sciences, Hamadan, Iran

Ofosua Adi-Dako
Department of Pharmaceutics, Faculty of Pharmacy and Pharmaceutical Sciences, College of Health Sciences, Kwame Nkrumah University of Science and Technology (KNUST), Kumasi, Ghana
School of Pharmacy, University of Ghana, Legon, Ghana

Kwabena Ofori-Kwakye and Mariam EL Boakye-Gyasi
Department of Pharmaceutics, Faculty of Pharmacy and Pharmaceutical Sciences, College of Health Sciences, Kwame Nkrumah University of Science and Technology (KNUST), Kumasi, Ghana

Samuel Frimpong Manso, Clement Sasu and Mike Pobee
School of Pharmacy, University of Ghana, Legon, Ghana

Siddhartha Maity and Biswanath Sa
Division of Pharmaceutics, Department of Pharmaceutical Technology, Jadavpur University, Kolkata 700032, India

Amit Kundu and Sanmoy Karmakar
Division of Pharmacology, Department of Pharmaceutical Technology, Jadavpur University, Kolkata 700032, India

Ahmed Mahmoud and Abdel Haleem Ali
Department of Pharmaceutics and Pharmaceutical Technology, College of Pharmacy, Taif University, Taif, Saudi Arabia
Department of Pharmaceutics and Industrial Pharmacy, Faculty of Pharmacy, Beni-Suef University, Beni-Suef, Egypt

Mayyas Mohammad Ahmad Al-Remawi
Department of Pharmaceutics and Pharmaceutical Technology, College of Pharmacy, Taif University, Taif, Saudi Arabia
Department of Pharmaceutics and Pharmaceutical Technology, Faculty of Pharmacy and Medical Sciences, Petra University, Amman, Jordan

Chandra Sekhar Patro and Prafulla Kumar Sahu
Raghu College of Pharmacy, Dakamarri, Visakhapatnam, Andhra Pradesh 531 162, India

Mei X. Chen, Kenneth S. Alexander and Gabriella Baki
Department of Pharmacy Practice, College of Pharmacy and Pharmaceutical Sciences, University of Toledo, 3000 Arlington Ave., Toledo, OH 43614, USA

Yuritze Alejandra Aguilar-López and Leopoldo Villafuerte-Robles
Departamento de Farmacia, Escuela Nacional de Ciencias Biológicas, Instituto Politécnico Nacional de México, Ciudad de México, Mexico

Upendra Nagaich, Neha Gulati and Swati Chauhan
Department of Pharmaceutics, Amity Institute of Pharmacy, Amity University, Noida, Uttar Pradesh, India

Wafa Al-Madhagi
Department of Pharmaceutical Chemistry, Faculty of Pharmacy, Sana'a University, Sana'a, Yemen
Department of Pharmacy, Faculty of Medicine and Health Sciences, Yemeni Jordanian University, Sana'a, Yemen

Ahmed Abdulbari Albarakani, Abobakr Khaled Alhag and Zakaria Ahmed Saeed
Department of Pharmacy, Faculty of Medicine and Health Sciences, Yemeni Jordanian University, Sana'a, Yemen

Nahlah Mansour Noman
Department of Pharmacy, Faculty of Medicine and Health Sciences, Thamar University, Dhamar, Yemen

Khaldon Mohamed
Department of Biomedical Science, Sana'a University, Sana'a, Yemen

Alka Sonkar, Anil Kumar and Kamla Pathak
Department of Pharmaceutics, Rajiv Academy for Pharmacy, Mathura, Uttar Pradesh 281001, India

Takahiro Murai
Graduate School of Pharmaceutical Sciences, Osaka University, 1-6 Yamadaoka, Suita, Osaka 565-0871, Japan

Norihito Kawashita and Tatsuya Takagi
Graduate School of Pharmaceutical Sciences, Osaka University, 1-6 Yamadaoka, Suita, Osaka 565-0871, Japan
Research Institute for Microbial Diseases, Osaka University, 3-1 Yamadaoka, Suita, Osaka 565-0871, Japan

Yu-Shi Tian
Graduate School of Information Science and Technology, Osaka University, 1-5 Yamadaoka, Suita, Osaka 565-0871, Japan

Siew Ling Ong, Siau Hui Mah and How Yee Lai
School of Biosciences, Taylor's University, No. 1 Jalan Taylor's, 47500 Subang Jaya, Malaysia

Muhammad Ali Sheraz, Syed Furqan Ahsan, Marium Fatima Khan, Sofia Ahmed and Iqbal Ahmad
Baqai Institute of Pharmaceutical Sciences, BaqaiMedical University, 51 Deh Tor, Toll Plaza, SuperHighway, Gadap Road, Karachi 74600, Pakistan

Hemant Kumar Nagar, Madan Lal Kurmi and Harinarayan Singh Chandel
Department of Pharmacology, Truba Institute of Pharmacy, Karond Gandhi Nagar, Bhopal, Madhya Pradesh 462038, India

Amit Kumar Srivastava
Department of Pharmacology, Sapience Bioanalytical Research Lab, Bhopal, Madhya Pradesh 462021, India

Rajnish Srivastava
Faculty of Pharmacy, Moradabad Educational Trust Group of Institutions, Moradabad, Uttar Pradesh 244001, India

Mahendra Singh Ranawat
Bhupal Nobles' College of Pharmacy, Udaipur, Rajasthan 313002, India

Dessalegn Asmelashe Gelayee
Department of Pharmacology, College of Medicine and Health Sciences, University of Gondar, Gondar, Ethiopia

Roshanak Alavi Moghadam, Mohsen Heidarpour and Amir Bahari Khoob
Trauma Research Center, Shahid Rajaee (Emtiaz) Trauma Hospital, Shiraz University ofMedical Sciences, Fars Province, Shiraz, Iran

Shahram Paydar
Trauma Research Center, Shahid Rajaee (Emtiaz) Trauma Hospital, Shiraz University ofMedical Sciences, Fars Province, Shiraz, Iran
Department of General Surgery, Shiraz University of Medical Sciences, Fars Province, Shiraz, Iran

Majid Akrami
Department of General Surgery, Shiraz University of Medical Sciences, Fars Province, Shiraz, Iran
Breast Diseases Research Center, Shiraz University of Medical Sciences, Fars Province, Shiraz, Iran

Amirreza Dehghanian
Trauma Research Center, Shahid Rajaee (Emtiaz) Trauma Hospital, Shiraz University ofMedical Sciences, Fars Province, Shiraz, Iran
Department of Pathology, School of Medicine, Shiraz University of Medical Sciences, Fars Province, Shiraz, Iran

Behnam Dalfardi
Student Research Committee, Shiraz University of Medical Sciences, Shiraz, Iran
Department of Internal Medicine, Shiraz University of Medical Sciences, Shiraz, Iran

Index